This book is to be returned on o.
the last date stamped belo

Coronary Heart Disease Prevention

For Churchill Livingstone:

Commissioning editor: Ellen Green
Project manager: Valerie Burgess
Project development editor: Mairi McCubbin
Design direction: Judith Wright
Project controller: Pat Miller
Copy editor: Sue Beasley
Indexer: Tarrant Ranger Indexing Agency
Sales promotion executive: Hilary Brown

Coronary Heart Disease Prevention

A Handbook for the Health Care Team

Edited by

Grace M. Lindsay BSc(Hons) RGN SCM RN MN
Lecturer in Nursing and Midwifery Studies, University of Glasgow, Glasgow, UK

Allan Gaw MB ChB MD PhD
British Heart Foundation Research Fellow and Honorary Senior Registrar in Clinical Biochemistry, Department of Pathological Biochemistry, Glasgow Royal Infirmary, Glasgow, UK

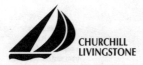
CHURCHILL LIVINGSTONE

NEW YORK EDINBURGH LONDON MADRID MELBOURNE SAN FRANCISCO TOKYO 1997

CHURCHILL LIVINGSTONE
Medical Division of Pearson Professional Limited

Distributed in the United States of America by Churchill
Livingstone Inc., 650 Avenue of the Americas, New York,
N.Y. 10011, and by associated companies, branches and
representatives throughout the world.

First published 1997

ISBN 0 443 05460 6

British Library of Cataloguing in Publication Data
A catalogue record for this book is available from the British
Library.

Library of Congress Cataloging in Publication Data
A catalogue record for this book is available from the Library
of Congress.

Note
Medical knowledge is constantly changing. As new
information becomes available, changes in treatment,
procedures, equipment and the use of drugs become
necessary. The editors / authors / contributors and the
publishers have, as far as it is possible, taken care to ensure
that the information given in this text is accurate and up-to-
date. However, readers are strongly advised to confirm that
the information, especially with regard to drug usage,
complies with latest legislation and standards of practice.

The
publisher's
policy is to use
paper manufactured
from sustainable forests

Printed in Singapore

Contents

Contributors

Gillian E. Armstrong BSc MCSP
Senior Physiotherapist, Cardiac Rehabilitation, Glasgow Royal
Infirmary University NHS Trust, Glasgow, UK
7. Lifestyle management: exercise

Paul Bennett PhD
Consultant Clinical Psychologist, Gwent Psychology and
Consultation Liaison Psychiatry Services, University of Wales, UK
8. Lifestyle management: behavioural change

Douglas Carroll BSc PhD
Professor of Applied Psychology, School of Sport and Exercise
Sciences, University of Birmingham, Birmingham, UK
8. Lifestyle management: behavioural change

Margaret Clubb RGN DipFP ATC/RCCTPDip
Practice Nurse, Eskbridge Medical Centre, Musselburgh, UK
14. Prevention in practice: the role of the nurse in the risk factor team

Joan Curzio PhD RGN
Project Leader, Research Initiative for Scotland, Glasgow Caledonian
University, Glasgow, UK. Formerly Nurse Researcher in Department
of Medicine and Therapeutics, University of Glasgow, Western
Infirmary, Glasgow, UK
4. Hypertension

Elizabeth Farish PhD FRCPath
Consultant Biochemist, Department of Biochemistry, Stobhill NHS
Trust, Glasgow, UK
13. Women and coronary heart disease

Allan Gaw MB ChB MD PhD
British Heart Foundation Research Fellow and Honorary Senior
Registrar in Clinical Biochemistry, Department of Pathological
Biochemistry, Glasgow Royal Infirmary, Glasgow, UK
3. *Cholesterol and lipoproteins*
10. *Lipid-lowering drug therapy*

Nicola S. Gilbert BSc(Hons) Nutrition SRD
Joint post as Lecturer in Nutrition, School of Biological Sciences,
University of Surrey and Dietitian at the Royal Surrey County and
St Luke's Hospitals NHS Trust, Surrey, UK
6. *Lifestyle management: diet*

Bruce A. Griffin BSc PhD
Lecturer in Nutritional Metabolism, School of Biological Sciences,
University of Surrey, Surrey, UK
6. *Lifestyle management: diet*

Elizabeth M. Keith RGN
Cardiac Rehabilitation Sister, Glasgow Royal Infirmary,
Glasgow, UK
12. *Cardiac rehabilitation*

Susan S. Kennedy BSc RGN SCM District Nurse
Nurse Co-ordinator, Shared-Care for Hypertension, Western
Infirmary, Glasgow, UK
4. *Hypertension*

Grace M. Lindsay BSc(Hons) RGN SCM RN MN
Lecturer in Nursing and Midwifery Studies, University of Glasgow,
Glasgow, UK
2. *Risk Factor Assessment*
13. *Women and coronary heart disease*

A. Ross Lorimer MD FRCP (Glasgow, London, Edinburgh)
Honorary Professor in Medicine, Consultant Physician and
Cardiologist Royal Infirmary, Glasgow, UK
1. *Coronary Heart Disease: pathology, epidemiology and diagnosis*

Gordon T. McInnes BSc MD GRCP FFPM
Senior Lecturer and Honorary Consultant Physician,

University Department of Medicine and Therapeutics, Western Infirmary, Glasgow, Glasgow, UK
11. Anti-hypertensive therapy

Doreen McIntyre MA(Hons) MPH PGCE
Co-ordinator Glasgow 2000, Greater Glasgow Health Board, Glasgow, UK
5. Lifestyle management: smoking

Keith G. Oldroyd MD(Hons) MRCP
Consultant Cardiologist, Hairmyres Hospital, East Kilbride, UK
9. Medical management of coronary heart disease

James Shepherd FRCPath FRCP
Professor, Department of Pathological Biochemistry, Royal Infirmary, Glasgow, UK
3. Cholesterol and lipoproteins

Ginny Styles BA(Hons)
Workplace Consultant; Glasgow 2000, Greater Glasgow Health Board, Glasgow, UK
5. Lifestyle management: smoking

Preface

Coronary heart disease (CHD) is the largest single cause of death and disability in the industrialized world. The modern health care team has an important function in the diagnosis and management of this disease, but, in addition, plays a key role in its prevention. Several modifiable risk factors for CHD are well recognized: principally smoking, hypertension and hyperlipidaemia. The assessment and correction of these risk factors by lifestyle and medical means is an enormous challenge to health care professionals today.

This book is designed to present the evidence and rationale for CHD risk factor management. It is written from a practical standpoint, focusing on the patient and providing useful advice for the practitioner. The book has not been targeted towards any single group within the large and diverse health care team that manages patients with this disease or those at increased risk of developing it. Instead, a broad approach has been taken with the inclusion of useful information for the different professions such as dietitians, physiotherapists, occupational therapists, clinical psychologists, physicians and nurses.

The book begins with an introductory chapter, which describes the nature of the disease. Other chapters focus on the three main correctable risk factors for CHD and their management. Also included are chapters on cardiac rehabilitation, women and CHD, and global risk assessment. The book concludes with a chapter specifically on the role of the nurse in acknowledgement of the fact that nurses are the single largest professional group in health care and, as such, are key figures in the prevention and management of this disease.

Each chapter includes case histories, practical exercises in order to help the reader translate theory into practice, and a summary of the chapter's key points as well as directions for further, more detailed reading.

By their very nature, the chapters overlap to some degree. While we have attempted to minimize this we have allowed some repetition of central issues in order to facilitate continuity and to reinforce these important points. What we have tried to do is equip the health care team with a working tool in the form of this handbook, which will provide, in a single volume, much of the practical information that is needed to tackle these problems successfully.

Glasgow 1997   G. M. L., A. G.

Coronary heart disease: pathology, epidemiology and diagnosis

A. Ross Lorimer

■ CONTENTS

EPIDEMIOLOGY

Coronary heart disease (CHD) is the single most important cause of death and, more importantly, the single biggest cause of premature death in modern, industrialized countries. In addition, it is an increasing cause of death in developing countries. In England and Wales, in 1991, 26% of all deaths were attributed to CHD and 2.5% of the National Health Service expenditure was taken up by CHD (DoH 1992) at a cost of £500 million per annum.

Throughout the world since 1979 all registered health events are coded using the International Statistical Classification of Diseases, Injuries and Cause of Death (ICD, ninth revision). For health events related to CHD, ICD numbers 410–414 are used. In most epidemiological studies, CHD events are defined by these ICD codes and this allows useful comparison between different populations.

The CHD mortality rates in 1994 for men and women in 32 countries are shown in Figure 1.1. There is clearly a wide variation in these rates, the highest being found in Eastern Europe, Northern Ireland and Scotland and the lowest rates in Spain, France and Japan. Mortality rates are generally much higher for men than women. This distinction is present at all ages but is less after the menopause. Coronary morbidity and mortality rates in

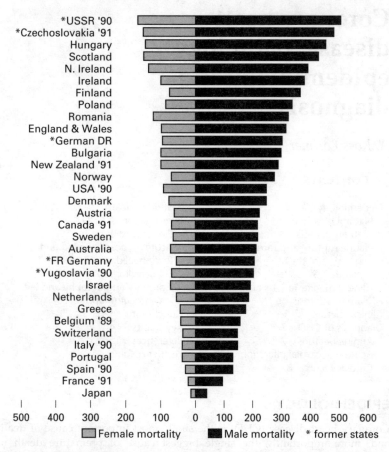

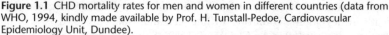

Figure 1.1 CHD mortality rates for men and women in different countries (data from WHO, 1994, kindly made available by Prof. H. Tunstall-Pedoe, Cardiovascular Epidemiology Unit, Dundee).

women generally lag behind those for men by about 10 years, but beyond the seventh decade in life become similar in men and women.

Between the years 1970 and 1985, world-wide trends in age-adjusted death rates for CHD in men show a dramatic decline of 50% in countries such as the USA, while countries such as Poland and Romania in the same period have shown marked increases of more than 70% (Uemura & Pisa 1988). Scotland has shown a fall of approximately 10–15% but remains near the top of the international league table of male and female CHD mortality (Tunstall-Pedoe 1994, personal communication). Over the last 10 years in Scotland both male and female rates of CHD have fallen although at a slower rate for women (Fig. 1.2).

CHD mortality rates per 100 000 population over last 10 years in Scotland

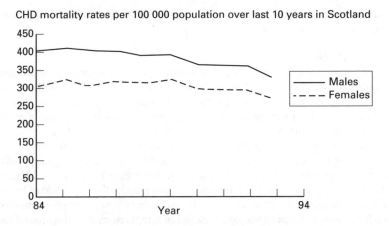

Figure 1.2 CHD mortality rates per 100 000 population over the last 10 years in men and women in Scotland (Registrar General for Scotland 1994).

In addition to geographical variation, CHD mortality rates are also influenced by ethnic origin and social class. Studies of different ethnic groups within the UK have demonstrated a higher than average rate within the South Asian community and a lower than average rate in those of Afro-Caribbean origin (Poulter 1993).

CHD mortality varies across different social classes. Rates in the most deprived groups are much greater than those seen in the affluent groups (OPCS 1986). It is interesting to note that the current relationship between affluence and CHD is a reversal of the previous situation. When CHD first emerged as an important cause of death it was seen predominantly in social class I. People in this group have made lifestyle modifications and diminished their risk of CHD but now, as the disease emerges in the Third World, it is once again those in social class I who are susceptible. This has important implications for both aetiology and treatment.

A search for the origins, cause and subsequent prevention of CHD has proceeded from early epidemiological studies of populations to prospective cohort studies where a population sample is identified, clinically assessed and then monitored for a number of years for signs of disease. The aetiology of CHD has therefore been the subject of intense study over the last five decades and many contributory or risk factors have been identified. These are discussed in detail in Chapter 2.

Natural history of atherogenesis

Atherosclerosis is a pathological process, which is defined as a focal, inflammatory fibro-proliferative response to multiple forms of endothelial injury. The response to injury hypothesis for the development of athero-sclerosis was formally proposed by Ross and his colleagues more than 20 years ago and has been refined and developed since. There are other hypotheses that try to explain the complex pathogenesis of the atherosclerotic plaque but none have been so widely accepted as that of a normal repair process gone awry.

Fatty streak

All infants have focal thickening of the coronary artery intima due to smooth muscle cell proliferation. Although this is an important hallmark of the developing atherosclerotic plaque, it is not unique to this condition as it is considered to be a simple adaptive response. The first lesions that may be recognized as truly atherosclerotic are called fatty streaks. These are small lesions that on gross inspection are hardly raised, and are caused by focal collections of foam cells within the intima. Necropsy studies (Stary 1989) reveal the presence of atherosclerotic plaques ranging in size from the fatty streak to larger plaques. The fatty streak lesion may be the precursor of larger atherosclerotic plaques but also may be an entirely reversible phenomenon. Such a belief comes from necropsy studies of infants from societies around the world where atherosclerosis as a cause of death is relatively rare. These infants, although unlikely to have died from CHD if they had lived to maturity, have many fatty streaks in their arteries.

Progression of the fatty streak to a larger more complex lesion is thought to occur due to two key processes. First the foam cells, engorged with lipid, begin to die and break down in the centre of the fatty streak. Release of their cytoplasmic contents leads to the presence of extracellular lipids and the secretion of growth factors as part of the inflammatory response (Fig. 1.3).

Smooth muscle cell migration and proliferation is the second process involved in the progression of the fatty streak. Smooth muscle cells push into the lipid-rich plaque where they divide and begin to synthesize a connective tissue matrix composed of elastic fibre proteins, collagen and proteoglycans. The increase in cell numbers and the laying down of collagenous matrix both serve to increase the bulk of the plaque, which now protrudes into the artery lumen and is referred to as a raised fibrolipid or advanced plaque. Such plaques are difficult to age but necropsy studies suggest that they take 10–15 years to develop (PDAY 1990). It is also believed that new fatty streaks are continually forming throughout adult life.

Plaque rupture and thrombosis

The dangers of the plaque lie both in its size and in its tendency to fissure and ulcerate. The final pathway to a major clinical event, such as an acute myocardial infarction (MI), is not clear but haemorrhage into an atheromatous plaque, rupture or fissuring of a plaque, or thrombosis on the surface of a plaque are mechanisms that are likely to be involved.

Davies and his colleagues (1985) have shown that in patients with crescendo angina and acute myocardial infarction, thrombus formation was an important, rapidly changing and dynamic process. Post-mortem studies have shown that coronary thrombi are nearly all related to the fissuring of the atheromatous plaque. The factors which determine whether thrombus does occur within the lumen are partially local, including the size and geometry of the intimal tear, whether lipid is extruded into the lumen itself, the degree

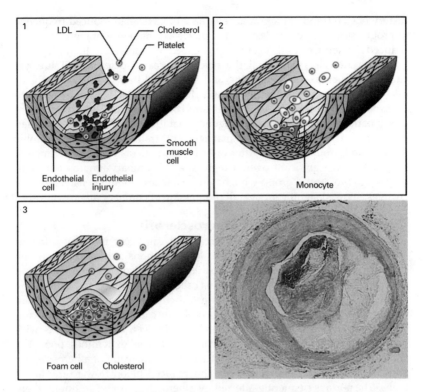

Figure 1.3 Development of atheroma in coronary arteries, with histopathological section (bottom right): LDL = low density lipoprotein. (Reproduced with permission from Gaw et al 1995.)

of stenosis, and blood flow rate at the site. Systemic factors such as the thrombotic or thrombolytic potential at the time will also play a part. Not all plaque fissuring will result in these dire consequences. The plaque may re-stabilize and heal over, but at a cost: the healed plaque will now be larger than before (Fuster et al 1992).

Regression of the atherosclerotic plaque

The concept of therapeutic intervention producing reversal or regression of atherosclerotic lesions originated in the 1940s. Post-mortem examinations on individuals who had suffered great weight losses prior to their death, revealed that the extent of plaque development in the aorta and coronary arteries was much less than expected. Many studies have been conducted to confirm and evaluate these observations.

Recently, the results from randomized, controlled clinical studies using different treatments for lowering cholesterol have been reported. In the Familial Atherosclerosis Treatment Study (Brown et al 1990), middle-aged men who had moderately elevated low density lipoprotein (LDL), a family history of CHD, and angiographic evidence of CHD, had reduced frequency of progression of coronary lesions and increased frequency of regression and reduced incidence of CHD events if prescribed lipid-lowering therapy.

In the Lifestyle Heart Trial the objective was to determine if lifestyle changes in diet, exercise, smoking and stress could affect coronary atherosclerosis. Patients with angiographically documented CHD were assigned to an experimental group or to a usual care control group. The experimental group patients were prescribed a regimen that included a low-fat vegetarian diet, smoking cessation, stress management training, moderate aerobic exercise and group support. After only 1 year, patients in the experimental group showed significant overall regression of coronary atherosclerosis in contrast to the control group who, having made less comprehensive lifestyle changes, showed significant overall progression of coronary atherosclerosis.

Clinical manifestations of atherosclerosis

Atherosclerosis is a pathological process that can occur in many different arteries. The most common clinical manifestations are seen when the coronary arteries are involved. Atherosclerosis can also affect the peripheral arteries resulting in leg muscle ischaemia called intermittent claudication. The patient will usually complain of calf muscle cramps when walking that are relieved by rest. The severity of this condition can vary from mild inconvenience to the very severe when there is pain even at rest. Patients with peripheral vascular disease may also complain of cold extremities, poor skin and ulceration or even gangrene, all of which are the result of atherosclerotic narrowing of the peripheral arteries and reduced blood flow to the lower limbs. The aorta is frequently affected by atherosclerosis and, although there is seldom complete occlusion of blood flow through this, the largest of our arteries, there can be serious clinical consequences. The atherosclerotic lesions weaken the aortic wall and can contribute to the development of aneurysms, particularly in the abdominal aorta. Rupture of an aortic aneurysm will result in sudden death. When the cerebral arteries are affected by atherosclerosis, the patient may suffer a spectrum of effects ranging from mild neurological disturbances such as reversible memory loss through transient ischaemic attacks (TIAs) to a fatal cerebrovascular accident. The precise clinical presentation of cerebrovascular disease depends on the area of the central nervous system deprived of blood.

The medical and surgical management of the atherosclerotic lesion itself rather than its clinical sequelae is relatively new. Surgical intervention by means of bypass grafting of stenosed vessels provides symptomatic relief but in itself does nothing to correct the underlying disease process, which will continue unabated. Such a dramatic and expensive intervention should always be accompanied by a careful atherosclerotic risk profile assessment and the correction of the major risk factors. This will only be possible with the cooperation of the patient, which in turn will depend on providing him or her with the facts.

As yet there is no way to obtain complete dissolution of atheromatous plaques but animal and human angiographic studies have demonstrated that powerful lipid-lowering drug therapy can halt the progression of such lesions and in many instances result in their regression with an improved clinical outcome for the patient. These observations place lipid-lowering drug treatments on a new therapeutic level. Previously, they were regarded as merely preventive measures to reduce the overall atherosclerotic risk of an individual; now they may be viewed as active anti-atherosclerotic treatments.

CLINICAL PICTURE

There are a number of clinical presentations of CHD. The most common of these are:

- sudden death
- myocardial infarction, which may be recognized or silent
- angina pectoris, which may be stable or unstable
- asymptomatic ischaemia.

Although it is convenient to consider these as different end points in the CHD process, it is important to remember that these conditions are inter-related and the individual patient can move from one group to another.

DIAGNOSIS OF CHD

Coronary heart disease (CHD) can present as angina pectoris, myocardial infarction, congestive heart failure or sudden death. The diagnosis of CHD is based on a combination of symptoms and signs (Box 1.1).

Angina pectoris

Angina pectoris is a symptom complex due to reversible myocardial ischaemia. The symptoms are those of chest pain or tightness which can radiate to one or both arms, to the throat or to the back. Pain is brought on by effort or emotion, or may occur spontaneously at rest. Patients with angina pectoris can be divided into clinical subgroups by symptoms. Those with stable angina have a reproducible pattern in terms of intensity and duration of pain and precipitating factors. Unstable angina includes those with recent onset of symptoms (less than 6 months) or a changing pattern often involving spontaneous pain at rest or with crescendo worsening of symptoms.

It must be remembered that angina pectoris is a symptom and not a diagnosis. It is most often due to underlying atherosclerotic CHD but can be due to other causes such as anaemia, thyroid dysfunction and aortic valve

---

Box 1.1 Angina pectoris: clinical presentation

- Lasts from 30 seconds to 20 minutes.
- Is precipitated by exertion or emotion.
- Is described by the patient as *pressing, squeezing, tightness* or *a weight.*
- Sometimes radiates to left arm, neck or lower jaw.
- Is relieved by rest or nitrates.

disease. Angina pectoris results from a transient imbalance of myocardial oxygen supply and demand.

The factors which influence demand are:

- heart rate
- contractility
- wall tension
- left ventricular volume.

The pathogenesis of angina is usually based on an underlying stenotic lesion of one or more coronary arteries. The concept that dynamic coronary obstruction is most commonly due to coronary vasoconstriction (spasm) has been re-examined (Maseri 1980), and the condition has been found to usually occur in association with underlying coronary atherosclerotic narrowing.

Although the diagnosis of angina is often straightforward, angina may be confused with other conditions, for example:

- musculoskeletal problems
- oesophagitis
- pericarditis
- pulmonary embolism.

Acute myocardial infarction

Acute myocardial infarction develops when myocardial ischaemia occurs for sufficient time to cause necrosis of a localized area of the myocardium. The initial reduction in myocardial blood flow may be secondary to:

- intracoronary thrombus—often associated with plaque fissure
- substantial haemorrhage with bleeding into an atheromatous plaque
- platelet aggregation in the presence of severe atheroma leading to reduced flow and perhaps thrombus.

Infarction may occur without total coronary artery occlusion when coronary flow falls as a result of severe hypotension. This can be associated with systemic haemorrhage or shock. Premonitory symptoms are common but their origin is often unrecognized. The pain of myocardial infarction is similar to that of angina pectoris but results from irreversible myocardial ischaemia. The pain does not subside with rest or nitrate therapy and may last for several hours. The intensity of pain gives no indication of the severity of the infarction. Indeed, particularly in the elderly, myocardial infarction may be 'silent' and present, not with pain, but with some other feature such as acute left ventricular failure. Accompanying symptoms are summarized in Box 1.2. Such symptoms are largely due to associated autonomic disturbance. Up to 50% of all deaths from MI occur within 2 hours of onset, mainly as a result of dysrhythmia. The majority of these deaths occur outside hospital.

Cardiac failure

Cardiac failure can be defined as 'a clinical state resulting from the inability of the heart to provide sufficient blood for tissue metabolic needs'. The clinical syndrome of cardiac failure has long been recognized but its management

Box 1.2 Symptoms associated with acute myocardial infarction

- Severe crushing central chest pain
- Dyspnoea
- Syncope
- Cold sweat
- Pallor
- Nausea
- Sudden death

remains a major problem. At least 25% of patients with cardiovascular disease have heart failure and the long-term prognosis is determined by the extent to which cardiac performance is impaired.

There have been recent major advances in our understanding of the patho-physiology of heart failure and its management. The role of angiotensin-converting enzyme (ACE) inhibitors has been especially important in improving symptoms and prognosis in those with impaired left ventricular function.

CHD is a major, although not the only, factor in depressing left ventricular function. Dyspnoea is the predominant feature due to increasing pulmonary vascular engorgement and decreased compliance of the left ventricle.

Sudden death

Reducing the rates of sudden death is an important challenge in cardiology. While prevention of sudden death is, of course, the ultimate aim, it is also important that resources are available to take advantage of the considerable advances that have been made in the resuscitation of those apparently 'dead'. These improvements have been largely due to the more widespread avail-ability of defibrillators and the training of paramedic personnel. In sudden cardiac death, 75% of subjects have evidence of CHD while other causes include cardiomyopathy, hypokalaemia and valvular disease. The mode of death is arrhythmic—usually ventricular fibrillation—and may occur both in the absence and presence of acute myocardial infarction (Cobb et al 1980). The development of ventricular fibrillation appears to be the end result of an interplay of electrical and mechanical factors related to acute myocardial ischaemia and cellular membrane instability.

INVESTIGATION OF CHD

Since angina is a symptom complex, objective confirmatory evidence for the diagnosis is usually sought. The severity of pain is not a guide to the severity of the disease. Minor coronary artery disease can be associated with severe chest pain and major coronary artery disease can have apparently mild symptoms.

Electrocardiography

The main initial investigation is electrocardiography. A resting electrocardiograph (ECG) should always be recorded. It may or may not be abnormal. Indeed, the resting ECG is normal in 50% of those with a history of possible angina. The resting ECG may show evidence of a previous infarction or changes representing ischaemia such as ST segment depression or T wave inversion (Fig. 1.4).

Exercise electrocardiography

Exercise (stress) testing helps to diagnose myocardial ischaemia. Stress testing by treadmill or bicycle ergometer is important both for making the diagnosis and establishing the degree of disability. It is essential to use a standard protocol. The best-known is that developed by Bruce in Seattle. The angle and speed of the treadmill are increased at regular intervals of 3 minutes. The total workload is easily calculated and the ECG monitored for the development of ST depression as an indicator of myocardial ischaemia.

Ischaemic changes developing within a few minutes of starting graded exercise can be an indication for more detailed investigation such as coronary angiography. Stress testing will allow the diagnosis of CHD to be made in a further 35% of patients.

The exercise stress test provides an objective non-invasive measure of a patient's cardiovascular capacity. It is widely available, easily repeated and has a low (but not absent) mortality and morbidity: mortality 1 : 20 000; combined morbidity and mortality 1 : 1000 (Stuart & Ellestad 1980). Experience and resuscitation equipment are required for those supervising exercise testing. The most straightforward uses of exercise testing are:

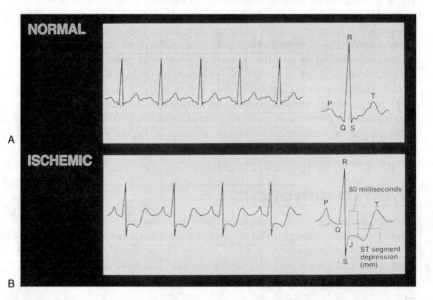

Figure 1.4 ECG tracings showing: (A) normal tracing and (B) acute myocardial ischaemia.

- clinical assessment
  —chest pain of unknown cause
  —stable angina
  —after myocardial infarction
- evaluation of treatment
  —medical therapy
  —after coronary artery bypass grafting
  —after myocardial infarction.

Exercise testing is recommended following myocardial infarction to help identify those at risk. A normal exercise test indicates a good prognosis. An exercise test limited by pain or by the development of ischaemic ECG changes or a dysrhythmia can identify those at risk and requiring further investigation. Many units undertake symptom-limited exercise testing just before discharge (usually 8 days post-infarct) and again at 6 weeks. Some patients with a positive test at discharge will have a negative test at 6 weeks. This may be the consequence of resolution of thrombus and vessel recanalization or development of collateral circulation. Others may develop ischaemic changes at 6 weeks when exercise performance has improved and the underlying ischaemia can be identified.

Acute myocardial infarction

The diagnosis of acute myocardial infarction is based on the combination of clinical symptoms and signs, ECG changes and enzyme changes.

The ECG changes of acute myocardial infarction occur in sequence and are known as sequential changes. In acute transmural or full-thickness infarction the changes are:

- ST segment elevation   day 1
- Q wave development   day 1–2
- Subsequent T wave inversion   day 3–4.

When MI does not involve the full thickness of the ventricle it is known as subendocardial MI. There are ST and T wave changes but Q waves do not develop. Transmural and subendocardial infarction are of equal clinical importance.

Cardiac enzyme changes

Intracellular enzymes are released when ischaemia disrupts cell membranes. Changes in cardiac enzymes after MI follow a characteristic pattern over time and are of considerable value in making a diagnosis (Fig. 1.5). The following enzymes are usually measured in the first 3 days following a suspected MI:

- total creatine kinase (CK)
- aspartate transaminase (AST)
- alanine transaminase (ALT)
- lactate dehydrogenase (LDH).

Increasingly important is *creatine kinase MB isoenzyme* (CKMB). CK levels

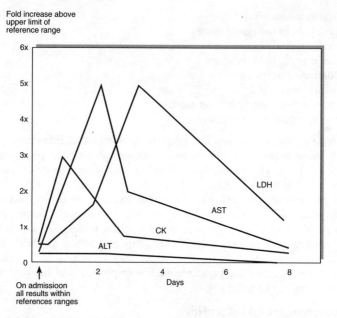

Fold increase above
upper limit of
reference range

On admissioon
all results within
references ranges

Days

Figure 1.5 Enzymes in serum following an uncomplicated myocardial infarction (reproduced with permission from Gaw et al 1995).

rise rapidly after muscle damage and peak in approximately 24 hours. This allows rapid diagnosis of a suspected MI.

AST is found in heart muscle and in the liver while ALT is predominantly found in the liver. Increased AST with a normal ALT indicates cardiac muscle damage while raised AST and ALT would point to liver damage as the cause of raised enzyme levels.

Sometimes a patient may only be seen 2–3 days after a possible infarction. The LDH enzyme will still be increased at this time when the others have returned to normal. The diagnosis of infarction can still be made with confidence.

CKMB is a specific isoenzyme found in cardiac muscle. A raised level implies cardiac damage whereas a raised total CK may follow muscle damage anywhere in the body. It will be raised for example following an intramuscular injection. CKMB measurements may well become increasingly used and increasingly valuable.

Radionuclide assessment

The use of radionuclides enhances the non-invasive detection of CHD. Radionuclides are injected intravenously and the gamma camera provides an image of the distribution of radioactivity. Information can be obtained at rest or after exercise. Technetium-99m tagged to red blood cells or to albumin is an isotope that initially remains largely within the blood pool and can be used to estimate the dynamic performance of the heart, especially left ventricular volume and contractility. Thallium-201 is an isotope that is taken up by the myocardium itself. The uptake reflects myocardial blood supply. The better the blood supply the higher the uptake of thallium.

Areas of ischaemia are areas of poor uptake and are detected as 'cold' areas on the myocardial image. Such areas may remain 'cold' at rest and indicate scar or infarct tissue. They may also, however, reperfuse and this indicates areas of reversible ischaemia that might benefit from revascularization. Nuclear cardiology is especially useful in assessing whether or not an intervention such as coronary angioplasty has been of benefit. Impaired myocardial perfusion if present can be detected without the need for invasive angiography.

Another important role for nuclear cardiology is when conventional exercise testing is not possible because of arthritis or peripheral vascular disease. The heart can be 'stressed' by pharmacological methods such as by injecting dipyridamole or dobutamine, which enhance differences in perfusion and again demonstrate 'cold' areas of impaired blood supply. Nuclear cardiology techniques are a useful adjunct to conventional exercise testing by ECG analysis but do not replace it.

Echocardiography

Cardiac ultrasound (echocardiography) is now established as a major non-invasive investigation. Initially used in the diagnosis of congenital and rheumatic heart disease, echocardiography is now a mainstay in the assessment of the consequences of CHD. It does not deal with the coronary circulation but with ventricular function. The ability of the heart muscle to contract can be observed and measured both in terms of localized areas and of global ventricular function. The terms used are:

- *Dyskinesis:* expansion or dilatation instead of contraction—usually an indication of an aneurysm
- *Akinesis:* absent contraction—this can be found when there is a large infarct or scar tissue
- *Hypokinesis:* diminished movement—often when there is impaired coronary blood flow.

Left ventricular function can be quantified in terms of ejection fraction (EF).

$$EF = \frac{\text{end diastolic volume} - \text{end systolic volume}}{\text{end diastolic volume}} \times 100$$

An EF is usually around 60–70%. Reduction in the ejection fraction to below 25% is associated with a poor prognosis following infarction. Regular echocardiograms can be a useful method of following progress and assessing effects of treatment.

Coronary angiography and left ventriculography

Cardiac catheterization allows radiographic visualization of the left ventricle and coronary arteries. Catheters are inserted into either the femoral artery (Judkin's technique) or brachial artery (Sones' technique) and manipulated retrogradely to the left ventricle. Injection of contrast medium and recording

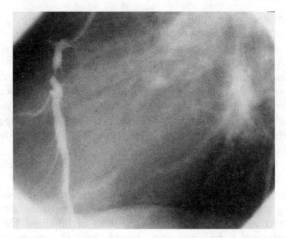

Figure 1.6 Coronary angiography: radio-opaque dye has been injected into the coronary arteries through a fine catheter inserted into the femoral artery in the groin and passed up to the aortic ring.

on video or film gives information on coronary artery anatomy (Fig. 1.6), left ventricular structure and function in terms of contractility. Selective coronary angiography in multiple projections remains the principal diagnostic study in selecting patients for coronary angioplasty or coronary bypass surgery, is still the most accurate index available for assessing prognosis in patients with angina pectoris and is probably still the final arbiter in studies of obscure chest pain.

CONCLUSIONS

The diagnosis of CHD can be reached through non-invasive means such as clinical history, and ECG tracings at rest and during exercise. More invasive investigations include angiography and radionuclide imaging techniques. CHD leads to a range of clinical consequences including angina, myocardial infarction, heart failure and sudden death.

■ KEY POINTS

• CHD is the greatest single cause of death in the industrialized world, occurring in both sexes, but presenting earlier in men. Rates are improving in some groups while worsening in others.

• It may present as sudden death, myocardial infarction, or angina pectoris with chest pain being the classic symptom.

• A good history is the most important aid in the diagnosis of angina but there are many other techniques available for the full evaluation of CHD.

• Angina pectoris is a symptom complex due to reversible myocardial ischaemia.

- The diagnosis of acute myocardial infarction is based on the combination of clinical symptoms and signs, ECG changes and enzyme changes.

- Cardiac ultrasound (echocardiography) is a major non-invasive investigation used in the assessment of the consequences of CHD.

- Cardiac catheterization allows radiographic visualization of the left ventricle and coronary arteries and is used to assess prognosis and treatment options in patients with CHD.

REFERENCES

Brown G, Albers J J, Fisher L D, Schaefer S M, Lin J T, Kaplan C, Zhao X Q, Bisson B D, Fitzpatrick V F, Dodge H T 1990 Regression of coronary artery disease as a result of intensive lipid-lowering therapy in men with high levels of apolipoprotein B. New England Journal of Medicine 323: 946–955

Cobb L A, Werner J A, Teobaugh J 1980 Sudden cardiac death. Modern Concepts in Cardiovascular Disease XLIX: 31–36

Davies M J, Thomas A 1985 Plaque fissuring—the cause of acute myocardial infarction, sudden ischaemic death and crescendo angina. British Heart Journal 53: 363–373

Department of Health (DoH) 1992 The health of the nation: a strategy for health in England. HMSO, London

Fuster V, Badimon L, Badimon J J, Chesebro J H 1992 The pathogenesis of coronary artery disease and the acute coronary syndromes (I). New England Journal of Medicine 326(4): 242–250

Gaw A et al 1995 Clinical biochemistry: an illustrated colour text. Churchill Livingstone, Edinburgh

Lerner D J, Kannel W B 1986 Patterns of coronary heart disease morbidity and mortality in the sexes: a 26 year follow-up of the Framingham population. American Heart Journal 111: 383–390

Maseri A 1980 Pathogenic mechanisms in angina pectoris. British Heart Journal 43(6): 648–660

Office of Population Censuses and Surveys (OPCS) 1986 Registrar General's decennial supplement on occupational mortality (1979–1983). HMSO, London

Office of Population Censuses and Surveys (OPCS) 1990 Mortality statistics, cause. Leaflet DH2 (17). HMSO, London

Pathological Determinants of Atherosclerosis in Youth (PDAY) Research Group 1990 A preliminary report of the Pathological Determinants of Atherosclerosis in Youth (PDAY) Research Group. Journal of the American Medical Association 264(23): 3018–3024

Pisa Z, Uemura K 1982 Trends of mortality from ischaemic heart disease and other cardiovascular diseases in 27 countries, 1968–1977. World Health Statistics Quarterly 35: 11–47

Poulter N 1993 The coronary heart disease epidemic: British and international trends. In: Poulter N, Sever P, Thom S (eds) Cardiovascular disease: risk factors and intervention. Radcliffe Medical Press, Oxford

Registrar General for Scotland 1994 Report of the Registrar General for Scotland. HMSO, Edinburgh

Stary H C 1989 Evolution and progression of atherosclerotic lesions in coronary arteries of children and young adults. Arteriosclerosis 9 (Suppl. 1): 119–132

Stuart R J Jr, Ellestad M H 1980 National survey of exercise testing facilities. Chest 77(1): 94–97

Thomas C et al 1992 Textbook and colour atlas of the cardiovascular system. Chapman & Hall Medical, London

Uemura K, Pisa Z 1988 Trends in cardiovascular disease mortality in industrialised countries since 1950. World Health Statistics Quarterly 41: 155–178

FURTHER READING

Braunwald E (ed) 1988 Heart disease: a textbook of cardiovascular medicine. W B Saunders, Philadelphia

Gaw A, Packard C J, Shepherd J 1994 Lipids and atherosclerosis. In: Bloom A L, Forbes C D, Thomas D P, Tuddenham E G D (eds) Haemostasis and thrombosis, 3rd edn. Churchill Livingstone, Edinburgh, ch 50: 1153–1168

Lorimer A R, Shepherd J (eds) 1991 Preventive cardiology. Blackwell Scientific Publications, Oxford

Ross R 1993 The pathogenesis of atherosclerosis: a perspective for the 1990s. Nature: 362: 801–809

Shepherd J (ed) 1987 Lipoprotein metabolism. Baillière's Clinical Endocrinology and Metabolism. Baillière Tindall, London

Swales J D (ed) 1994 Textbook of hypertension. Blackwell Scientific Publications, Oxford

Risk factor assessment

Grace M. Lindsay

INTRODUCTION

The importance of underlying risk factors in the treatment and management of coronary heart disease (CHD) is captured in the following quotation: 'Coronary disease does not really begin with crushing chest pain, pulmonary edema, shock, angina or ventricular fibrillation, but rather with the more subtle signs like a poor coronary risk profile' (Kannel 1976).

The subtlety of the poor coronary risk profile alludes to the sub-clinical nature of many of the risk factors so that active steps have to be taken in order to reveal their presence. Estimation of risk is an integral part of preventing premature CHD, particularly because there is now sound evidence that effective intervention can not only decrease risk but also halt the continued development of atherosclerosis, or even reverse the process. This chapter addresses the concept of CHD risk, its assessment, interpretation and role in the prevention of CHD.

RISK

The terms 'risk' or 'risk factor' are used often but sometimes without the meaning being clear. The word 'risk' originates from the French *risque* and is a fairly modern addition to the English language. Collinson & Dowie (1980) report that the word did not enter the language until the mid-17th century and then appeared in anglicized spelling in insurance transactions during the second quarter of the 18th century.

One of the immediate difficulties that arises when trying to define risk is that it has both a technical definition, e.g. risk assessment or hazard management, and a strong colloquial usage. In common use the word 'risk' is associated with the chances of loss rather than gain. The Oxford English Dictionary definition of risk includes 'hazard, chance of bad consequences, loss etc.'. The consideration of risk in decision-making is to recognize that the future can never be known with certainty and, at best, comes with a range of possibilities. Risk and uncertainty are often used interchangeably. Both concepts can be defined as being basically a problem of lack of information about future events that might arise. Knight (1933) distinguishes between the two concepts by arguing that *risks* are future outcomes to which it is possible to attach probabilities, whereas *uncertainty* is a situation where a probability cannot be ascribed. CHD risk factor assessment is concerned with the nature of risk, where probabilities can be ascribed to outcome and where modification of risk can have a beneficial effect on outcome.

The term 'risk factor' is widely used to describe those characteristics found in individuals that have been shown in observational epidemiological studies, autopsy studies, metabolic studies and genetic studies to relate to the subsequent occurrence of CHD.

In global terms, risk factor categories cover personal, lifestyle, biochemical and physiological characteristics, some of which are modifiable while others are not.

Risk factor hypothesis

A search for the origins, cause and subsequent prevention of CHD has proceeded from early descriptive epidemiological studies of populations (Keys 1980) to prospective cohort studies. In the latter, a population sample is identified, clinically assessed and then monitored for a number of years for signs of disease (Dawber et al 1951, Multiple Risk Factor Intervention Trial Research Group 1982). One of the first major prospective studies to monitor and document incidence of CHD was started in the small community of Framingham in the United States (Dawber et al 1951). As stated by Shaper et al (1985), it has 'become synonymous with the risk factor concept and is the source of much of our knowledge about the risk of CHD in individuals'.

Quantifying the risk

Statistical techniques have been used to estimate the strength of association between risk factors and the likelihood of developing CHD. There are two main approaches: univariate analysis and multivariate analysis.

Univariate analysis. This seeks to test the effect of one variable at a time on subsequent risk of disease. An association must be interpreted with care because many factors are related or dependent on each other, e.g. with increased obesity there is an associated increase in blood pressure. To evaluate whether a risk factor is exerting an effect in its own right, the more complex multivariate analysis must be employed.

Multivariate analysis. This tests the effect of several risk factors at the same time and estimates the strength of the relationship. It also tests whether the relationship is independent of the effects of some other variables or dependent on them. Examination of risk factor 'dependence' is concerned with the search for aetiology. However, it is important to remember that even if a risk factor can be explained by its relationship to another factor (dependent) for an individual such an increased risk factor still contributes to increased CHD risk.

Relative and absolute risk

A further complexity in interpretation of risk of CHD for the individual depends on whether the risk is quoted in *absolute* terms or *relative* to other individuals or other factors.

Absolute risk defines the expected rate of CHD events for any given combination of age, gender, and other risk factors. *Relative risk* is the ratio between the absolute risk in an individual and the absolute risk in someone of the same age and gender who has no other CHD risk factors.

Relative risk is therefore comparative in nature and it can be applied in grading risk within groups of individuals. For example, a young person smoking will have a high relative risk compared to an age and gender matched non-smoker but will have a low absolute risk. In contrast, with rising age absolute risk increases and relative risk falls, because in old age CHD is more common even in the absence of major CHD risk factors.

Identification of risk factors

The Framingham Study (Dawber et al 1951) began in the 1940s and was designed to generate information that would help in the early detection and prevention of CHD. The study started with a small number of male and female volunteers (740) in 1948 and has subsequently grown into a major prospective trial. Follow-up of the recruits, and in some cases their offspring, is still ongoing today and data from the study have given investigators valuable information about the relationship between various risk factors and CHD. It is also notable because it is one of the few large epidemiological studies of CHD that has included women in its cohort.

Several other prospective population studies were initiated in the United States in the 1950s and 1960s and a summary of their results has been published in the final report of the Pooling Project (Pooling Project Research Group 1978). Along with the Seven Countries Study (Keys 1980), they indicate factors that seem to predict a major part of the subsequent CHD. These were documented as level of blood pressure, serum cholesterol, relative weight and ECG abnormalities.

The web of causation for heart disease is complex and, as more experience of the disease process was gained, it became apparent that more factors than had already been documented had a role to play. While a multitude of factors have been potentially associated with CHD, St George (1983) reviewed the

---

Box 2.1 CHD risk factors

Lifestyle
- Tobacco smoking
- Diet high in saturated fat and calories, low in fruit and vegetables, high in sugar
- Physical inactivity
- Stress
- Excess alcohol
- Obesity

Biochemical or physiological
- Elevated plasma cholesterol
- Elevated BP
- Low plasma HDL-cholesterol
- Elevated plasma triglyceride
- Diabetes mellitus
- Thrombogenic factors

Personal
- Age
- Gender
- Family history (first degree)
- Personal history

---

literature and quantified the number of well-documented risk factors to be of the order of 20. However, in practice, attention focuses on the factors presented in Box 2.1. In terms of clinical practice it is useful to consider risk factors as either modifiable or immodifiable as detailed in Box 2.2.

Box 2.2 Major CHD risk factors routinely assessed in clinical practice

Modifiable
- Smoking
- Elevated plasma cholesterol
- Elevated BP
- Obesity
- Physical inactivity
- Excess alcohol
- Stress

Immodifiable
- Family history of CHD
- Personal history of CHD
- Diabetes mellitus
- Age
- Gender

RISK FACTORS FOR CORONARY HEART DISEASE

Three important, independent and modifiable risk factors have received particular attention, namely cigarette smoking, hyperlipidaemia and hypertension, with the weight of evidence suggesting a causal relationship with CHD. Because of their importance in the aetiology of CHD, separate chapters are devoted to each, namely Chapters 3, 4 and 5 respectively. The evidence for the association of other risk factors is less strong, but clearly demonstrates a link with the development of CHD; these will now be considered in more detail.

Age and gender

CHD increases with age in both men and women. It is rare in the first two decades of life, becoming more prevalent after the age of 30 and much more marked in males than in females below the age of 60 years. Beyond 60 years, CHD in females increases at an accelerated rate and after the seventh decade the rate approaches that in males (Fig. 2.1). It is unclear whether atherosclerosis is a result of the ageing process per se, or the cumulative effect of the known risk factors exerting their effect over time.

Epidemiological studies reveal that women are relatively protected against CHD while premenopausal and that this protection is less evident in the postmenopausal years. Interpretation of risk factors in females, the effects of

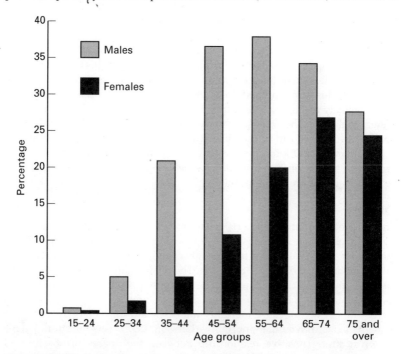

Figure 2.1 CHD death rates as a percentage of all deaths in men and women at different ages in Scotland, 1994 (data kindly provided by Prof. H. Tunstall-Pedoe).

hormonal status and the role of hormonal replacement therapy will be dealt with in more depth in Chapter 13.

Family history

A significant family history is considered to be present if CHD is diagnosed in first-degree relatives before the age of 60 years. The clustering of risk factors such as hypertension, diabetes and obesity is also common. Most of these groupings are a result of interactions between genetic factors and environmental influences so it is difficult to determine the relative effect of genetic factors, except in those with familial hypercholesterolaemia. Familial hypercholesterolaemia, in its heterozygous form, occurs in about 1 in 400–500 of the population with the homozygous form being extremely rare. It is thought that the genetic component of CHD risk is likely to be the result of the influence of many genes, i.e. polygenic, rather than the result of a single gene effect. In practice, the importance of recognizing a positive family history of CHD is so that other individuals at high risk can be identified and therefore made a priority for CHD risk factor assessment and management (Neufeld & Goldbourt 1983).

Physical activity

Long-term physical activity is known to be important in maintaining body weight and muscle tissue, in lowering blood pressure and in raising high density lipoprotein (HDL) cholesterol. Experimental studies using angiography in primates (Kramsch et al 1981) indicate that aerobic exercise reduces the severity of atherosclerosis even in the presence of an atherogenic diet. Indirect measures of ischaemia using electrocardiograph (ECG) treadmill testing have demonstrated a favourable response to physical training. Moreover, using this same methodology, men who were less physically fit were twice as likely to suffer a myocardial infarction than their fitter counterparts (Peters et al 1993). The exercise level required to improve a patient's risk factor profile has not been fully established but an excess energy expenditure of approximately 2000 kilocalories per week is thought to provide the same protection as that observed in athletes (Milvy & Seigel 1981). Exercise will be discussed in more detail in Chapter 7.

Obesity

The precise role of obesity as a risk factor for CHD is uncertain although there is general consensus on its adverse effects on both health and longevity. Body mass index (BMI) calculated from weight/height^2 has been recommended as the best estimate of obesity (Bray 1979). The relationship between obesity and all-cause mortality is 'J-shaped'. The thinnest people show some excess risk compared to those who are 'normal' or slightly overweight, but with increasing obesity all-cause mortality increases and this is largely due to an increase in cardiovascular mortality (Larsson 1992). Several studies have shown a strong positive relationship between the degree of obesity and presence of hypertension, hypertriglyceridaemia, hyperinsulinaemia and low levels of HDL-cholesterol. Central obesity, which is associated with increased intra-abdominal fat mass, has a particularly adverse effect on these risk factors and the actual risk of CHD.

Stress

Some consider stress to be an important risk factor, none more so than the patient who has suffered a myocardial infarction. The difficulty of assessing stress lies in defining what is 'stress', for an activity that may be stressful for one person may be regarded as a positive challenge to another. The possible mechanisms by which stress exerts its negative effects on CHD risk have been cited as increases in blood pressure, heart rate, increased plasma cholesterol levels and adverse effects on coagulation and fibrinolysis (Johnston 1993). In lifestyle counselling, it is important to include an assessment of the level of stress perceived by patients. Individualized strategies to reduce stress can improve patient well-being greatly.

Thrombogenic factors

Fibrinogen is an important factor in controlling blood coagulation. Elevated plasma levels of fibrinogen have been shown to be a risk factor for a CHD event (Kannel et al 1987). In addition, other haemostatic factors such as factor VII and plasminogen activator inhibitor have been associated with increased CHD risk. However, in current clinical practice these measurements are not widely performed and are rarely used in routine CHD risk factor assessment.

Increased propensity for platelet aggregation has been found to be associated with an increased risk of CHD events (Elwood et al 1991). Unfortunately the methods used for measuring this parameter have not been fully established, so yet again this risk factor cannot be used in overall risk assessment. However, compelling evidence from clinical trials of patients with established CHD have demonstrated beneficial effects of anti-platelet drugs, particularly aspirin. Comparing the results of several trials of aspirin usage, the Antiplatelet Trialist Collaboration group (1994) concluded that in patients with CHD the use of low-dose aspirin (75–150 mg) reduces future CHD events by one-quarter. It is important to note that these findings cannot, with present knowledge of risk and benefits, be extrapolated to advocating use of aspirin in a healthy population to reduce the risk of CHD events.

Diabetes mellitus

Both insulin-dependent diabetes mellitus (IDDM) and non-insulin-dependent diabetes mellitus (NIDDM) are associated with markedly increased risk of CHD, peripheral vascular disease and cerebrovascular disease (Pyörälä et al 1987). Diabetes mellitus is a particularly strong cardiovascular risk factor in women and has been shown to diminish the relative protection against atherosclerotic disease that the female hormones confer (Pyörälä et al 1987).

The mechanism by which diabetes mellitus exerts its effect on the atherogenic process is not clear. Diabetics have been shown to have a two- to fourfold increase in risk of CHD compared to the general population and indeed CHD is the leading cause of death in diabetic patients. De Fronzo & Ferrannini (1991) have documented the following mechanisms through which diabetes mellitus may act. These are principally mediated via elevated plasma insulin levels:

- adverse effect on lipid profile leading to hypertriglyceridaemia and increased levels of the atherogenic low density lipoprotein (LDL) cholesterol
- proliferation of smooth muscle cells and the production of various growth factors
- increased transport of cholesterol into smooth muscle cells
- increased glycosylation of lipoproteins and endothelial matrix components.

In patients with IDDM, good metabolic control has been able to maintain plasma lipids and blood pressure levels within normal limits (Krolewski et al 1987).

NIDDM is associated with more profound abnormalities in cardiovascular risk factors (Pyörälä et al 1987). Therefore it should not be regarded as a milder or less-threatening condition with less-serious consequences in terms of CHD risk. The approach to CHD risk reduction should be multifaceted, addressing all the major risk factors of hypertension, smoking and hyperlipidaemia. Since weight control has been shown to improve glucose control, a weight-reducing and lipid-lowering diet are recommended in addition to a diet which maintains carbohydrate balance.

MULTIPLE RISK FACTORS

a single risk factor ... is not sufficiently sensitive to identify all individuals at high risk of coronary heart disease

(Assmann & Schulte 1990)

It has gradually become more evident that CHD mortality could not be explained solely on the basis of the effect of single risk factors. Analysis of existing data to examine the effects on CHD mortality when more than one risk factor is present revealed that the risk factors interacted synergistically, i.e. in a multiplicative rather than an additive manner, to increase markedly the risk of CHD (Grundy 1986). Observational and intervention studies in populations were conducted to examine the effect of multiple risk factors on subsequent risk of CHD.

The USA Multiple Risk Factor Intervention Trial (Neaton et al 1984) shows that male 5-year CHD death rates per 1000 were 17.4 when the individual was a smoker, had diastolic blood pressure of greater than 90 mmHg and a cholesterol level greater than 6.5 mmol/l. In contrast, when an individual was a non-smoker, had a diastolic blood pressure less than 90 mmHg and a cholesterol level of less than 6.5 mmol/l then the rate was much lower at 2.4 per 1000.

In the British Regional Heart Study, Shaper et al (1985) collected data on middle-aged men over a period of 2 years, and examined the relationship between CHD risk factors and the rate of CHD events at a 5-year follow-up. The aim of this study was to see if it was possible to identify men at high risk of CHD. The parameters that were used as indices of risk were smoking, mean blood pressure, previous diagnosis of CHD and diabetes, family history of CHD, ECG evidence of CHD and plasma total cholesterol. A score was developed on the basis of these risk factors and it was found that the top fifth of the score distribution identified 59% of men who subsequently had a major CHD event. It was also evident that the bulk of CHD incidence does not occur in those individuals who lie at the upper end of any single risk factor distribution, but rather in those individuals who have moderate elevations in a number of risk factors.

Data from the Framingham Study, described above, also show how steeply CHD risk rises when combinations of risk factors are present (Castelli 1984). Similar trends can be seen in men and women living in the West of Scotland. Male smokers in Renfrew and Paisley with cholesterol greater than 6 mmol/l (top 40% of distribution) and diastolic pressure greater than 97 mmHg (top 20% of distribution) had a fourfold higher CHD mortality than men who did not smoke, whose cholesterol was less than 6 mmol/l and diastolic blood pressure less than 97 mmHg. The relative risk for women with multiple risk factors was even greater, although this probably reflects the fact that absolute rates for low-risk women were lower than for low-risk men (Isles et al 1989).

Evidence from trials which have sought to evaluate the impact on CHD mortality of attempts to change multiple risk factors have been mixed (McCormick & Skrabanek 1988). One of the first of these trials was carried out in Oslo (Hjermann 1983) and focused on changes in cholesterol and smoking in men aged 40–49 of whom 70% were smokers and had elevated cholesterol levels (7–9.5 mmol/l). The subjects were randomly assigned to an intervention or a control group, intervention taking the form of dietary and anti-smoking advice. After 5 years the results indicated a successful change of both risk factors in the intervention group compared with the control group and that the rate of fatal and non-fatal CHD events was reduced by 45%. However, as in many other intervention studies, there was no significant reduction in all-cause mortality.

The second of the trials was carried out in the United States and was the Multiple Risk Factor Intervention Trial (Cutler et al 1985). It was most notable because of its size, having recruited more than one-third of a million high-risk men (age range 35–57 years). From these men, a cohort of 12 866 men was selected on the basis of their CHD risk and randomized to usual care or intervention. Intervention was in the form of lifestyle changes to lower cholesterol, stop smoking and reduce weight, and drug treatment for hypertension. Over an average 7-year follow-up period risk factor levels declined in both groups, but to a greater extent in the intervention group. Mortality from CHD was reduced in both groups but, disappointingly, there was no significant difference in CHD mortality between the two groups. Explanations for this have included:

- the adverse affects of anti-hypertensive treatment on lipids in the intervention group
- the fact that the control group were aware of their 'high-risk' status

influenced their own health-related behaviour in such a way as to lower their risk factor status
- the 'un-blinding' of control individuals to the intervention programme of the treatment group who in many cases came from the same occupational environment.

Other studies involving population intervention programmes have been able to show modest reductions in CHD mortality in response to reduction in levels of risk factors (Puska et al 1983, Farquhar et al 1977, Kornitzer et al 1983). Therefore multiple risk factor intervention has been advocated as the best approach to reducing the incidence of CHD.

Risk factor screening strategies

Because CHD and the related risk factors are common in the western world and resources are limited, it is important to define priorities in screening so that those individuals likely to gain the greatest benefit from intervention are identified. The highest priority should be given to those patients with established CHD and other atherosclerotic vascular disease. This will include patients with angina, and those who have suffered a myocardial infarction, or have undergone percutaneous transluminal coronary angioplasty (PTCA) or coronary artery bypass grafting (CABG). These groups should not be overlooked in the belief that their risk factors have already been corrected. It has been shown that modifiable risk factors are present in such high-risk individuals (Lindsay et al 1995).

The next groups of individuals to tackle are those asymptomatic subjects with one or more major CHD risk factors. This includes subjects with hyper-cholesterolaemia, hypertension, diabetes or a family history of premature CHD and smokers and the obese.

The final individuals to be considered are all healthy 18- to 65-year-old males and females, using the guidelines for screening provided in *The New Health Promotion Package* (BMA 1993).

RISK FACTOR SCORING TOOLS

In order to take into account the effect of several CHD risk factors in their assessment of an individual's global risk, scoring systems have been designed, based on data from epidemiological studies. These systems are used to calculate the marginal contribution of a given risk factor to overall risk of CHD with various additive or multiplicative weights assigned to the various factors. The cumulative score does not aim to provide a precise risk indicator for a disease of such complexity but it does provide the health care practitioner with a better estimation of overall risk where several risk factors are present. Three different forms of scoring systems are reviewed.

Risk factor calculator

The 'Infarct Risk Calculator Spirit' (Fig. 2.2) is produced by Boehringer-Mannheim and has been developed to assist in the provision of an objective overall risk of a myocardial infarction in an individual patient. It is based on

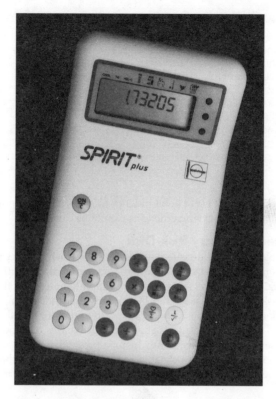

Figure 2.2 Boehringer-Mannheim Infarct Risk Calculator Spirit (reproduced by permission of Boehringer-Mannheim).

results of the ongoing 'Prospective Cardiovascular Munster Study' which began in 1979 (Assmann & Schulte 1989). Nine parameters are included in its estimation of risk and these are listed in Box 2.3.

After entering the value of all nine parameters, the probability of suffering a myocardial infarction within 4 years is calculated and displayed as a percentage. In addition to this numerical estimation of risk, the calculator also provides a quantitative evaluation in terms of high, medium or low risk. The estimation takes into account a wide range of factors so from this perspective it is good. Providing a numerical value for risk that can be interpreted by the patient is very useful, particularly when a new score, based on the patient making changes, may be calculated so that the patient can see the improvement in risk factor status, e.g. a new score can be given that anticipates stopping smoking. One of the disadvantages is that the evaluation of smoking does not take into account number of cigarettes smoked or length of time as a smoker. In addition, all nine parameters may not be available at a routine screening clinic, e.g. triglycerides must be measured in a fasting sample. The manufacturers state that the calculator can still be used by entering 'normal' values for the missing data; however, this may interfere with the validity of

---

Box 2.3 CHD risk factors considered in the infarct risk calculator

- Total plasma cholesterol
- Plasma triglycerides
- Plasma HDL-cholesterol
- Blood pressure
- Smoking (Y/N)
- Age
- Diabetes mellitus
- Angina
- Family history (myocardial infarction in relatives under 60 years old)

---

the scoring system and it is not good practice to guess values of physiological measurements for patients when the tests cannot be carried out.

The Dundee Coronary Risk-Disk

This is a simple circular slide rule device (Fig. 2.3) which places patients in a rank order from 1 (high risk) to 100 (low risk) based on their relative position in the general population, from a score that integrates the three major, modifiable risk factors of smoking, blood pressure and serum cholesterol (Tunstall-Pedoe 1991). It is based on a prospective study of middle-aged men followed for a 5-year period (Rose et al 1983). It focuses on modifiable risk factors alone, excluding gender, family history, presence of CHD and diabetes mellitus. Although these immodifiable risk factors cannot be changed they must affect the interpretation of risk from any other factors and should be

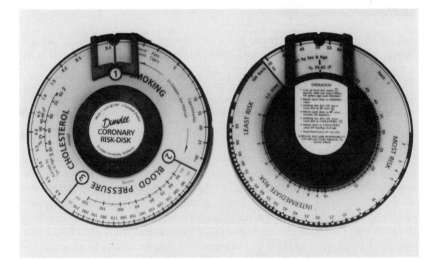

Figure 2.3 Dundee Coronary Risk-Disk (reproduced by permission of Prof. H. Tunstall-Pedoe).

taken into account along with the predictive score using the Risk-Disk. The risk assessment is given in terms of relative risk, i.e. the risk compared to another individual of the same age.

Actual values of the three risk factors are used, avoiding assessment of individual risk factors by cut-off points. However, there are many factors that are not included, for instance BMI or HDL-cholesterol. Therefore other factors must be considered along with the score obtained from the disk. Again the limitation of using results based on experience gained solely in men is present in this tool. The Risk-Disk has been endorsed by the Coronary Prevention Group and by the British Heart Foundation.

The British Regional Heart Study: GP Score

A scoring system based on the British Regional Heart Study, has been developed to identify men and postmenopausal women at high risk of myocardial infarction, for use in general practice by doctors or nurses. It is based on the belief that prediction of cases of major CHD can be improved by assessing the combined effects of several risk factors and the presence of pre-existing disease. A questionnaire was administered asking people to recall any chest pain they have experienced in response to various activities. The score is calculated from the formula outlined in Box 2.4. The score is interpreted in terms of risk of CHD in a 5-year period as set out in Table 2.1.

The score does not include a cholesterol measurement but the authors suggest that the score is used as a basis for deciding who should have their level measured. Neither does it take into account the number of cigarettes smoked, justifying this on the results from the British Regional Heart Study which found, of the indices of smoking, that 'years smoking' was the one

---

Box 2.4 Scoring algorithm for the British Regional Heart Study: GP Score

7 × years of smoking cigarettes
+ 6.5 × mean blood pressure (mmHg)
+ 270 if the individual recalls a diagnosis of CHD
+ 150 if there was evidence of angina in the health questionnaire
+ 85 if either parent had died of CHD
+ 150 if diabetic

Table 2.1 Interpretation of scores obtained using the British Regional Heart Study: GP Score

Score reference range	Risk of CHD event in 5 years
High risk: > 1000	1 in 10
900–999	1 in 25
Average: 800–899	1 in 30
700–799	1 in 100
Low risk: < 700	1 in 250

which most strongly correlated with risk of CHD. There is a more detailed score developed from the data from the same study, taking into account age, a cholesterol measurement and an electrocardiograph. When evaluated, the top fifth of score distribution identified 59% of the men who subsequently had a CHD event during the following 5 years, compared to 53% of men using the simplified score detailed above.

The Joint European Guidelines

These most recent guidelines (Pyörälä et al 1994) published have been produced jointly by the Task Force of the European Society of Cardiology, European Atherosclerosis Society and European Society of Hypertension. This collaboration demonstrates the growing consensus in risk factor evaluation and it is likely that these recommendations will gain wider acceptability. The guidelines endorse assessment of the total burden of CHD risk that an individual is exposed to rather than considering solely the effect of single risk factors such as smoking, hypertension or hyperlipidaemia in isolation. This approach acknowledges previously discussed concepts, i.e. aetiology is multifactorial, risk factors have a multiplicative effect and global risk factor assessment should be practised. It has also made an important step forward in providing separate assessment for men and women in recognition of the different profile of CHD in relation to gender. The aim of these recommendations is to summarize from the clinical perspective those most important issues in CHD prevention that there is good agreement on and thereby to give practitioners the best possible advice, thus facilitating their work in CHD prevention.

In assessing CHD risk status in an individual, the presence or absence and severity of each individual risk factor has to be considered. Age, gender, systolic blood pressure, smoking status and plasma total cholesterol level are included in the risk evaluation. In addition, the assessment recommends that patients with CHD, a strong family history of premature CHD, diabetes mellitus or low HDL-cholesterol levels be considered at higher risk. The guidelines are based on a risk function derived from the Framingham Study (Anderson et al 1991) and predict a person's absolute 10-year risk of a coronary event expressed as percentage chance (Fig. 2.4). An individual's absolute risk of developing a coronary event in the following 10 years is found by entering the relevant measurement into the chart and identifying the grade of risk category. The percentage chance is given in the key. The chart can be used·to predict the change in overall risk status as a result of changing any risk factor. The effect of increasing risk with age can be clearly followed using the chart. In general, even low-risk subjects should be offered healthy lifestyle advice to maintain their low-risk status. Advice should be intensified with increasing risk and a level of 20% chance of an event in the next 10 years should signal intensive risk modification efforts.

The risk assessment, although fairly comprehensive, does omit diastolic blood pressure, which may be a limitation, and factors such as family history, diabetes and low HDL-cholesterol levels are given a broad 'increased risk' status without inclusion in a quantifiable way in the risk function.

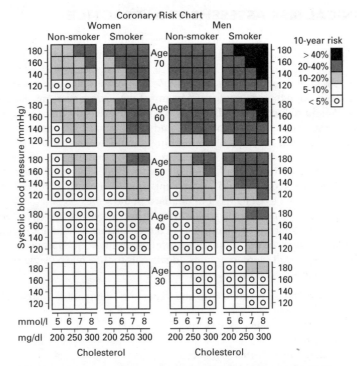

Coronary Risk Chart

To find a person's absolute 10-year risk of a CHD event, find the table for his/her sex, age and smoking status. Inside the table, find the cell nearest to their systolic blood pressure (mmHg) and cholesterol (mmol/l or mg/dl).

To find a person's relative risk, compare his/her risk category with other people of the same age. The absolute risk shown here may not apply to all populations, especially those with a low CHD incidence. Relative risk is likely to apply to most populations.

The effect of changing cholesterol, smoking status or blood pressure can be read from the chart.

The effect of lifetime exposure to risk factors can be seen by following the table upwards. This can be used when advising younger people.

Risk is at least one category higher in people with overt cardiovascular disease. People with diabetes, familial hyperlipidaemia or a family history of premature cardiovascular disease are also at increased risk.

Risks are shown for exact ages, blood pressures and cholesterols. Risk increases as a person approaches the next category.

The tables assume HDL cholesterol to be 1.0 mmol/l in men (39 mg/dl) and 1.1 mmol/l (43 mg/dl) in women. People with lower levels of HDL cholesterol and/or with triglyceride levels above 2.3 mmol/l (200 mg/dl) are at higher risk.

Cholesterol: 1 mmol/l = 38.67 mg/dl.

Figure 2.4 Coronary risk chart derived from epidemiological data from the Framingham Study produced as part of the Joint European Guidelines of the European Society of Cardiology, European Atherosclerosis Society and the European Society of Hypertension (reproduced with permission from Pyörälä et al 1994).

CLINICAL RISK ASSESSMENT IN PRACTICE

CHD risk factor scoring devices are based on information gathered in populations and may require additional information in order to fully assess CHD risk at the individual level. In practice, other risk factors such as alcohol intake, stress and lack of physical exercise and obesity are also taken into account, although they do not feature in any of the scoring systems discussed above. Weight reduction in individuals who are overweight helps to control blood pressure and plasma cholesterol, and aids mobility. Documentation of excess alcohol and subsequent counselling should be carried out because of its possible effects on blood pressure, weight and triglyceride levels. Therefore management should be tailored to the individual factors as revealed in the screening and assessment process including those factors known to be linked to CHD risk but not used in the score.

In summary, all risk factor scores should be viewed as merely offering guidelines and a means of identifying in a quantifiable way an individual's CHD risk. They provide a quantifiable means of monitoring improvements in risk status as a result of interventions. Ideal goals for lifestyle behaviours and CHD risk factors can be summarized as:

- a diet, low in fat and high in fruit and vegetables, compatible with ideal body weight
- plasma cholesterol levels of less than 5.2 mmol/l
- regular exercise
- the avoidance of all forms of tobacco
- blood pressure levels of 130/80 or below.

In general, interventions should be aimed towards such ideals. When dealing with moderate elevations in several risk factors, because of the nature of risk interaction, modest reductions in more than one risk factor are likely to reduce risk more than aggressive reduction of a single risk factor.

■ KEY POINTS

- The aetiology of CHD is multifactorial and is described in terms of 'risk factors'.
- The term 'risk factor' is widely used to describe those characteristics found in individuals that relate to the subsequent occurrence of CHD.
- Absolute risk defines the expected rate of CHD events for any given combination of age, gender, and other risk factors.
- Relative risk is the ratio between the absolute risk in an individual compared to the absolute risk in someone of the same age and gender who has no other CHD risk factors.
- Key factors that increase risk of CHD have been established.
- Risk factors interact in a multiplicative manner to greatly increase risk.
- Identifying high-risk individuals is the priority in screening strategies.

- Global risk factor assessment should be practised.
- Risk factors have a multiplicative effect.
- A scoring system is a clinical tool that enables an individual to be placed in a category of risk by assessing the effect of multiple risk factors.
- Scoring systems are useful in monitoring intervention programmes to reduce risk.
- Clinical guidelines based on best practice may be integrated into patient care through risk factor scoring systems.

Case Study 2.1

At the 'well person' clinic you are about to undertake a CHD risk factor assessment. Use the European Guidelines to help guide your assessment of risk and the advice that you can offer the following individual:
A 52-year-old male who is currently smoking 20 cigarettes a day, and has a systolic blood pressure of 158 mmHg and a non-fasting plasma cholesterol of 6.8 mmol/l.

Questions
1. Using the coronary risk chart in Figure 2.4, what is his absolute 10-year risk of a CHD event?
2. What further assessments would you make and what advice would you give?
3. The patient returns after 3 months and has managed to stop smoking, his systolic blood pressure is 154 mmHg and plasma cholesterol 7.1 mmol/l. Has his absolute 10-year risk of a CHD event changed?

Answers
1. Minimum estimate of the 10-year risk is 20–40%.
2. Assess: BMI; alcohol intake; family history; history of diabetes mellitus; diastolic blood pressure; physical activity.
   Advise the patient:
   — to stop smoking
   — to change diet to reduce fat intake and increase intake of fruit and vegetables and energy to achieve ideal body weight
   — to achieve recommended levels of physical activity.
3. Minimum estimate of the 10-year risk is 10–20% representing a reduction by half in risk. Congratulate patient! BMI within 10% of ideal limits. Diastolic blood pressure 86 mmHg. Further investigation of cholesterol elevation is required.

PRACTICAL EXERCISE

From your database of patient records, identify patients who are at high risk of CHD or have had a CHD event:

- What numbers have had a full CHD risk factor assessment?
- Do any high-risk or CHD patients have uncorrected CHD risk factors?

REFERENCES

Anderson K M et al 1991 An updated coronary risk profile: a statement for health professionals. Circulation 83: 356–362

Antiplatelet Trialist Collaboration 1994 Collaborative overview of randomized trials of antiplatelet therapy—I: Prevention of death, myocardial infarction, and stroke by prolonged antiplatelet therapy in various categories of patients. British Medical Journal 308: 81–106

Assmann G, Schulte H 1989 Results and conclusions of the Prospective Cardiovascular Munster (PROCAM) Study. In: Assmann G (ed) Lipid metabolism disorders and coronary heart disease. MMV Medizin, Verlag, Munchen

Assmann G, Schulte H 1990 Modelling the Helsinki Heart Study by means of a risk equation obtained from the PROCAM Study and the Framingham Heart Study. Drugs 40 (Suppl. 1): 13–18

Bray G A 1979 Obesity in America. Publication No. (NIH) 79-359. US Department of Health, Education and Welfare, Washington, DC

British Medical Association (BMA) 1993 The new health promotion package. General Medical Services Committee. British Medical Association, London

Castelli W P 1984 Epidemiology of coronary heart disease: the Framingham Study. American Journal of Medicine 76(2A): 4–12

Collinson J, Dowie D 1980 Concepts and classifications. Unit 1 of U201, Risk: a second level university course. Open University Press, Milton Keynes

Cutler J A, Neaton J D, Hulley S B, Kuller L, Paul O, Stamler J 1985 Coronary heart disease and all-cause mortality in the Multiple Risk Factor Intervention Trial: subgroup findings and comparison with other trials. Preventive Medicine 14: 293–311

Dawber T R, Meadows G F, Moore F E 1951 Epidemiological approaches to heart disease: the Framingham Study. American Journal of Public Health 41: 279–286

De Fronzo R A, Ferrannini E 1991 Insulin resistance. A multifaceted syndrome responsible for NIDDM, obesity, hypertension, dyslipidaemia and atherosclerotic cardiovascular disease. Diabetes Care 14: 173–194

Elwood P C, Renaud S, Sharp D S, Beswick A D, O'Brien J R, Yarnell J W 1991 Ischaemic heart disease and platelet aggregation. The Caerphilly Collaborative Heart Disease Study. Circulation. 83: 38–44

Farquhar J W, Maccoby N, Wood P D, Alexander J K, Breitrose H, Brown B W, Haskell I V, McAlister A L, Meyer A J, Nash J D, Stern M P 1970 Community education for cardiovascular health. Lancet i: 1192–1195

Grundy S M 1986 Cholesterol and heart disease: a new era. Journal of the American Medical Association 256: 2849–2858

Hjermann I 1983 A randomised primary preventive trial in coronary heart disease: the Oslo Study. Preventive Medicine 121: 181–184

Isles C G, Hole D J, Gillis C R, Hawthorne V M, Lever A F 1989 Plasma cholesterol, coronary heart disease and cancer in the Renfrew and Paisley survey. British Medical Journal 298: 920–924

Johnston D W 1993 The current status of the coronary prone behaviour pattern. Journal of Sociological Medicine 86: 406–409

Kannel W B 1976 Some lessons in cardiovascular epidemiology from Framingham. American Journal of Cardiology 37: 269–282

Kannel W B, Wolf P A, Castelli W P and D'Agnostino R B 1987 Fibrinogen and risk of cardiovascular disease. Journal of the American Medical Association 258: 1183–1186

Keys A 1980 Seven Countries Study: a multivariate analysis of death and coronary heart disease. Harvard University Press, Cambridge MA

Knight F H 1933 Risk, uncertainty and profit. Houghton, Mifflin, Boston

Kornitzer M, De Backer G, Dramaix M 1983 Belgian Heart Disease Prevention Project: incidence and mortality results. Lancet i: 1066–1070

Kramsch D M, Aspen A J, Abramowitz B M, Kreimendahl T, Hood W B Jr 1981 Reduction of coronary atherosclerosis by moderate conditioning in monkeys on an atherogenic diet. New England Journal of Medicine 305: 1483

Krolewski A S, Kosinski E J, Warram J H et al 1987 Magnitude and determinants of coronary heart disease in juvenile-onset, insulin-dependent diabetes mellitus. American Journal of Cardiology 59: 750–755

Larsson B 1992 Obesity and body fat distribution as predictors of coronary heart disease. In: Marmot M, Elliot P (eds) Coronary heart disease epidemiology. From aetiology to public health.: Oxford University Press, Oxford, pp 233–241

Lindsay G M, Tait G W, Carter D, Lorimer A R, Shepherd J, Smith L N, Gaw A 1995 Modifying cardiovascular risk factors after CABG. Audit in General Practice 13(6): 13–17

McCormick J, Skrabenek P 1988 Coronary heart disease is not preventable by population interventions. Lancet i: 839–841

Milvy P, Seigel A J 1981 Physical activity levels and altered mortalities from CHD with emphasis on marathon running: a critical review. Cardiovascular Reviews and Reports 2: 233–236

Multiple Risk Factor Intervention Trial Research Group 1982 Multiple Risk Factor Intervention Trial: risk factor changes and mortality results. Journal of the American Medical Association 248: 1465–1477

Neaton J D, Kuller L H, Wentworth D, Borhani N D 1984 Total and cardiovascular mortality in relation to cigarette smoking, serum cholesterol concentration, and diastolic blood pressure among Black and White males followed up for five years. American Heart Journal 108: 759–769

Neufeld H N, Goldbourt U 1983 Coronary heart disease: genetic aspects. Circulation 67(5): 943–954

Peters P K, Cady L D, Bischoff D B 1983 Physical fitness and subsequent myocardial infarction in healthy workers. Journal of the American Medical Association 249: 3052–3056

Pooling Project Research Group 1978 Relationship of blood pressure, serum cholesterol, smoking habit, relative weight abnormalities to incidence of major coronary events. Journal of Chronic Diseases 31: 201–306

Puska P, Nissinen A, Salanen J T, Toumilchto J 1983 Ten years of the North Karelia Project: results with community-based prevention of CHD. Scandinavian Journal of Social Medicine 11: 65–68

Pyörälä K, Laakso M, Uusitupa M 1987 Diabetes and atherosclerosis: an epidemiologic view. Diabetes/Metabolism Review 3: 463–524

Pyörälä K, De Backer G, Graham I, Poole-Wilson P, Wood D 1994 Prevention of coronary heart disease in clinical practice. Recommendations of the Task Force of the European Society of Cardiology, European Atherosclerosis Society and European Society of Hypertension. European Heart Journal 15: 1300–1331

Rose G, Tunstall-Pedoe H, Heller R F 1983 United Kingdom Heart Disease Prevention Project: incidence and mortality results. Lancet i: 1062–1065

Shaper A G, Pocock S J, Walker M, Phillips A N, Whitehead T P, Macfarlane P W 1985 Risk factors for ischaemic heart disease: the prospective phase of the British Regional Heart Study. Journal of Epidemiology and Community Health 39: 197–209

St George D P 1983 Is coronary heart disease caused by environmentally induced chronic metabolic imbalance? Medical Hypotheses 12: 283–296

Tunstall-Pedoe H 1991 The Dundee coronary Risk-Disk for management of change in risk factors. British Medical Journal 303: 744–747

FURTHER READING

Gotto A M Jr, Farmer J A 1992 Risk factors for coronary artery disease. In: Braunwald W (ed) Heart disease: a textbook of cardiovascular medicine, 4th edn. W B Saunders, Philadelphia, ch 37: 1125–1160

Lorimer A R, Shepherd J (eds) 1991 Preventative cardiology. Blackwell Scientific Publications, Oxford

Thompson G R, Wilson P W 1992 Coronary risk factors and their assessment. Science Press, London

Cholesterol and lipoproteins

Allan Gaw   James Shepherd

■ CONTENTS

INTRODUCTION

There are three main coronary heart disease (CHD) risk factors over which we, as individuals, have any control. These are abnormal plasma lipid concentrations or dyslipidaemia, hypertension and smoking. This chapter will deal in detail with the first of these. To discuss the role of cholesterol and lipoproteins in the development of CHD we must first be clear of the definitions of a number of terms. The most commonly used of these are defined in Box 3.1.

THE LINK BETWEEN LIPIDS AND CHD

Lipids were first implicated in the development of atherosclerosis almost 150 years ago when cholesterol was noted to be present in atheromatous lesions in arteries. However, it was not until the early years of the 20th century that the important association between dietary cholesterol and atherosclerotic lesions was confirmed experimentally. The Russian researcher Anitschkow and his colleagues (1913) fed egg yolk to rabbits and observed the development of lesions in their aortae, identical to the atherosclerotic lesions in man.

Box 3.1 Definitions

Lipid. Any substance that is insoluble in water but soluble in apolar solvents, such as ether or chloroform, is a lipid. Cholesterol and triglyceride belong to the lipid family of compounds.

Cholesterol. A white, odourless substance that is insoluble in water. Cholesterol is composed of 27 carbon atoms in the form of four interconnecting rings with a short tail. It is found only in animal cells; plants do not possess the ability to manufacture cholesterol.

Cholesteryl ester. That form of cholesterol in which a fatty acid is attached to its third carbon through an ester bond. This is the storage form of cholesterol that is found inside cells and that is carried in the core of lipoproteins.

Triglyceride. Also called triacylglycerol, a member of the lipid family in which three fatty acids are attached to a glycerol backbone through ester bonds.

Apolipoproteins. These are special proteins that are present in lipoproteins. They are named by letters and numbers and each has a specific structural or metabolic function.

Fatty acid. This type of molecule consists of a string of carbon atoms whose length and degree of saturation varies. Saturated fatty acids are those where all the positions in the carbon string are occupied or saturated with hydrogen atoms. A monounsaturated fatty acid is one where a single position in the carbon string is unsaturated, i.e. two adjacent carbon atoms are missing one hydrogen atom and are joined by a double bond. Polyunsaturated fatty acids have two or more of these double bonds in their string of carbon atoms.

Phospholipids. Usually contain a glycerol backbone, two fatty acids, and a third polar component in which a chemical compound is attached to the glycerol through its phosphorus component. Phospholipids act as detergent molecules and are usually visualized as having two hydrophobic or water-hating tails with a single hydrophilic or water-loving head.

Lipoprotein. A complex of proteins called apolipoproteins and lipids, such as cholesterol, cholesteryl esters, triglyceride and phospholipids. Lipoproteins are responsible for transporting lipids between various organs of the body.

As this work progressed, Anitschkow became convinced that there could be 'no atheroma without cholesterol'.

In the 'Seven Countries Study', Keys (1980) found that the incidence of CHD was high in countries where median cholesterol levels were high and correspondingly low in countries where median cholesterol levels were low. This trend was also documented more recently by Marmot & Mann (1987). Even within populations, higher levels of blood cholesterol were associated with higher rates of CHD mortality (Rose & Shipley 1986).

Using this evidence the so-called cholesterol hypothesis was formulated. This stated that elevated plasma levels of cholesterol were causally related to the development of CHD and by lowering the plasma cholesterol we would reduce the CHD risk.

Evidence to support the view that cholesterol is causally linked to the development and progression of atherosclerosis and CHD mortality has come from major intervention trials, which have aimed to test this cholesterol hypothesis. The two most recent and largest are the Scandinavian Simvastatin Survival Study (4S) (1994) and the West of Scotland Coronary Prevention Study (Shepherd et al 1995). These studies together with other major trials are discussed in detail below.

If we choose to attempt to lower the plasma cholesterol of an individual we must first have some concept of what constitutes a raised plasma cholesterol. With most laboratory measurements a report is issued, which is accompanied by a reference range to allow interpretation of the results. These reference ranges are constructed by measuring the blood levels of the substance in question in a large number of apparently healthy subjects. The mean is determined and the reference range is taken as the mean plus or minus 2 standard deviations, thus, by definition, encompassing 95% of the population.

If we do this with plasma cholesterol, we obtain a wide range of values which include those higher values that we know to confer an increased risk of CHD. Why is this? The key to understanding this apparent paradox is to remember that the reference range is not a normal range in a clinical sense, but is in fact chosen arbitrarily to include 95% of the population in the 'normal' category. The individuals used to construct the range were apparently healthy but many of those individuals will have poor CHD risk profiles and will ultimately develop and die from CHD. We cannot conclude therefore, if a patient's plasma cholesterol falls within a reference range, that they are safe. It is much better, in cases such as this where we are dealing with a relatively silent risk factor, that we measure the significance of our plasma cholesterol levels against a different yardstick.

The concept of action limits has been widely adopted for assessing the risk associated with plasma cholesterol. Intervention guidelines by the British Hyperlipidaemia Association (Shepherd et al 1987) classify levels of cholesterol in the range less than 5.2 mmol/l as associated with the lowest level of risk, 5.2–6.5 mmol/l as low to moderate risk, 6.5–7.8 mmol/l as moderate to high risk and levels greater than 7.8 mmol/l as very high risk, with management strategies depending on the presence of other risk factors for CHD. More recently published joint intervention guidelines by the European Societies of Cardiology and Hypertension and the European Atherosclerosis Society present management strategies depending on the level of plasma total cholesterol and the presence of other risk factors for CHD (Pyörälä et al 1994). These guidelines do not define cut-off cholesterol values for different levels of risk but rather view lipid-related CHD risk as a continuum, which is strongly influenced by other risk factors such as gender, smoking, hypertension and personal history of CHD.

Several studies have been conducted in order to measure the prevalence of hyperlipidaemia in the community. A survey of cholesterol levels in a sample of 12 092 British men and women, aged 25–59, years revealed that two-thirds had levels above 5.2 mmol/l (Mann et al 1988). In Scotland, as part of the MONICA (monitoring of trends and determinants in cardiovascular disease) studies for the World Health Organization, cholesterol levels were measured in 10 450 men and women in 1984–86 (Tunstall-Pedoe et al 1989). In that country, 75% of the group had cholesterol levels greater than 5.2 mmol/l. Both studies were conducted in large samples across the UK and offer compelling evidence that hyperlipidaemia is highly prevalent in our community, although these figures do not grade the severity of the problem.

Given that plasma lipid levels are intimately and causally related to CHD risk, any attempt to modify that risk must take account of the mechanisms that control plasma lipid and lipoprotein levels. There follows a brief discussion of lipoprotein metabolism and a description of the structure and function of the plasma lipoproteins.

LIPOPROTEIN METABOLISM

Lipids are important sources of energy, of essential synthetic precursors and cellular components. Because of this a complex system has evolved to solve the problems of transporting lipids around the body in the aqueous environment of the plasma. This system depends on the packaging of neutral lipids (cholesteryl esters and triglyceride) with specific proteins and polar lipids (phospholipids and cholesterol) to create multimolecular particles called lipoproteins. The most widely used system of nomenclature defines four main classes of lipoprotein on the basis of their density and these are shown in Table 3.1. They are:

- chylomicrons
- very low density lipoprotein (VLDL)
- low density lipoprotein (LDL)
- high density lipoprotein (HDL).

In the interpretation and understanding of CHD risk the two lipoproteins, LDL and HDL, play a key role. The total cholesterol in the plasma is approximately distributed as follows: 60–70% transported as LDL and 20–30% as HDL. The significance of the relative amounts of these lipoproteins lies in the attributed protective properties of HDL and the atherogenic potential of LDL. Although the exact mechanism for these effects has not been fully elucidated, there is evidence from a number of prospective studies to indicate that HDL is a protective factor for CHD risk independently of other risk factors (Betteridge 1989) and that the correlation between total cholesterol and CHD is almost entirely due to the concentration of LDL in the plasma (Kannel et al 1971).

The major organs involved in lipid metabolism are the gut and the liver. Together these organs are responsible for the majority of lipoprotein synthesis and breakdown. Regulation of lipid transport is exerted through several agencies: apolipoproteins with specific signalling and cofactor functions, specific cell-surface lipoprotein receptors, intravascular enzymes that break

Table 3.1 The plasma lipoproteins

Lipoprotein	Main apolipoproteins	Function
Chylomicrons	B_{48}, A-I, C-II, E	Largest lipoprotein. Synthesized by gut after fatty meal. Main carrier of dietary lipid
Very low density lipoprotein (VLDL)	B_{100}, C-II, E	Synthesized in liver. Main carrier of endogenously produced triglyceride
Low density lipoprotein (LDL)	B_{100}	Generated from VLDL in the circulation. Main carrier of cholesterol
High density lipoprotein (HDL)	A-I, A-II	Smallest but most abundant. Protective function. Returns cholesterol to liver for excretion from peripheral tissues

down lipids, and transfer proteins that all act together to maintain cholesterol and triglyceride homeostasis. Malfunction of these regulatory factors may cause or contribute to the development of dyslipidaemia and in turn atherosclerosis. An overview of lipoprotein metabolism illustrating the roles that each plays in lipid transport is given in Figure 3.1.

Lipoprotein metabolism may be thought of as three interconnected and interdependent cycles. These are:

• the exogenous lipid pathway which deals with the transport and utilization of dietary lipids
• the endogenous pathway, which deals with the transport and utilization of lipids produced in the liver
• the reverse cholesterol transport pathway which serves to return cholesterol from the peripheral tissues to the liver where it can be excreted in the bile.

All three pathways are centred on the liver, which is the key organ in lipoprotein metabolism, although all organs in the body are in some way involved, either as consumers or producers of the plasma lipoproteins and the regulatory factors that control their metabolism.

Exogenous lipid pathway

Daily we eat about 0.5 g of cholesterol and about 100 g of triglyceride. Under normal circumstances, most dietary triglyceride is absorbed, but only about half of the dietary cholesterol is taken up, the remainder being lost in the faeces (Norum et al 1983). Within the cells lining the gut, the dietary lipids are packaged into large chylomicrons. These appear in abundance in the intestinal mucosal cells following a meal and are secreted into lacteals within

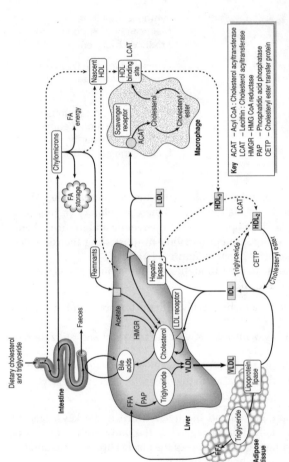

Figure 3.1 Lipoprotein metabolism. Following its absorption, dietary fat is packaged into large, triglyceride-rich chylomicron particles within the enterocyte and secreted into the circulation. There, lipolysis reduces the particle's triglyceride core and makes redundant part of its surface coat, which is shed to high density lipoprotein (HDL). The remnants produced in the process are rapidly assimilated by a receptor-mediated mechanism in the liver. In the fasting state, very low density lipoprotein (VLDL) replaces chylomicrons as the major triglyceride transporter and the liver dominates lipoprotein metabolism. Cholesterol and triglyceride elaborated in this organ are released into the plasma where they are subject to tissue lipolysis. This degrades them to low density lipoprotein (LDL) via an intermediate species (IDL). The LDL is removed by receptors present on the liver and peripheral tissues. When these are saturated, alternative scavenger receptor pathways become dominant. Interchange of lipids between circulating lipoprotein particles is facilitated by the plasma enzyme lecithin : cholesterol acyltransferase (LCAT) and cholesterol ester transfer protein (CETP) both of which participate in the process of reverse cholesterol transport from peripheral sites to the liver, where the sterol is excreted.

the wall of the small bowel. These large lipoprotein particles reach the bloodstream via the thoracic duct. In the circulation their triglyceride is gradually removed by the action of the enzyme lipoprotein lipase. This enzyme is present in the capillaries of a number of tissues, predominantly adipose tissue and skeletal muscle. As the chylomicron loses its triglyceride core the particle becomes smaller and deflated with folds of redundant surface material. These particles, now called chylomicron remnants, are taken up by the liver, where their cholesterol content may be used for cell membrane synthesis, as the building blocks for bile salts, or may be excreted into the bile. The liver provides the only route by which cholesterol leaves the body in significant amounts.

The metabolism of chylomicrons is depicted schematically in Figure 1, which emphasizes the bi-functionality of the process: the delivery of dietary triglyceride to skeletal muscle and adipose tissue, and of cholesterol to the liver.

Endogenous lipid pathway

Lipids synthesized in the liver have several fates (Norum et al 1983, Packard & Shepherd 1986). First, a significant proportion of the cholesterol and triglyceride is exported in VLDL, the major vehicle for endogenous triglyceride transport. Secondly, lipid surplus to requirements may be stored, temporarily, within the hepatocyte; and, thirdly, the liver cell has the unique ability to eliminate cholesterol into the bile, either unchanged or following oxidation to bile acids (Dietschy & Wilson 1970). These compounds, produced by the liver and secreted into the gut to aid digestion, are reabsorbed in the terminal ileum and extracted from the portal blood by the liver, thus returning to their site of origin in this 'enterohepatic circulation'.

Clearly, medical or surgical interruption of the enterohepatic circulation of bile acids will have profound effects on hepatic lipid metabolism. Such therapeutic manoeuvres can therefore be used to advantage in the management of hypercholesterolaemia, as discussed in Chapter 10.

After secretion into the bloodstream the VLDL synthesized by the liver undergoes the same form of delipidation as chylomicrons by the action of lipoprotein lipase. This results again in the formation of smaller triglyceride-poor particles and the VLDL remnants are called IDL. After further delipidation these particles become LDL. LDL may be removed from the circulation by the high affinity LDL receptor route or by other less well-defined scavenger receptor routes. The latter are thought to be important at high plasma LDL levels as the main way in which cholesterol is incorporated into atheromatous plaques.

Reverse cholesterol transport pathway

The key lipoprotein in this cycle is the HDL particle. These lipoproteins are the smallest of the lipoproteins yet the most numerous and are derived from both liver and gut. From the discovery that plasma HDL levels are associated with protection from coronary heart disease (reviewed in Gordon et al 1989) came the concept that this lipoprotein acts as a vehicle to transport cholesterol from peripheral tissues to the liver. The necessity for such a mechanism is unquestionable since cholesterol cannot be broken down to any significant extent in humans or animals and must therefore be excreted intact via its major organ of elimination, the liver. HDL has the capacity to acquire cholesterol from cells in vitro as an initial step in the 'reverse cholesterol transport pathway'. The cholesterol in HDL is taken up either directly by the liver, or indirectly by being transferred to other circulating lipoproteins, which then return it to the liver. Thus HDL acts as a cholesterol shuttle, removing the lipid from the peripheral tissues and returning it to the liver. This process is thought to be anti-atherogenic, and an elevated plasma HDL-cholesterol level has been shown to confer a decreased risk of CHD on an individual.

THE LDL RECEPTOR

Familial hypercholesterolaemia (FH), the autosomal codominant trait that occurs in its heterozygous form in 1 in 500 of the population, is associated with high levels of LDL-cholesterol in the plasma and premature coronary heart disease and is known to arise because of a defect in the LDL receptor. Since its discovery, more than 150 different mutations of the LDL receptor have been described (Hobbs et al 1990) which are responsible for FH. Recent observations suggest that similar and equally deleterious effects may result from defects in its primary ligand, apoB-100. This is most commonly seen in a condition called familial defective apoB-100 which is due to a mutation, present again at a level of approximately 1 in 500 of the population (Innerarity et al 1990). Such changes in apoB sequence appear to be of real clinical significance and further mutations are currently being sought.

The discovery and characterization of the LDL receptor has become the paradigm of lipoprotein research and was the result of the efforts of Brown & Goldstein (1987). This molecule is a single transmembrane glycoprotein that recognizes and interacts with lipoproteins containing apoB or apoE.

We know from extensive experiments on cultured cells that the activity of LDL receptors is regulated by variation in the intracellular cholesterol content. When the requirement for cholesterol is increased, receptor synthesis is stimulated and LDL uptake promoted. Conversely, in times of excess, receptor expression is diminished and LDL assimilation suppressed. Extrapolation of these concepts to man has enlightened our understanding of the regulation of LDL metabolism and provided an explanation for the actions of a number of cholesterol-lowering drugs (see Ch. 10). Bile acid sequestrant resins such as cholestyramine promote faecal sterol excretion and in consequence deplete the liver of cholesterol. The organ responds both by up-regulating synthesis of cholesterol from acetate and by increasing the number of LDL receptors on liver cell membranes. The latter of course produces the desired pharmacological action of the drug by promoting receptor-mediated clearance of LDL from the circulation (Shepherd et al 1980). A similar end result is also achieved by inhibition of cholesterol synthesis in the liver using the competitive inhibitors of HMG CoA reductase, which is the enzyme controlling the rate-limiting step in cholesterol synthesis (Bilheimer et al 1983).

LIPOPROTEINS AND ATHEROSCLEROSIS

The build-up of the atherosclerotic plaque, so pivotal to the development of clinical CHD, has been discussed in Chapter 1. Here we shall focus on the role of lipoproteins in that complex pathological process.

Detailed electron microscopic studies have shown that in cholesterol-fed non-human primates the earliest sign of a developing atherosclerotic plaque is focal infiltration of the arterial wall by cells of the monocyte/macrophage series. When examined in culture, these cells are able to internalize and store cholesteryl esters (Brown & Goldstein 1983). The source of this lipid in vivo has been the topic of a large body of research. Plasma LDL, the most abundant cholesterol transporter, does not generate these deposits. However, modified LDL particles do have this ability (Hoff & Morton 1987) and can turn the tissue macrophage into the large lipid-filled foam cell so characteristic of the atheromatous lesion. These modified lipoprotein particles differ from the normal lipoprotein by being oxidized and thus more negatively charged.

A number of observations support the hypothesis that oxidized LDL is important in the development of atheromatous plaques. Firstly, there is immunological evidence for the presence of oxidized LDL in atheromatous lesions (Yla-Herttuala et al 1989). Secondly, LDL isolated from atherosclerotic plaques (Goldstein et al 1981), is electronegative and produces foam cell transformation in vitro. And, thirdly, Carew and his colleagues (1987) have attributed the protective action of the drug probucol to its ability to scavenge free radicals and limit the rate of LDL oxidation, rather than to its lipid-lowering properties. When the drug was administered to Watanabe rabbits, LDL uptake into atherosclerotic lesions fell by 65% while a comparative group given alternative lipid-lowering drugs showed no improvement.

Thus, plasma lipoproteins may enter the artery wall and there contribute lipid to the evolving atheromatous lesion.

EVIDENCE FOR THE ROLE OF CHOLESTEROL IN CHD

A large number of studies have investigated the cholesterol hypothesis over the last three decades. In the early studies using a variety of intervention strategies, many of which are now obsolete, there was only partial success and some very disappointing results, particularly from the large WHO trial which is outlined below. With the introduction of improved lipid-lowering drugs several large-scale trials have been conducted, which now provide us with a portfolio of positive results

WHO trial

This was the first major primary prevention trial to test the cholesterol hypothesis and used the oldest member of the fibrate drug family, clofibrate (Committee of Principal Investigators 1978). This multicentred placebo-controlled trial reported limited lipid-lowering efficacy. More importantly, however, deaths from non-cardiac causes were higher in the treatment group. Although no single cause of death was identified, there was an excess of deaths from gastrointestinal tract malignancy and associated with cholecystectomy.

These findings, coupled with the relatively poor clinical efficacy of clofibrate (Levy et al 1972) and the increased bile lithogenicity reported with its use (Coronary Drug Project Research Group 1977), have made the drug clofibrate obsolete and prompted the development of derivatives of this compound and their examination as potential lipid-lowering drugs. This exercise has been fruitful and has provided the clinician with a range of agents with improved efficacy and safety which are discussed in Chapter 10.

Lipid Research Clinics Coronary Primary Prevention Study

After the WHO trial the first major study to be undertaken was that conducted by the Lipid Research Clinics in the United States (Lipid Research Clinics Program 1984). This was a multicentre, randomized, double-blind study involving 3806 middle-aged men with primary hypercholesterolaemia. The participants were followed for an average of 7.4 years. Those treated with the bile acid sequestrant drug, cholestyramine showed an 8.5% reduction in total cholesterol, a 12.6% reduction in LDL-cholesterol, a 3% rise in HDL-cholesterol and a 4.5% rise in triglyceride, over the placebo-treated control group. These lipid and lipoprotein changes were further enhanced in those who had adhered to the prescribed 24 g/day dosage. The drug-induced lipid changes were associated with a 24% fall in definite CHD deaths and a 19% fall in non-fatal MI. Incidence rates of new positive exercise ECGs, angina and coronary artery bypass grafts were significantly reduced by 25%, 20%, and 21% respectively in the sequestrant-resin-treated group. These findings provided the stimulus for other groups to investigate the clinical efficacy of lipid-lowering therapy and, since 1984, several major intervention trials have been published.

Helsinki Heart Study

The next major study confirmed the clinical efficacy of one of the fibrates, gemfibrozil. The Helsinki Heart Study (Frick et al 1987), a randomized, double-blind, placebo-controlled trial designed to test the drug in reducing the risk of coronary heart disease was conducted in Finland. A group of over 4000 middle-aged men (40–55 years) with primary dyslipidaemia (non-HDL-cholesterol ≥ 5.2 mmol/l) were recruited. Half received gemfibrozil, 600 mg twice daily, while the others received a placebo. Gemfibrozil therapy was associated with reductions in triglyceride of 35%, in LDL-cholesterol of 11%, and an increase in high density lipoprotein (HDL) cholesterol of 11%. The cumulative rate of cardiac end points (fatal and non-fatal myocardial infarctions combined) at 5 years was 27.3/1000 in the gemfibrozil-treated group and 41.4/1000 in the placebo group: a reduction in CHD of 34% (p < 0.02). Further analyses of the Helsinki Heart Study data (Manninen et al 1988, 1992) have provided more detail on the relationship between the lipid changes and incidence of CHD. The success of gemfibrozil in reducing CHD events was related not only to its ability to lower LDL-cholesterol but also to its effect of raising HDL-cholesterol (Manninen et al 1988). Manninen and his colleagues (1992) went on, using subgroup analysis, to identify a high-risk group of subjects. These individuals were found to have an LDL/HDL-cholesterol ratio > 5 and plasma triglyceride > 2.3 mmol/l. This group profited most from gemfibrozil therapy in the Helsinki Heart Study with a 71% lower incidence of CHD events than the corresponding placebo subgroup. We may hypothesize that if a similar intervention trial were designed only to include this high-risk group in sufficient numbers, thereby preventing the dilutional effect seen by including all hypercholesterolaemic subjects, the clinical efficacy of the fibrate in reducing coronary morbidity would be dramatic.

Despite obvious difficulties in the interpretation of extended follow-up studies to major clinical trials, the recently published 8.5-year follow-up of the Helsinki Heart Study (Heinonen et al 1994) provides further supportive evidence for a beneficial effect on CHD risk attributable to fibrate therapy.

Scandinavian Simvastatin Survival Study

Perhaps the most convincing evidence of all for the benefits of cholesterol-lowering therapy comes from the 4S study (Scandinavian Simvastatin Survival Study Group 1994), which is the first major secondary prevention trial using an HMG CoA reductase inhibitor or statin. In this study almost 4444 men and women with CHD were given either simvastatin, 20–40 mg/day or a placebo over an average 5-year period.

The drug-treated group enjoyed a 25% fall in plasma total cholesterol, a 35% fall in plasma LDL-cholesterol, a 10% fall in plasma triglyceride and an 8% increase in plasma HDL-cholesterol. The primary end point in this study was survival and those that received the lipid-lowering drug were 30% less likely to die from any cause and 42% less likely to die from CHD (Fig. 3.2). Importantly, there was no excess of deaths from non-cardiac causes such as suicide or accident, finally putting to rest the misconception that lipid-lowering drug therapy per se was associated with these phenomena. When the results of 4S are extrapolated to patient care it is estimated that if 100 patients with CHD are treated for 6 years with simvastatin we expect to save 4 of the 9 patients who would otherwise die from CHD, prevent 7 of the 21 expected non-fatal MIs and avoid 6 of the 19 anticipated CABG or angioplasty procedures. These are impressive results by any standard, and already many patterns of clinical practice are changing in this country and abroad.

West of Scotland Coronary Prevention Study

The West of Scotland Coronary Prevention Study (Shepherd et al 1995) is the most recent of the major lipid-lowering drug trials. The design of this study was similar to that of both the Helsinki Heart study and the Lipid Research Clinics study in that it was a double-blind, randomized, placebo-controlled primary prevention trial of a lipid-lowering drug. A group of 6595 men aged between 45 and 64 years in the West of Scotland, who had an average baseline total cholesterol of 7.0 mmol/l were recruited. The study group was randomized in equal numbers to treatment with placebo or with the HMG

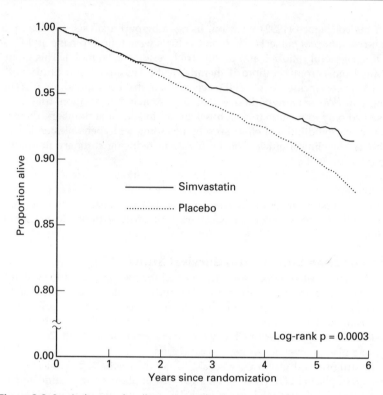

Figure 3.2 Survival curves for all-cause mortality. In the 4S study, 4444 patients with CHD were randomized to receive either the lipid-lowering drug simvastatin or a placebo. Over the course of the study the death rates in the two groups diverged after the first 18 months of therapy and progressively separated. By the end of the study 5 years later, the investigators could claim a very highly significant improvement in both all-cause and CHD mortality. (Redrawn with permission from Scandinavian Simvastatin Survival Study Group 1994.)

CoA reductase inhibitor, pravastatin, 40 mg nocte. This study is essentially a primary prevention trial in that at the time of randomization the participants had no evidence of previous myocardial infarction. However, it should be noted that 5% of the participants had evidence of mild angina. These individuals were randomized equally to treatment and placebo groups. All subjects were given smoking and dietary advice throughout the study.

After an average treatment period of 5 years, pravastatin therapy resulted in a 20% reduction in plasma total cholesterol in the treatment group. There was a 26% fall in plasma LDL-cholesterol, a 12% fall in plasma triglyceride and a 5% increase in plasma HDL-cholesterol.

The principal study end points were:

1. CHD death plus non-fatal myocardial infarction
2. CHD death
3. non-fatal myocardial infarction.

Importantly, no increase in non-cardiovascular mortality was observed in the pravastatin-treated goup and as a result all-cause mortality was reduced by 22%.

This study extends and confirms the important findings of 4S by demonstrating again that the statins are effective drugs in altering the lipid profile beneficially and without adverse effects. Furthermore, in this primary prevention group the use of pravastatin resulted in a marked improvement in the CHD risk status of the participants, decreasing their risk of fatal or non-fatal myocardial infarction by 31% (Fig. 3.3).

When we take together the results of these four major trials, and the many others which have not been discussed due to lack of space, we are no longer in any doubt that the cholesterol hypothesis as outlined above is an hypothesis no more. Lowering plasma total cholesterol and more specifically LDL-cholesterol reduces the risk of subsequent coronary events in those men and women who have pre-existing CHD and in high-risk men who have no overt evidence of disease. Some questions remain, of course, but these should not inhibit us from the active screening and management of lipid risk factors in these groups or, as has been the case in the past, give us the excuse for inactivity.

CLINICAL DISORDERS OF LIPID METABOLISM

Disorders of lipoprotein metabolism are among the commonest metabolic diseases seen in clinical practice. In addition to their important role in the

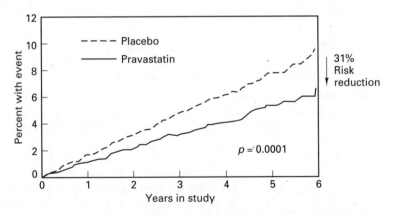

Figure 3.3 Survival curves for coronary mortality. In the West of Scotland Coronary Prevention Study, 6595 middle-aged men were randomized to receive either placebo or pravastatin (40 mg at night). These curves show the Kaplan–Meier analysis of the time to a definite non-fatal myocardial infarction or death from CHD, according to treatment group, over the course of the study. Note the curves continuously diverge throughout the study, culminating in a highly significant difference between the pravastatin treatment group and the placebo control group. (Redrawn with permission from Shepherd et al 1995.)

Table 3.2 Some examples of specific genetic causes of hyperlipidaemia

Disease	Genetic defect	Fredrickson	Risk
Familial hypercholesterolaemia	Reduced numbers of functional LDL receptors	IIa or IIb	Increased risk of CHD
Familial hypertriglyceridaemia	Possibly single gene defect	IV or V	? Increased risk of CHD
Familial combined hyperlipidaemia	Possibly single gene defect	IIa, IIb, IV or V	? Increased risk of CHD
Lipoprotein lipase deficiency	Reduced levels of functional lipoprotein lipase	I	Increased risk of pancreatitis

development of CHD some lipid disorders have other consequences; most notably, acute pancreatitis, failure to thrive in infants, neurological disorders and the development of cataracts.

There is currently no satisfactory comprehensive classification of lipoprotein disorders. Genetic classifications have been attempted but are becoming increasingly complex as different mutations are discovered. Some of the recognized genetic causes of hyperlipidaemia are shown in Table 3.2. Until the advent of gene therapy and/or specific substitution therapy, genetic classifications, while biologically sound, are unlikely to prove very useful in clinical practice. Today, most lipoprotein disorders are simplistically classified as being:

- primary, when the disorder is not due to an identifiable underlying disease
- secondary, when the disorder is a manifestation of some other disease.

Primary hyperlipidaemia

The Fredrickson or World Health Organization classification is the most widely accepted for the primary lipoprotein disorders. This classification, shown in Table 3.3, relies on the findings of analysis of the patient's plasma, rather than genetics. It is therefore a phenotypic rather than genotypic classification. This has a number of consequences. Patients with the same underlying genetic defect may fall into different groups, or may change grouping as their disease progresses or is treated. However, the major advantage of using this classification is that it is very widely known and gives some guidance to management. It is also important to realize that the six different classes of hyperlipoproteinaemia defined in the Fredrickson classification are not equally common in the population. Types I and V are rare, while types IIa, IIb and IV are very common. Type III hyperlipoproteinaemia, also known as familial dyslipoproteinaemia, is intermediate in frequency, occurring in about 1/5000 of the population.

Table 3.3 Fredrickson (WHO) classification of hyperlipoproteinaemia. This system is based on the appearance of a fasting plasma sample after standing for 12 hours at 4°C and analysis of its cholesterol and triglyceride content

	Normal	Type I	Type IIa	Type IIb	Type III	Type IV	Type V
Lipoprotein	N	+ CM	+ LDL	+ LDL + VLDL	+ IDL	+ VLDL	+ CM + VLDL
Total cholesterol	N	N or +	+	+	+	N or +	N or +
Triglyceride	N	++	N	+	+	+	++
LDL-cholesterol	N	N or –	+	+	N or –	N	N
HDL-cholesterol	N	N or –	N or –	N or –	N or –	N or –	N or –

Key: CM = chylomicrons; N = normal; + = increased; – = decreased

Secondary hyperlipidaemia

Hyperlipoproteinaemia is a well-recognized consequence of a number of diseases which divide broadly into two categories. On the one hand there is a group of clinically obvious diseases such as renal failure, nephrotic syndrome and cirrhosis of the liver in which an abnormal plasma lipid profile is to be expected. On the other hand there are a number of relatively covert conditions in which the hyperlipidaemia or its consequences may be the presenting feature. These conditions include hypothyroidism, diabetes mellitus and alcohol abuse. Perhaps the most common form of hyperlipidaemia in the population is that due to diet. This is discussed more fully in Chapter 6. This form of hyperlipidaemia may exist in isolation but is very often superimposed on some underlying genetic defect or defects.

Physical signs of hyperlipidaemia

The physical signs of hyperlipidaemia are not specific for any particular disease and may sometimes be present in normolipidaemic subjects. An example of the latter would be the arcus senilis, which when present in the young patient is a good indicator of an abnormal lipid profile, but which is very common in the elderly and then of no clinical significance. Tendon xanthomas, which present as firm lumps usually on the extensor tendons of the feet (Achilles tendon) elbows or hands, are particularly associated with FH but do occur in other forms of hyperlipidaemia.

Measuring plasma lipids and lipoproteins

The causal association between certain forms of hyperlipidaemia and the development of CHD is the main stimulus for the measurement of plasma lipids and lipoproteins in clinical practice. The most common aberrant lipid profile linked with atherogenesis and an increased risk of CHD is an elevated plasma LDL-cholesterol level, but increasingly it is being recognized that individuals with low plasma HDL-cholesterol and hypertriglyceridaemia are also at increased risk.

Blood for plasma lipid analysis may be collected into plain containers or into containers with the anticoagulant, ethylene diamine tetra-acetic acid (EDTA). Tubes containing heparin should not be used. A range of different analyses may be performed on this sample by the biochemistry laboratory, increasing in complexity from a simple total cholesterol measurement to a full lipoprotein analysis and perhaps even DNA analysis. If all that is required is a total cholesterol measurement the sample does not need to be a fasting one. If plasma triglyceride or lipoprotein cholesterol measurements are also required then the patient should have been instructed to fast. It is very important that patients should have the meaning of the term 'fasting' explained to them clearly, with an emphasis that they should eat and drink nothing except water for 12 hours prior to the blood sampling.

Most commonly a total cholesterol and triglyceride will be generated from the blood sample, and in addition an HDL-cholesterol may be provided. As well as these measured values, the LDL-cholesterol may be calculated from the Friedewald formula below if the three other parameters are known.

$$\text{LDL-cholesterol (mmol/l)} = \text{total cholesterol} - \text{HDL-cholesterol} - 0.45 \times \text{triglyceride (mmol/l)}.$$

The accuracy with which the LDL-cholesterol is estimated using this formula is relatively poor due to the summation of different analytical errors, but it does provide some useful information. It is important to note, however, that the Friedewald formula should not be used if the plasma triglyceride is greater than 4.0 mmol/l.

The most comprehensive and expensive analysis is known as a beta quantification where the total cholesterol, triglyceride, VLDL-cholesterol, LDL-cholesterol and HDL-cholesterol will be provided. In most circumstances this full lipoprotein profile is not necessary and patients can be adequately managed with total cholesterol, triglyceride and HDL-cholesterol measurements with, or without, a calculated LDL.

As with all blood chemistries there are a number of factors that affect the results of plasma lipid levels reported from the biochemistry laboratory. There is a natural biological variation from day to day and week to week in patients which must be taken into account when interpreting the results of serial samples. Similarly, there is a degree of analytical imprecision which will result in slightly different values reported even if the same blood sample is measured in the same laboratory on different days. Because of these sources of variation, both biological and analytical, it is important to take account of the results from more than one sample for lipid analysis before any action is taken. It is recommended in the Joint European Guidelines (Pyörälä et al 1994) that at least three measurements should be carried out on three separate samples before management decisions are made.

Another potentially important consideration in the analysis of blood lipids is the increasing use of desk top analysers and the advent of home cholesterol test kits. The former comprise test strips to which are applied a drop of capillary blood from a finger stab. The results are read and displayed using a small portable analyser such as a Reflotron. These assay systems are used in outpatient clinics, in primary care settings and at risk factor assessment sessions in the community. The accuracy and precision of the analysers can be very good. However, in common with all laboratory analyses conducted outside the main laboratory, there is sometimes a disregard by operators of the need for careful maintenance of the equipment and proper storage of the test strips. Clearly, the results obtained if maintenance, storage and operating procedures are not followed properly will be less than ideal.

Home cholesterol test kits are available from most pharmacies and although expensive are the preferred option for some individuals; usually those who are simply curious about their CHD risk status. A formal laboratory assessment of plasma lipids is recommended in any individuals who present concerned about the results they have obtained from self-use of these kits.

■ KEY POINTS

- Lipoproteins are complexes of lipids and proteins which facilitate lipid transport around the body.
- Lipoprotein metabolism can be thought of as three interconnected cycles centred on the liver.
- The Fredrickson (WHO) classification is the most commonly used system to classify hyperlipidaemias.
- Many primary hyperlipidaemias are due to defined genetic defects, while others remain as yet uncharacterized.
- Secondary causes of hyperlipidaemia include hypothyroidism, diabetes mellitus, liver disease and alcohol abuse.
- Elevated plasma LDL-cholesterol and decreased plasma HDL-cholesterol are associated with increased risk of CHD.
- By lowering plasma cholesterol we can reduce a patient's risk of CHD. This has been proven conclusively in men and women with established CHD and in high-risk men without overt CHD.
- In assessing the lipid-related CHD risk status of a patient, up to three separate blood samples should be taken and analysed before important management decisions are taken.
- Interpretation of lipid-related risk should always be part of a global CHD risk factor assessment.
- A fasting blood sample is required if triglyceride or lipoprotein measurements are requested. However, if only a total cholesterol measurement is requested a random sample is sufficient.
- The accuracy and reliability of lipid assays performed outside the laboratory depend on the operator following the test procedures closely and on the proper maintenance and storage of equipment.

Case Study 3.1

A 42-year-old man comes to see you after his 39-year-old brother dies of an acute MI. He is understandably concerned and wants advice. On questioning, he states that he is a non-smoker and that for exercise he plays golf every Sunday. On closer questioning about his family history, he reveals that his father died of an MI aged 50, his mother is 68 years old and well, his sister is aged 44 and is asymptomatic, his brother aged 40 has a 1-year history of angina, and his own two sons are 17 and 15, both healthy.

On examination, his blood pressure is 135/90 mmHg. His body mass index is 26. The results of blood tests taken on a fasting sample are as follows:

Total cholesterol—8.6 mmol/l
Triglyceride—2.1 mmol/l
HDL-cholesterol—0.95 mmol/l
Glucose—5.0 mmol/l.

Questions

Consider this man's overall risk of CHD. On the basis of his plasma lipid values what would his Fredrickson classification be? Does his history suggest any possible specific diagnosis? How should the man be managed? What advice would you offer him regarding his family?

Answers

In view of this man's very poor family history for CHD and his hypercholesterolaemia he is undoubtedly a high-risk patient. His hypercholesterolaemia would be consistent with a classification of Fredrickson type IIa hyperlipoproteinaemia. If his triglyceride had also been raised he would have fitted the type IIb or type IV depending on the appearance of his plasma.

The very strong family history of premature CHD coupled with the isolated very elevated plasma cholesterol, which in view of the low HDL-cholesterol will be due to an increased plasma LDL-cholesterol (calculated LDL-cholesterol = 6.7 mmol/l), this man is likely to have familial hypercholesterolaemia.

The patient's hyperlipidaemia should be confirmed by repeat sampling. If confirmed, he should be offered lifestyle advice with emphasis on dietary modification in an attempt to lower his plasma cholesterol level. In patients with FH this is unlikely to result in normalization of lipid levels and he is a candidate for lipid-lowering drug therapy. Assuming he has normal hepatic function and no other contraindications, the drug of first choice would be a statin. His surviving brother and his sister should have their CHD risk factors formally assessed with particular attention to their plasma lipid profile. His sons should also be screened as they have a 50% chance of inheriting his faulty LDL receptor gene.

This patient may already have early ischaemic changes and should be considered for referral to the cardiology clinic, where a resting ECG, chest X-ray and exercise test could be performed.

PRACTICAL EXERCISE

If blood samples are to be taken from a patient for plasma lipoprotein measurement the importance of fasting cannot be overemphasized. In practice many inappropriately timed blood samples are sent to the laboratory and much time and money is wasted. Consider, then, how and when you take blood from patients for these assays. What information is given to your patients regarding fasting, e.g. do you have an explanatory leaflet and if not, should you have one? When is the clinic where such blood samples are taken? Ideally it should be in the morning to allow patients to come fasting: if it is in the afternoon or evening how could you reorganize things to improve your service?

REFERENCES

Anitschkow N 1913 Uber die Veranderungen der Kaninchenaorta bei experimenteller Cholesterinsteatose. Beitrage zur pathologisten Anatomie und zur allgemeinen Pathologie 56: 379–404

Betteridge D J 1989 High density lipoprotein and coronary heart disease. British Medical Journal 298: 974–975

Bilheimer D W, Grundy S M, Brown M S, Goldstein J L 1983 Mevinolin and colestipol stimulate receptor-mediated clearance of low density lipoprotein from plasma in familial hypercholesterolemia heterozygotes. Proceedings of the National Academy of Sciences USA 80: 4124–4128

Brown M S, Goldstein J L 1983 Lipoprotein metabolism in the macrophage. Annual Review of Biochemistry 52: 223–261

Brown M S, Goldstein J L 1987 The LDL receptor. In: Gallo L L (ed) Cardiovascular disease. Plenum Press, New York, pp 87–91

Carew T E, Schwenke D C, Steinberg D 1987 Antiatherogenic effect of probucol unrelated to its hypocholesterolemic effect: evidence that antioxidants in vivo can selectively inhibit low density lipoprotein degradation in macrophage-rich fatty streaks and slow the progression of atherosclerosis in the Watanabe heritable hyperlipidemic rabbit. Proceedings of the National Academy of Sciences USA 84: 7725–7729

Committee of Principal Investigators 1978 A cooperative trial in the primary prevention of ischaemic heart disease using clofibrate. British Heart Journal 10: 1069–1118

Coronary Drug Project Research Group 1977 Gall bladder disease as a side effect of drugs influencing lipid metabolism. New England Journal of Medicine 296: 1188–1190

Dietschy J M, Wilson J D 1970 Regulation of cholesterol metabolism. New England Journal of Medicine 282: 1128–1138

Frick M H, Elo O, Haapa K et al 1987 Helsinki Heart Study: primary-prevention trial with gemfibrozil in middle-aged men with dyslipidemia. New England Journal of Medicine 317: 1237–1245

Goldstein J L, Hoff H F, Basu S K, Brown M S 1981 Stimulation of cholesteryl ester synthesis in macrophages by extracts of atherosclerotic human aortas and complexes of albumin / cholesteryl esters. Atherosclerosis 1: 210–216

Gordon D J, Probstfield J L, Garrison R J et al 1989 High-density lipoprotein cholesterol and cardiovascular disease. Four prospective American studies. Circulation 79: 8–15

Heinonen O P, Huttunen J K, Manninen V et al 1994 The Helsinki Heart Study: coronary heart disease incidence during an extended follow-up. Journal of Internal Medicine 235: 41–49

Hobbs H H, Russell D W, Brown M S, Goldstein J L 1990 The LDL receptor locus in familial hypercholesterolemia—mutational analysis of a membrane protein. Annual Review of Genetics 24: 133-170

Hoff H F, Morton R E 1987 Uptake of LDL sized particles extracted from human aortic lesions by macrophages in culture. In: Gallo L L (ed) Cardiovascular disease. Plenum Press, New York, pp 87–91

Innerarity T L, Mahley R W, Weisgraber K H et al 1990 Familial defective apolipoprotein B-100: a mutation of apolipoprotein B that causes hypercholesterolemia. Journal of Lipid Research 31: 1337–1349

Kannel W B, Castelli W, Gordon T, McNamara D J 1971 Serum cholesterol, lipoproteins, and the risk of coronary heart disease. The Framingham Study. Annals of Internal Medicine 74: 1–12

Keys A 1980 Seven Countries Study: a multivariate analysis of death and coronary heart disease. Harvard University Press, Cambridge MA

Levy R I, Fredrickson D S, Shulman R, Bilheimer D W, Breslow J L, Stone N J, Lux S E, Sloan H R, Krauss R M, Herbert P N 1972 Dietary and drug treatment of primary hyperlipoproteinemia. Annals of Internal Medicine 77: 267–294

Lipid Research Clinics Program 1984 The Lipid Research Clinics Coronary Primary Prevention Trial results. I. Reduction in incidence of coronary heart disease. Journal of the American Medical Association 251: 351–364

Mann J I, Lewis B, Shepherd J, Winder A F, Fenster S, Rose L, Morgan B 1988 Blood lipid concentrations and other cardiovascular risk factors: distribution, prevalence and detection in Britain. British Medical Journal 296: 1702–1706

Manninen V, Elo O, Frick M H et al 1988 Lipid alterations and decline in the incidence of coronary heart disease in the Helsinki Heart Study. Journal of the American Medical Association 260: 641–651

Manninen V, Tenkanen L, Koskinen P et al 1992 Joint effects of serum triglyceride and LDL cholesterol and HDL cholesterol concentrations on coronary heart disease risk in the Helsinki Heart Study. Implications for treatment. Circulation 85: 37–45

Marmot M G, Mann J I 1987 Epidemiology of ischaemic heart disease. In: Fox K M (ed). Ischaemic heart disease. Lancaster University Press, Lancaster

Norum K R, Berg T, Helgerud P, Drevon C A 1983 Transport of cholesterol. Physiological Reviews 63: 1343–1397

Packard C J, Shepherd J 1986 Cholesterol 7α hydroxylase: involvement in hepatobiliary axis and regulation of plasma lipoprotein levels. In: Fears R, Sabine J R (eds) Cholesterol 7α hydroxylase. CRC Press, Boca Raton FL, pp 147–165

Pyörälä K, De Backer G, Graham I, Poole-Wilson P, Wood D 1994 Prevention of coronary heart disease in clinical practice. Recommendations of the Task Force of the European Society of Cardiology, European Atherosclerosis Society and European Society of Hypertension. European Heart Journal 15: 1300–1331

Rose G, Shipley M 1986 Plasma cholesterol concentrations and deaths from coronary heart disease: 10 year results of the Whitehall Study. British Medical Journal 293: 306–307

Scandinavian Simvastatin Survival Study Group 1994 Randomised trial of cholesterol lowering in 4444 patients with coronary heart disease: the Scandinavian Simvastatin Survival Study (4S). Lancet 344: 1383–1389

Shepherd J, Packard C J, Bicker S, Lawrie T D V, Morgan H G 1980 Cholestyramine promotes receptor-mediated LDL catabolism. New England Journal of Medicine 302: 1219–1222

Shepherd J, Betteridge D J, Durrington P, Laker M, Lewis B, Mann J, Miller J P, Reckless J P D, Thompson G R 1987 Strategies for reducing coronary heart disease and desirable limits for blood lipid concentrations: guidelines of the British Hyperlipidaemia Association. British Medical Journal 295: 1245–1246

Shepherd J, Cobbe S M, Ford I, Isles C G, Lorimer A R, Macfarlane P W, McKillop J H, Packard C J 1995 Prevention of coronary heart disease with pravastatin in men with hypercholesterolaemia. New England Journal of Medicine 333: 1301–1307

Tunstall-Pedoe H, Smith W C S, Crombie I K, Tavendale R 1989 How-often-that-high graphs of serum cholesterol. Findings from the Scottish Heart Health and Scottish MONICA Studies. Lancet 1 (March 11): 540–542

Yla-Herttuala S, Palinski W, Rosenfield M E et al 1989 Evidence for the presence of oxidatively modified low density lipoprotein in atherosclerotic lesions of rabbit and man. Journal of Clinical Investigation 84: 1086–1095

FURTHER READING

Durrington P N 1989 Hyperlipidaemia: diagnosis and management. Wright, London

This is an excellent book covering all aspects of clinical lipidology and would be a good resource for those wishing to take the subject further.

Gaw A, Packard C J, Shepherd J 1994 Lipids and atherosclerosis. In: Bloom A L, Forbes C D, Thomas D P, Tuddenham E G D (eds) Haemostasis and thrombosis, 3rd edn. Churchill Livingstone, Edinburgh, ch 50: 1153–1168

This is a recent and much more detailed description of lipoprotein metabolism by the authors.

Gaw A, Cowan R A, O'Reilly D St J, Stewart M J, Shepherd J 1995 Clinical biochemistry: an illustrated colour text. Churchill Livingstone, Edinburgh

This textbook includes useful fully illustrated sections on lipids and coronary heart disease.

Quiney J R, Watts G F 1989 Classic papers in hyperlipidaemia. Science Press, London

This book presents reprints of all the major papers detailing the story of the cholesterol hypothesis from its earliest days.

ACKNOWLEDGEMENTS

Portions of this work were carried out under the tenure of British Heart Foundation Grants FS 92001 and FS 94001, and SOHHD Grant K/MRS/50/C2310.

Hypertension

Joan L. Curzio   Susan S. Kennedy

4

INTRODUCTION

Despite being one of the most systematically researched topics, hypertension (high blood pressure) remains an enigma. Hypertension has traditionally been defined as the blood pressure above which intervention has been shown to reduce risk (Pickering 1968). However, no definitive cut-off point has been discovered.

In this chapter we will cover the epidemiology, physiological definition, measurement, assessment, diagnosis and follow-up care of hypertension, keeping in mind that it cannot be viewed or cared for in isolation. Hypertension is just one of the factors that increases an individual's risk of coronary and cardiovascular disease (MacMahon et al 1990). Therefore, hypertension care needs to be part of an integrated multiple risk factor reduction programme.

It is estimated that 90% of individuals with chronically raised blood pressure have 'essential hypertension', that is, without known cause. This is the entity being dealt with in this chapter. However, when assessing anyone with elevated blood pressure, it must be kept in mind that upwards of 10% of patients will have a diagnosable and treatable cause for their chronically elevated blood pressure, i.e. secondary hypertension (Box 4.1). All assessment protocols need to include screening for these conditions with referral to a specialist centre for diagnosis and treatment.

EPIDEMIOLOGY

Epidemiological surveys indicate that the risk of coronary heart disease and cerebrovascular disease increases continuously with increasing blood pressure; the higher an individual's blood pressure the higher the risk, the

---

Box 4.1 Causes of secondary hypertension

- Renal disease:
  —glomerulonephritis
  —pyelonephritis
  —polycystic kidneys
  —renal infarction
- Renal artery stenosis
- Phaeochromocytoma
- Primary aldosteronism
- Adrenal adenoma
- Cushing's syndrome
- Coarctation of aorta
- Late polio or encephalitis
- Drug induced:
  —oral contraceptives
  —steroids
  —carbenoxalone
  —monoamine oxidase inhibitors

---

lower the blood pressure the lower the risk (MacMahon et al 1990) regardless of sex (Isles et al 1992).

Blood pressure levels vary in different populations and by social class. There are racial differences in the occurrence of hypertension; for example, Black Africans who live in westernized societies have higher blood pressure and more strokes than their Caucasian counterparts. An example of the cultural differences that occur is seen in Africa with Black Africans who have moved to westernized cities having higher blood pressures than Black Africans who continue to live in a rural setting. Blood pressure rises as people grow old in westernized societies, but again not in rural, undeveloped ones. Finally, there is a genetic component and it has been found that there are 'hypertensive' families (Bulpitt 1985).

It has also been noted that individuals with more than one cardiovascular risk factor (i.e. hypertension, hyperlipidaemia, cigarette smoking, family history, etc.) are at greater risk from the combination of factors. A synergy between factors appears to be present, increasing the risk well above that which is attributed to the factors singly (Kannel et al 1986). Unfortunately, it also seems that if one cardiovascular risk factor is present, that individual is more likely to have other risk factors and therefore be at higher risk. This clustering effect has been noted in westernized populations from Australia (MacMahon et al 1985) and the USA (Criqui et al 1986).

There are a number of other independent risk factors. The ones of most importance to a community health care team, that add to cardiovascular risk, include the presence of cardiovascular disease in a first-degree relative, particularly occurring at a younger age. Left ventricular hypertrophy (LVH), enlargement of the left ventricle of the heart on an electrocardiogram (ECG), or indications of ischaemia or previous coronary event on ECG or by history are also significant (Bulpitt 1985).

Several factors have been identified, not as independent cardiovascular risk factors, but as factors which have been shown to increase blood pressure. These include excess weight, alcohol and sodium intake (Bulpitt 1985).

Finally, there is evidence that lowering these risk factors is beneficial. The results from hypertension trials are strong, particularly in regards to the reduction of cerebrovascular mortality (Collins et al 1990). The trials to reduce hypertension in the elderly have also demonstrated significant reductions in coronary heart disease mortality (MRC 1992). Lowering weight lowers blood pressure in the obese (Berchtold et al 1982) and decreasing alcohol intake has also been shown to decrease blood pressure (MacMahon & Norton 1986). The level of salt reduction required to have significant effects on blood pressure is difficult to achieve and maintain (Wood 1986), but there is value in reduction of excessive salt intake (Stein & Black 1993).

The foregoing is only a brief summary of the epidemiological evidence for the role hypertension and related factors play in cardiovascular disease and its reduction. An in-depth review of coronary heart disease risk can be found in Chapter 2. This evidence is presented as justification for the non-pharmacological (described in this chapter) and the pharmacological treatment of hypertension (described in Ch. 11).

WHAT IS BLOOD PRESSURE?

Blood pressure is the pressure in the arterial system, which waxes and wanes as the heart beats. It also varies from beat to beat. The maximum pressure, i.e. systolic blood pressure, occurs as the left ventricle empties into the aorta, and the resting pressure, i.e. diastolic blood pressure, is as the ventricle fills. The major determinants of blood pressure are cardiac output, i.e. the amount of blood expelled by the left ventricle in 1 minute of pumping, and peripheral resistance, which is determined by the tone or tension of the vascular musculature and the diameter of the vessels in the periphery.

This pressurized system is dynamic, reacting with increases and decreases in pressure to a number of stimuli, each of which either affects the cardiac output or peripheral resistance or both. These stimuli include the release or inhibition of adrenaline, noradrenaline, renin, angiotensin, aldosterone, endothelin, etc. It is of paramount importance to comprehend these basic physiological influences as they form the basis for modern anti-hypertensive pharmacological intervention (Ch. 11).

CONTRIBUTION TO CORONARY HEART DISEASE PATHOGENESIS

The mechanisms whereby hypertension contributes to coronary heart disease pathogenesis are complex and remain somewhat unclear. However, much work is going on and evidence is accumulating for not one cause but a number of multifactorial defects.

In hypertension the structure and functioning of the vasculature is modified. In many hypertensives, the vascular wall is thickened with a decreased internal diameter, thus increasing peripheral resistance (Swales 1994). Cholesterol-rich deposits have a greater chance of blocking these narrower vessels and constriction is more likely to lead to vasospasm in them.

There are functional changes in the endothelial lining of the arteries which may also increase the likelihood of vasospasm. Decreased production and/or availability of vasorelaxing substances and an increase in vasoconstrictor substances have also been reported in hypertension. The vasodilator nitric oxide has received a lot of attention recently in this regard (Loscalzo 1995).

Finally, platelet adhesion, platelet activation and platelet aggregation may also be increased in hypertension (Luscher 1990). Such increases can promote thrombus formation.

MEASURING BLOOD PRESSURE

The importance of accurately measuring blood pressure cannot be over-emphasized. In hypertension, the level of an individual's blood pressure will determine diagnosis, if treatment is required, whether treatment is adequately controlling blood pressure and if additional or alternative treatment is necessary. Measurement needs to be standardized as repeated measurements must be reliable for comparison to be meaningful.

The observer needs to start with a review of the equipment to be used for measurement, and then progress to an understanding of the effects of physical and environmental factors (Box 4.2), before progressing to the actual measurement. The mercury sphygmomanometer, as first designed by Rivi Rocci in 1888, is a simple and elegant design. The robustness of this device is outstanding with its basic functioning easy to assess. Aneroid sphygmomanometers are useful and popular with community staff due to their portability. Unfortunately they require frequent 6-monthly calibration as they can loose accuracy due to a leaking diaphragm, or stretched spring.

Further specific equipment information for mercury and aneroid sphygmomanometers can be found in Box 4.3. There is an accompanying exercise to provide readers with an opportunity to assess their own equipment (Box 4.4). An example of an appropriate setup for blood pressure measurement can be seen in Figure 4.1.

Electronic or semi-automatic blood pressure measuring devices would appear at first to resolve the difficulties of manually measuring blood pressure as discussed in this section. Innumerable models from a number of manufacturers have been found wanting over the years. Standards for validating such devices have become much more rigorous in recent years (O'Brien et al 1993). Even though several newer models have met these validation standards, there is no prohibition on manufacturers from changing a model or producing newer models with a different specification.

Additional blood pressure measurements obtained outside of the clinical setting, either by the use of a home sphygmomanometer or a 24-hour ambulatory blood pressure monitor, can provide additional information about the variability of an individual's blood pressure. In addition to the aforementioned problems with equipment validation and calibration, home

---

Box 4.2 Factors that affect blood pressure measurement (compiled from O'Brien & O'Malley 1991)

Global factors
- Digit preference
- Observer bias
- Defence reaction
- Beat-to-beat variability
- Auscultatory gap

Factors causing overestimation of BP
- Cuff bladder too narrow
- Cuff applied loosely
- Bladder not centred over artery

- Mercury column slopes away from vertical (usually due to damaged hinges)
- Too rapid deflation of mercury column during measurement
  —overestimates diastolic BP
- Hearing impaired or eartips not forward
  —overestimates systolic BP
- Arm held below heart level

Factors increasing BP
- Talking
- Standing
  —slight increase in diastolic BP

- Arm unsupported, causing isometric exercise of limb
- 'White coat hypertension'

Factors causing underestimation of BP
- Cuff bladder too wide (less of a problem)
- Leaks in tubing
- Heavy pressure on stethoscope over artery
  —underestimates diastolic BP

- Too rapid deflation of mercury column during measurement
  —underestimates systolic BP
- Hearing impaired or eartips not forward
  —underestimates systolic BP
- Arm held above heart level

Factors decreasing BP
- Rest
- Standing
  —slight decrease in systolic BP
  —marked decrease in some elderly people and those taking alpha-blocking drugs

---

blood pressure monitoring requires each patient to be carefully taught. A double-headed stethoscope can be quite helpful. Regular review of equipment and technique is also required.

Ambulatory blood pressure monitoring can help to identify 'white coat hypertension', i.e. the occurrence of raised blood pressure only in the presence of health care personnel. The long-term epidemiological significance of ambulatory blood pressure measurement has yet to be established. Finally, the cost of ambulatory blood pressure monitoring equipment puts it out of reach of most general practices, particularly when compared with lower-cost alternatives such as self- or home measurements.

Box 4.3 Blood pressure equipment maintenance (compiled from: O'Brien & O'Malley 1991)

Briefly check equipment each time you use it. It is more likely that you will notice when it needs repair or maintenance.

Mercury sphygmomanometer
Check:
1. Hinges—they should be tight, allowing the mercury column to be straight in an upright position.
2. Mercury column—is the column clean, are the markings clear, and does the mercury rest at zero?
3. Tubing and connectors—check for cracks and loose/leaky connections.
4. Cuff—is it clean? When was the last time the cover was washed? Is the Velcro full of lint? (This can be cleared with a suede brush.) Is it the right size for the patient's arm?
5. Bulb—check for cracks, air leaks.
6. Inflation valve—can it be shut completely and opened slowly to allow for controlled deflation? Can you inflate it to above 200 mmHg in 3–5 seconds and deflate at a rate of 2–3 millimetres per second? (The control release valve is the commonest source of error in the system.)
7. Service—check when last serviced, note next date of service. Mercury sphygmomanometers should be checked once a year by a trained technician. It is not recommended for health professionals to handle mercury; it is a poison. (Some drug companies provide sphygmomanometer calibration and service free of charge. Alternatively, medical supply firms do it for a small fee.)

Aneroid sphygmomanometer
Check:
1. Tubing and connectors—check for cracks and loose/leaky connections.
2. Cuff—is it clean? When was the last time the cover was washed? Is the Velcro full of lint? (This can be cleared with a suede brush.) Is it the right size for the patient's arm?
3. Bulb—check for cracks, air leaks.
4. Inflation valve—can it be shut completely and opened slowly to allow for controlled deflation? Can you inflate it to above 200 mmHg in 3–5 seconds and deflate at a rate of 2–3 millimetres per second?
5. Dial—check that it zeros. Do not use one with a stop pin at zero. If gauge is outwith the zero range, DO NOT USE, have it serviced even if a service is not due.
6. Service—check when last serviced, note next date of service. Aneroid sphygmomanometers should be checked 6-monthly by a trained technician. Their calibration should be regularly compared against a mercury column using a Y-connector. (Some drug companies provide sphygmomanometer calibration and service free of charge. Alternatively, medical supply firms do it for a small fee.)

Other problems with aneroids: vacuum between diaphragms is hard to maintain, and the mechanical moving parts require regular lubrication.

Stethoscope
Check:
1. Tubing—keep as short as possible.
2. Ear pieces—are they clean and are they tilted forward when you use them? Do they fit you properly?
3. Head—use good quality diaphragm.

Box 4.4 Exercise: assessment of manual sphygmomanometer

Please assess the equipment you have available to use.

1. Sphygmomanometer
Please specify type:

_____ Mercury _____ Aneroid Other (please specify) _____
Please describe condition and circle response where appropriate:
Cuff tubing: _____ Cracks? Y / N
Machine tubing: _____ Cracks? Y / N
Bulb: _____ Cracks? Y / N
Cuff sizes available (mm × mm): _____

_____

Cuff covering type: Velcro or wrap around? _____
Cuff condition: _____
If mercury sphygmomanometer, condition of column (please circle):
Is oxidation present? Y / N   Markings legible? Y / N
Does it rest at zero? Y / N   If not, what is resting level? _____ mmHg
If box type, is lid held at 90° when open? Y / N

Date last calibrated: _____ Maintenance cycle: _____

Testing
Can the release valve be opened and shut smoothly? Y / N
Can you control deflation smoothly? Y / N
Does the system maintain pressure and not deflate prior to releasing valve? Y / N
Can it be inflated to 200 mmHg within 3–5 seconds? Y / N (please do twice to confirm)
Can it be deflated at 2–3 mmHg per second? Y / N (please do twice to confirm results)
Does the mercury return to zero after deflation? Y / N If no, does it after flick of lid? Y / N

2. Stethoscope
Type: diaphragm or bell tubing: _____ Cracks? Y / N
Length: _____ Ear piece condition: _____

3. Scales
Type: _____
Date last calibrated: _____ Maintenance cycle: _____

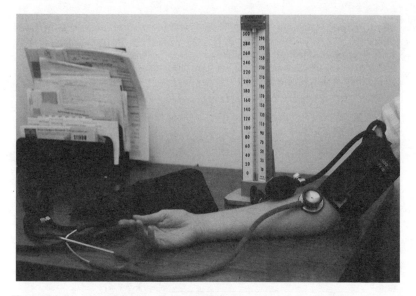

Figure 4.1 Accurate blood pressure measurement requires well-maintained equipment with the patient and equipment positioned correctly (see Box 4.5).

Recommendations for the manual measurement of blood pressure have evolved over the years in response to research. A brief summary of the British Hypertension Society's (BHS) recommended technique is given in Box 4.5. Unfortunately, work indicates that the knowledge and skills of many health care professionals in the measurement of blood pressure are lacking (McKay et al 1990, Feher et al 1992). Efforts have been made to improve this situation. The BHS produced a video and accompanying pamphlet (Petrie et al 1990) and training programmes have been set up and evaluated (O'Brien et al 1991). Ultimately, the responsibility for understanding the correct technique for the measurement of blood pressure lies with the individual practitioner.

MANAGEMENT OF HYPERTENSION

In the 1970s the 'Rule of Halves' was coined to describe the follow-up management of hypertension. Within a population, for example a group of patients in a health centre, 50% of those with hypertension would be known; of this identified group, 50% would be treated; and, of the treated group, only 50% would have blood pressure at a normal level. In other words, of all hypertensive patients, only about 12.5% were satisfactorily managed. In 1990 a Scottish group described the situation in Scotland in relationship to the 'Rule of Halves'. In their survey more patients were identified as hypertensive, but still only 12–14% were well controlled (Smith et al 1991).

Identification

As essential hypertension is symptomless, screening for high blood pressure is necessary. Over 75% of adults attend their general practitioner at least once

Box 4.5 Method recommended by the BHS for the manual measurement of blood pressure by mercury sphygmomanometer (Petrie et al 1990)

Positioning of patient and equipment
1. Explain procedure to patient.
2. Have patient in comfortable position with arm supported, in a warm environment with tight or restrictive clothing removed.
3. Apply cuff of appropriate size (to encompass approximately 80% of upper arm), with tubing superiorly, with the centre of the bladder over the brachial artery and the lower edge 2–3 cm above the antecubital fossa.
4. Ensure that the manometer is at eye level and within 3 feet of you.

Estimation of systolic blood pressure
1. Palpate brachial or radial pulse.
2. Inflate cuff until pulsation vanishes (systolic pressure).
3. Deflate cuff and record reading.

Measurement of systolic and diastolic pressure
1. Place stethoscope gently over maximal pulsation of brachial artery.
2. Inflate cuff to 30 mmHg above estimated systolic pressure.
3. Reduce pressure at rate of 2–3 mmHg per second or per heart beat.
4. Systolic blood pressure is noted when repetitive, clear tapping sounds appear for two consecutive beats.
5. Diastolic blood pressure is noted when repetitive sounds disappear.
6. Record reading.

every 3 years and this type of opportunistic screening has been shown to be successful (Barber et al 1979). This includes patients aged 65 years and over with otherwise good life expectancy. Opportunities for checking blood pressure present frequently, and such opportunities should be taken, using the recommended method for taking blood pressure as described. Furthermore, recording the level in a standard, prominent place within each patient's notes aids future assessment. Blood pressure measurement requires to be repeated over time and a suggested guideline to follow for such a programme is given in Table 4.1.

Assessment

This period of monitoring blood pressure can be used to assess patients for other cardiovascular risk factors and evidence of damage to organs susceptible to prolonged high blood pressure or periods of severe hypertension. These target organs include the brain in the form of cerebrovascular accidents (strokes) and transient ischaemic attacks. The heart can experience left ventricular hypertrophy, ischaemia, or heart failure. The peripheral blood vessels are more readily affected by formation of atheroma leading to claudication. Aneurysms which can develop and lead to dissection are rare, but more common in the hypertensive patient. The eyes can develop retinopathy and the kidneys chronic renal failure.

The baseline examination with investigations (Box 4.6) should be conducted at a return appointment to assess individuals found to have

Table 4.1 Follow-up as determined by level of blood pressure

Classification	Blood pressure level	Follow-up timescale
Normal blood pressure	< 160/90 mmHg	Repeat measure within 3–5 years
Mild/moderate hypertension	Diastolic blood pressure 90–110 mmHg	Repeat measure every 2–4 weeks for 3 visits
Moderate/severe hypertension	Diastolic blood pressure 110–120 mmHg	Repeat measure every 2 weeks for 3 visits
Severe hypertension	Diastolic blood pressure > 120 mmHg	No delay
Isolated systolic hypertension	Diastolic blood pressure < 90 mmHg and systolic blood pressure > 160 mmHg	Repeat measure every 2–4 weeks for 3–6 months

Box 4.6 Baseline procedures and investigations to be recorded

- History of cardiovascular risk factors. Note:
  —smoking status
  —alcohol intake
  —level of exercise
  —type of diet.
- Family history. Note:
  —cardiovascular disease (including MI, stroke)
  —renal disease.
- Past medical and drug history.
- Height and weight
  —calculate body mass index: $\dfrac{\text{weight (kilograms)}}{\text{height (metres)}^2}$
- Blood pressure and pulse rate.
- Physical examination including:
  —fundoscopy
  —radio-femoral delay
  —carotid and abdominal bruits
  —peripheral pulses.
- Test urine for:
  —protein
  —glucose
  —blood.
  (Send mid-stream urine for culture and sensitivity testing if blood and/or protein show up on reagent strips.)
- Blood sample for:
  —urea and electrolytes
  —creatinine
  —gamma GT
  —urate
  —random cholesterol
  —glucose.
- Arrange for 12-lead electrocardiograph and have it reported.

borderline, mild, or moderate hypertension. The appointment is best made when both the general practitioner and practice nurse are available, and when a venous blood sample can be sent promptly to a laboratory for analysis. The patient should be asked to bring a sample of urine.

There is a rationale for the examination and investigations suggested. Physical examination done by the doctor will most frequently be normal. Nevertheless rare signs of secondary causes could be present. Also, by looking in the eye for fundal changes (fundoscopy), evidence of target organ changes can be observed. Serious fundal changes such as exudates, flame haemorrhages or oedema of the optic disc (papilloedema) can indicate malignant hypertension. This condition is serious and requires treatment in hospital.

Urinalysis using reagent strips is easy to perform and worth taking the time to ask the patient to give a specimen of urine at the surgery if one is not brought to the appointment. This is because proteinuria and haematuria suggest underlying renal disease and should be investigated further. If a reagent strip shows glucose in the urine, diabetes should be considered. Hypertension with diabetes potentiates the risk of renal disease, so good control of both diabetes and hypertension should be sought.

Biochemical testing of blood is helpful to exclude several secondary causes of hypertension and identify other cardiovascular risks such as raised cholesterol and glucose. Also, a creatinine level can be used as an indicator of kidney function and thus target organ damage.

An electrocardiogram (ECG) gives information on the state of the heart. This provides a baseline for future comparison and assessment. In the patient with hypertension, an abnormal ECG tracing can be a guide to the presence of LVH, strain, and ischaemia. LVH is a powerful indicator of cardiovascular risk, independently of blood pressure. Therefore blood pressure control is vital in these patients. Thus the results of this initial physical examination and accompanying investigations as outlined above will help to determine the management of patients with hypertension.

General management

Once hypertension is diagnosed, the aim of treatment is to reduce the risk of end-organ damage. Non-pharmacological treatment to lower blood pressure includes achieving ideal body weight, avoidance of excessive alcohol intake, improving overall level of fitness, and reducing added salt to food (Table 4.2). Other lifestyle modifications which help to reduce the risk of cardiovascular disease are firstly not to smoke and secondly to improve the diet by reducing saturated fat intake and increasing fibre and vitamin C content.

As patients have no symptoms, time should be taken to explain why it is that they are being asked to make, in some cases, major changes to their lifestyles with no obvious short-term benefit to themselves. Research in the field of behavioural change is extensive. Many models have been developed to try to help us understand the complex nature of our actions but none have been able to fully explain human behaviour. We are all aware that despite much counselling and teaching, many people still fail to stop smoking, lose

Table 4.2 Effect of non-pharmacological intervention

Non-drug therapy	Effect on BP	Effect on risk
Normalizing glucose	No effect	Reduces risk
Normalizing cholesterol	No effect	Reduces risk
Stopping smoking	No effect	Reduces risk ++
Losing weight	Lowers BP*	Maybe
Decreasing alcohol intake	Lowers BP†	Maybe
Decreasing salt intake	Lowers BP‡	Maybe
Increasing exercise	Lowers BP	Reduces risk

* Weight reduction of 1 kg can drop BP by 2 mmHg.
† Reducing alcohol consumption to within the recommended units/week.
‡ Reducing salt to 6 g/day has less pronounced effect in mild hypertension and therefore remains controversial. Patients should be advised not to add salt at the table and avoid very salty foods.

weight, etc. Thus if a patient, after a reasonable amount of time and effort, is unable to make these suggested changes and blood pressure continues at an unsatisfactory level, then drug treatment should be initiated. If a patient does make all of these changes and yet fails to lower blood pressure to a satisfactory level, drug treatment should also be initiated (Ch. 11).

There are many booklets for patients on hypertension and associated cardiovascular risk factors, but care should be taken to review them for suitability. It is important that patients are given consistent advice by the health care team, and it is tailored to the level that they can best assimilate. Patients who have bought a home blood pressure device may also need help with interpreting the results obtained and maintaining the machine.

The following guidelines are suggested as a basis for a blood pressure clinic protocol which would also enable audit to be carried out. The protocol should include the methods to be used to:

- measure blood pressure
- advise and counsel patients on non-pharmacological methods of reducing cardiovascular risk
- provide education for patients regarding the benefits of long-term follow-up and compliance
- prescribe anti-hypertensive drug therapy after a period of monitoring as necessary
- follow up all patients and complete an annual review
- document care either by using a computer and/or card registration system.

These guidelines are based on recommendations from specialists in hypertension at a national (Sever et al 1993) and international level (WHO/ISH 1993). Each health care team will need to devise its own protocol based on these national and international guidelines, taking into consideration local constraints and conditions. Protocols need to be revised at regular intervals to incorporate any newly published research studies.

Follow-up visits

Routine follow-up visits can be organized in nurse-run clinics but a doctor needs to be available for advice. At each visit weight and blood pressure should be measured and recorded. A history of current general health should be sought along with an assessment of compliance and side effects. Any abnormalities detected need to be investigated.

In a nurse-run clinic the flow chart in Figure 4.2 suggests guidelines for when to refer the patient to a doctor. Patient education on aspects of

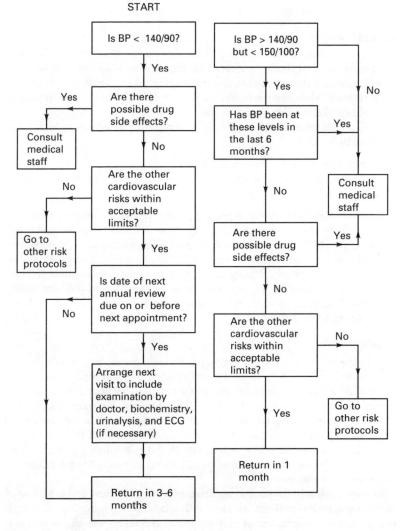

Figure 4.2 Flow chart for the follow-up of treated hypertensive patients.

hypertension and drug treatment, can be continued along with discussion of achievable targets for reducing other cardiovascular risks if present. A return appointment with a minimum frequency of 6-monthly is suggested for well-controlled patients, i.e. with a BP less than 140/90 mmHg. However, if systolic blood pressure is 140–160 mmHg or diastolic blood pressure is 91–95 mmHg then a 3-month return visit is suggested so that treatment change can be considered if blood pressure is still high. Similarly, if systolic blood pressure is greater than 160 mmHg or diastolic blood pressure is greater than 95 mmHg, give a 1-month return visit to assess treatment change if blood pressure is still elevated and if end-organ damage is present. Untreated patients can be scheduled in a similar way.

Annual review

The purpose of an annual review is to monitor the target organs for change. If present for the first time, a review of the management of blood pressure and other cardiovascular risk factors should be undertaken. It may be necessary to institute more stringent measures such as an increase in drug treatment or referral to a stop-smoking programme.

The procedures necessary to annually monitor for the effects of high blood pressure include:

- urinalysis for protein, glucose and blood
- a venous blood sample to test for urea and electrolytes, creatinine, urate, glucose, cholesterol and gamma GT.

If the initial ECG is normal, repeating it every 3–5 years can pick up serious changes. Keep in mind that it may be clinically indicated to repeat this earlier, e.g. with the occurrence of chest pain. The progression and regression of LVH can be monitored by serial ECG, as echocardiograms (ultrasound assessment of the heart), although a far more sensitive assessment of LVH are not readily available to hypertensive patients cared for in the community. A physical examination including fundoscopy ensures review with the physician in a nurse-run clinic.

Audit

In this chronic condition the long-term follow-up care by the health team requires to be of a high standard. By setting standards and considering targets for blood pressure reduction, protocols can be developed to encourage optimum care. Studies have shown that this can be most successfully achieved by including adequately trained nursing staff using an agreed protocol with recall facilities for patients who fail to attend (Silverberg et al 1982, Kenkre et al 1985). In a practice of 2500 it is estimated that 162 nurse hours/year are employed managing 225 mild, 25 moderate, and 3 severe hypertensive patients.

Regular review of the patient registration system for those lost to follow-up helps to identify patients at risk and who need prompting. Carefully completing documentation of each patient at annual review allows access to data either in the form of a log book, card system or computer program. An evaluation of all or part of the data from completed annual reviews can be made. Mean clinic blood pressures, weights or any risk factor can be monitored over the years. A sample set of forms to facilitate these activities is shown in Figure 4.3. In this way aspects of patient care can be reviewed and discussed with all members of the health care team.

Suggestions for referral to a specialist hypertension clinic

Most patients with essential hypertension will be able to be managed in general practice. However, there are situations where an individual is at

Patient details				Identification No:		
Name:		Title:		Sex: M/F	DOB / /	
Address:				Telephone No:		

Family history	Problem list	Date recorded
Mother: Father: Siblings:	Active:	
Smoking habits		
Drinking habits	Inactive:	

Previous treatment				Problem check list
Treatment name	Max. daily dose	Start date	Stop date	(Please tick any of the following which have occurred and are not listed above. Please ring A for active and I for inactive and add date.)

Date

☐ Cerebrovascular accident   A I
☐ Myocardial infarction   A I
☐ Ischaemic heart disease   A I
☐ Symptomatic angina   A I
☐ Peripheral vascular disease   A I
☐ Renal   A I
☐ Airways disease   A I
☐ Diabetes   A I
☐ Overweight   A I
☐ Anxiety   A I
☐ Social/psychological problems   A I
☐ Drug sensitivity   A I

Current treatment
(All treatment including oral contraceptive pill, NSAIDs etc.)

Treatment name   Total daily dose   Start date

Figure 4.3 Hypertension record sheets: (A) patient details.

Name: ....   Identification No: ....

Date					
Blood pressure systolic diastolic pulse					
Body mass index weight (kg) height (m)					
Urine dipstix glucose protein blood					
Blood test sodium potassium urea creatinine urate cholesterol glucose					
ECG date report					
Symptoms e.g. dyspnoea on effort, oedema, chest pain (please update)					

Treatment complications: please indicate whether complication is still present and name suspected drug.

Problem	Drug	First noted	Still present

Note: diastolic BP should be phase V measured in the right arm with a mercury sphygmomanometer and with the patient seated.

Figure 4.3 Hypertension record sheets: (B) annual review.

significantly increased cardiovascular risk, either from the disease itself, such as malignant phase hypertension, or secondary cause, such as phaeochromocytoma. Then referral to a specialist hypertension clinic is warranted.

Malignant phase hypertension presents with bilateral retinal haemorrhages or exudates with or without papilloedema. Phaeochromocytoma can cause great swings in blood pressure with the patient complaining about excessive changes in mood, anxiety and possibly night time sweats and flushing. Many

Patient name: ....   Identification No: ....

Treatment:

Date	Weight	BP + pulse	Check compliance	Blood tests	Well-being (include risk factor changes)

Figure 4.3 Hypertension record sheets: (C) follow-up record.

of the other secondary causes (Box 4.1) also require hospital referral at least for initial assessment.

Reasons for considering referral are if the patient is under 35 years of age, has uncontrolled BP despite full doses of two or three agents, abnormal and/or unexplained laboratory investigations, clinical findings suggesting possible secondary hypertension, or hypertension in the presence of other chronic conditions, e.g. diabetes.

Summary

The success or failure of the management of hypertension depends upon the following four Rs:

• *Register*—screening population to identify those at risk from high blood pressure and setting up a register.
• *Recall*—checking the total population regularly, recalling those lost to follow-up, and those previously identified as borderline.
• *Review*—regularly reviewing those diagnosed as hypertensive in a methodical manner, monitoring blood pressure control, target organ damage, compliance with treatment for non-pharmacological as well as pharmacological treatment.
• *Record*—document follow-up care, which allows for the assessment of interventions not only for an individual patient, but for the overall success within the care setting.

The hypertension literature is vast and by necessity, this chapter has covered much of it superficially. However, effort has gone into crystallizing relevant points for the practical follow-up of patients found to have high blood pressure. The reader is directed to the further reading list for more in-depth knowledge of many of the points raised. The challenge for community-based clinical care teams is to improve on the 'Rule of Halves'.

■ KEY POINTS

• Hypertension is only one of a number of cardiovascular risk factors and should not be treated in isolation, but as part of a multiple risk factor strategy.

• Blood pressure lowering has been shown to decrease cerebrovascular risk and, in the elderly, coronary heart disease mortality.

• It is the responsibility of practitioners to ensure that they have the knowledge and training to measure blood pressure accurately.

• Secondary causes can occur in 10% of patients with hypertension. Therefore protocols should include screening and referral for specialist assessment.

• The general practice team is in a key position to improve on the identification, follow-up and control of essential hypertension in the community.

• Hypertension should only be diagnosed after thorough assessment of blood pressure over time.

• All identified hypertensive patients should be assessed and followed over the long term using an established protocol developed using national and international guidelines.

• Other cardiovascular risk factors should be identified and interventions instituted where possible.

• Non-pharmacological treatments for hypertension should always be considered prior to and along with drug treatment.

- Patient education should be individualized and included whenever possible.
- Long-term follow-up should include assessment of end-organ damage on a regular basis, generally annually.
- The effectiveness of the protocols and strategies that are developed can only be assessed by regular audit.

Case Study 4.1

A 49-year-old man comes to the general practitioner for travel immunization. The practice nurse sees him and takes the opportunity to check his blood pressure. It is 154/96 and his body mass index is 28. There is no previous history of high blood pressure but his father has angina and his mother recently had a stroke aged 78 years. He has never smoked and used to play a lot of football, but now takes little exercise. He is married and works shifts as a controller in the fire service. At present, he is looking forward to his holiday in Greece in 3 months' time and is keeping well.

Questions
1. This patient needs to have his blood pressure rechecked; how soon would you offer him another appointment?
2. What could he do before his next visit to try to reduce his blood pressure?

Answers
1. I would discuss the level of blood pressure and reassure him that this is only one reading when he was coming for a painful procedure. It is not an immediate problem but one that should not be ignored, so it is important to check his blood pressure again in 4 weeks' time. If the blood pressure is still elevated at this level at the next two visits, 1 month apart, he should be given an appointment for a baseline physical examination by the general practitioner and initial investigations (routine biochemistry and cholesterol, urinalysis and an ECG).
2. He should consider his diet and exercise patterns. As he is overweight, he should reduce his calorie intake, taking foods high in fibre and vitamin C. I would also check how much salt he takes, e.g. in convenience food and snacks. I would discuss how much alcohol and coffee he takes. He has a sedentary job so exercise could be a problem and needs to be addressed. He need not worry that this might prevent him from going on holiday.

REFERENCES

Barber J H, Beevers D G, Fife R et al 1979 Blood pressure screening in general practice. British Medical Journal 278(1): 843–846

Berchtold P, Jorgens V, Kemmer F W, Berger M 1982 Obesity and hypertension: cardiovascular response to weight reduction. Hypertension 4 (Suppl. III): III-50–III-55

Bulpitt C J (ed) 1985 Handbook of hypertension volume 6: epidemiology of hypertension. Elsevier Science Publishers, Amsterdam

Collins R, Peto R, MacMahon S et al 1990 Blood pressure, stroke, and coronary heart disease. Part 2, short-term reductions in blood pressure: overview of randomised drug trials in their epidemiological context. Lancet 335: 827–838

Criqui M H, Cowan L D, Heiss G, Haskell W L, Laskarzewski P M, Chambless L E 1986 Frequency and clustering of nonlipid coronary risk factors in dyslipoproteinemia: the Lipid Research Clinics Program Prevalence Study. Circulation 73 (Suppl. I): I40–I50

Feher M, Harris-St John K, Lant A 1992 Blood pressure measurement by junior hospital doctors—a gap in medical education? Health Trends 24(2): 59–61

Isles C G, Hole D J, Hawthorne V M, Lever A F 1992 Relation between coronary risk and coronary mortality in women of the Renfrew and Paisley survey: comparison with men. Lancet 339: 702–706

Kannel W B, Neaton J D, Wentworth D et al 1986 Overall and coronary heart disease mortality rates in relation to major risk factors in 325,348 men screened for the MRFIT. American Heart Journal 112: 825–836

Kenkre J, Drury V W M, Lancashire R J 1985 Nurse management of hypertension clinics in general practice assisted by computer. Family Practice 2: 17–22

Loscalzo J 1995 Nitric oxide and vascular disease. New England Journal of Medicine 333: 251–253

Luscher T F 1990 Functional abnormalities of the vascular endothelium in hypertension and atherosclerosis. Scandinavian Journal of Clinical Laboratory Investigations 50 (Suppl. 199): 28–32

McKay D W, Campbell N R C, Parab L S, Chockalingam A, Fodor J G 1990 Clinical assessment of blood pressure. Journal of Human Hypertension 4: 639–645

MacMahon S W, Norton R N 1986 Alcohol and hypertension: implications for prevention and treatment. Annals of Internal Medicine 105: 124–126

MacMahon S W, Macdonald G J, Blacket R B 1985 Plasma lipoprotein levels in treated and untreated hypertensive men and women: the National Heart Foundation of Australia Risk Factor Prevalence Study. Arteriosclerosis 5: 391–396

MacMahon S, Peto R, Cutler J et al 1990 Blood pressure, stroke, and coronary heart disease. Part 1, prolonged differences in blood pressure: prospective observational studies corrected for the regression dilution bias. Lancet 335: 765–774

Medical Research Council Working Party 1992 Medical Research Council trial of treatment of hypertension in older adults: principal results. British Medical Journal 304: 405–412

O'Brien E, O'Malley K (eds) 1991 Handbook of hypertension. Volume 14: blood pressure measurement. Elsevier, Amsterdam

O'Brien E, Mee F, Tan K S, Atkins N, O'Malley K 1991 Training and assessment of observers for blood pressure measurement in hypertension research. Journal of Human Hypertension 5: 7–10

O'Brien E et al 1993 The British Hypertension Society protocol for the evaluation of blood pressure measuring devices. Journal of Hypertension 11 (Suppl. 2): s43–s62

Petrie J, Jamieson M, O'Brien E T, Little W A, Padfield P, de Swiet M 1990 Videotape: Blood pressure measurement. British Medical Journal Publications, London

Pickering G 1968 High blood pressure, 2nd edn. J & A Churchill, London

Sever P, Beevers G, Bulpitt C et al 1993 Management guidelines in essential hypertension: report of the second working party of the British Hypertension Society. British Medical Journal 306: 983–987

Silverberg D S, Baltuch L, Hermoni Y, Eyal P 1982 Control of hypertension in family practice by the doctor–nurse team. Journal of the Royal College of General Practitioners 32: 184–186

Smith W C S, Lee A J, Crombie et al 1991 Control of BP in Scotland: the rule of halves. British Medical Journal 302: 1057–1060

Stein P P, Black H R 1993 The role of diet in the genesis and treatment of hypertension. Medical Clinics of North America 77(4): 831–847

Swales J D 1994 Overview of essential hypertension. In: Swales J D (ed) Textbook of hypertension. Blackwell Scientific Publications, Oxford

Wood C (ed) 1986 Dietary salt and hypertension: implications for public health policies. Round Table Series Number 5. Royal Society of Medicine Services, London

World Health Organization/International Society of Hypertension 1993 Guidelines for the management of hypertension. Journal of Hypertension 11: 905–918

FURTHER READING

Beevers D G, MacGregor G A 1988 Hypertension in practice. Martin Danitz, London

This textbook covers all aspects of hypertension in some depth. The text is easy to read and well referenced. There are also many excellent illustrations which help to explain some of the more complex issues. The last section is on management issues in special circumstances which includes the elderly and pregnant patients. Although written for doctors, this is essentially a practical and thorough guide which is quite suitable for other health professionals interested in increasing their knowledge of this subject.

O'Brien E T, Beevers D G, Marshall H J 1995 ABC of hypertension. BMJ Publishing Group, London

This is a relatively short but concise book aimed primarily for use by health professionals who are not specialists in the field of hypertension. There is an emphasis in the early chapters on the correct measurement of blood pressure and screening procedures. The latest edition includes the current guidelines for the management of hypertension. This book is highly recommended for nurses monitoring hypertension in general practice.

Tudor Hart J 1993 Hypertension—community control of high blood pressure, 3rd edn. Radcliffe Medical Press, Oxford

The recent edition includes many current topics such as audit and HRT. This is a more traditional style academic book than the previous two and the longest. It is to be recommended because it is written by a general practitioner and therefore tends to exhibit a better insight into the mechanisms of follow-up and recording of information than the other two.

Lifestyle management: smoking

Ginny Styles   Doreen McIntyre

5

■ CONTENTS

INTRODUCTION

Smoking is the chief avoidable cause of premature death and ill health in the world. The World Health Organization estimates that world-wide, 3 million people die from smoking every year and if current smoking patterns persist tobacco will kill 10 million smokers every year (WHO 1991). In the UK, 111 000 people die prematurely from smoking-related diseases (HEA 1993). One in four of these smoking-related deaths is from coronary heart disease (CHD) and cigarette smoking is responsible for at least 20% of all deaths from CHD (OPCS 1991).

FACTS AND FIGURES

In 1948, when the first surveys of smoking rates were undertaken by the tobacco companies, 82% of men smoked, a peak in male smoking prevalence. Since the late 1950s there has been a steady decline in this rate.

Smoking prevalence amongst women peaked much later at 45% in the late 1960s and has declined more slowly since then (Wald & Nicolaides-Bauman 1991).

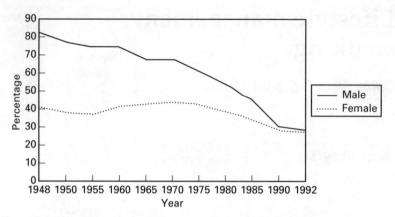

Figure 5.1 Percentages of men and women who smoke 1948–1992.

In 1972 when the OPCS started to collect smoking prevalence data, 52% of men and 41% of women aged 16 and over smoked. By 1992, this figure had dropped to 29% of men and 28% of women (OPCS 1994), but over the last 10 years the rate of decline has slowed (see Fig. 5.1).

WHAT IS SMOKING?

Tobacco was first brought to Britain from America in the 16th century by Sir Walter Raleigh. Cigarettes as we know them were introduced in the late 19th century, and by the turn of the 20th century largely replaced other forms of tobacco use such as snuff, chewing tobacco and cigars. The introduction of cigarettes is important from the point of view of health because unlike other previous forms of tobacco use, the cigarette smoke is inhaled. Cigarettes are also portable and tobacco smoking became a social and everyday phenomenon rather than ceremonial and formal.

Tobacco smoke contains some 4000 chemicals in the form of particles and gases. 60 of these substances are known or suspected carcinogens (IARC 1986). In the USA, the Environmental Protection Agency (1992) has classified tobacco smoke as a class A carcinogen along with asbestos, arsenic and radon gas.

The three main poisons in tobacco smoke are:

- *Tar*. A solid irritant, tar coats the lungs, blocks the airways and causes emphysema and lung cancer.
- *Nicotine*. Nicotine is a highly addictive toxic substance which diffuses into the bloodstream very quickly, providing a quick fix for the smoker. One cigarette contains about 1 mg of nicotine, which if taken intravenously could be fatal. Nicotine has a variety of adverse effects, many of which contribute to the development of CHD.
- *Carbon monoxide (CO)*. Carbon monoxide is absorbed via the lungs into the bloodstream where it binds to haemoglobin, replacing oxygen. The level of CO in a smoker's body depends on the number of cigarettes smoked and how they are smoked. Carbon monoxide causes heart and arterial disease.

Other poisons in tobacco smoke include formaldehyde, ammonia and benzene.

SMOKING AND HEALTH

As early as the 1920s, doctors noticed an increase in the frequency of lung cancer especially in patients who smoked heavily. But it was not until the 1950s that widespread awareness of the problem developed following studies by Doll & Hill (1950) on smoking and lung cancer.

A recent report by Doll et al (1994) updated 40 years' observation of 35 000 British doctors. It concluded that about half of all smokers will be killed by their smoking. Of those killed in middle age the average loss of life expectancy is 20–25 years.

The main diseases caused by smoking are lung cancer and CHD. 26% of smokers die from lung cancer and 25% from CHD. Other forms of cardio-vascular disease and emphysema are the other main causes of smoking-related deaths (15% each) (OPCS 1991).

Smoking has also been linked to cancers of the mouth, oesophagus, larynx, bladder and pancreas. Stroke, chronic bronchitis, and circulatory problems may also be caused by smoking. More recently published research has found links to premature menopause, complications in pregnancy, impotence, premature ageing and reduced fertility.

Passive smoking

Passive smoking is breathing other people's tobacco smoke. Tobacco smoke consists of sidestream smoke from the burning tip of the cigarette and mainstream smoke that has been inhaled and then exhaled by the smoker. 85% of tobacco smoke in a room is sidestream smoke which contains a higher proportion of toxic gases (US Department of Health and Human Services 1986).

As well as the short-term effects of passive smoking such as eye irritation, headaches, sore throats and coughing, research has found longer-term, more serious health risks. The British Government's Independent Scientific Committee on Smoking and Health (ISCSH 1988) found an increased risk of lung cancer in non-smokers exposed to passive smoking of between 10 and 30%.

Smoking and coronary heart disease

Smoking is one of the three main modifiable 'risk factors' for CHD, and nicotine and carbon monoxide have been identified as the main culprits. The death rate for all cardiovascular disease for smokers is two to three times that of non-smokers and between 35 and 40% of these deaths occur before retirement age (Royal College of Physicians 1983).

Smoking is associated with both aspects of atherosclerosis; it promotes the development of lesions, thus creating sites susceptible to blockage, and promotes the occurrence of triggering events that lead to blockages (US Department of Health and Human Services 1989).

Evidence has more recently linked passive smoking with CHD. In the short term, passive smoking decreases the ability of the heart to receive and process oxygen. In the longer term, it promotes the build-up of plaque and the development of atherosclerotic lesions (Wells 1994). In a review of recent literature, Glantz & Parmley (1995) concluded that passive smoking reduces the ability of the blood to deliver oxygen to the myocardium and reduces the ability of the myocardium to use the oxygen it does receive effectively. The study reports that the effects of passive smoking on the cardiovascular system are a result not of a single component in tobacco smoke but of many elements including carbon monoxide and nicotine.

Benefits of quitting

Approximately 12 million adults, 26% of the population in the UK, are ex-smokers (OPCS 1992). Therefore, people do stop smoking and the US Surgeon General's review of evidence (US Department of Health and Human Services 1990) found both significant short- and longer-term benefits of doing so.

Short-term benefits of quitting

As soon as a smoker stops smoking the body starts to cleanse itself of tobacco poisons. Within 8 hours the nicotine levels will be reduced by half and within 24–48 hours the carbon monoxide level will be down to that of a non-smoker. The oxygen level gradually returns to normal and the heartbeat slows.

The lungs start to clear of tar, the cilia recover and the ex-smoker feels less wheezy and breathless. Within a few weeks the senses of smell and taste improve, teeth are whiter and breath fresher.

Longer-term benefits of quitting

The longer-term benefits to cardiovascular risk are very considerable and these benefits occur at all age groups and at all stages of cardiovascular disease.

The excess risk of CHD from smoking reduces by half within 1 year of stopping smoking. After 15 years, the risk reverts to about the same level as that of someone who has never smoked. As would be expected, the level to which the risk drops varies between individuals and depends on how long the person smoked, how heavily he or she smoked and the other risk factors present.

For an individual who already has heart disease or who has had a heart attack, giving up smoking reduces the risk of premature death or another heart attack by up to 50% or more.

The review found that for lung cancer, smokers who quit after less than 20 years can reasonably expect their risk of developing lung cancer to fall to that of a lifelong non-smoker after approximately 10 years' cessation.

WHY DO PEOPLE START SMOKING?

In order to advise patients who smoke and help them in any attempt to stop, it is important to have an understanding of smoking; why people start, why they continue and why they decide to stop. Your understanding can then help to facilitate smokers' own understanding of their smoking behaviour and ultimately help them to stop.

Until about the age of 10, children accept the fact that smoking is bad for health. But as they approach adolescence, many of these children start smoking.

This may be the result of:

• *Peer pressure.* Adolescence is a time of change, from recognition as a family member to identification with the peer group, when it is important to be popular and liked by the right people. Smoking can lead to acceptance by peers and an increased feeling of maturity.

• *A desire to rebel.* Smoking is an adult behaviour not allowed in children and it is an act of defiance to those in authority. A smoking parent is a model for the child, but an over-zealous attitude by the parent can often spark an anti-authoritarian reaction in the child.

• *Out of curiosity or suggestibility.* UK tobacco advertising uses humour and puzzles to portray cigarettes as interesting and stylish. Children particularly enjoy this type of advertising.

However, no two smokers are the same. Individuals start smoking for different reasons and most smokers are not able to pinpoint any single reason why they started smoking. It is usually a combination of the above factors.

WHY DO SMOKERS CONTINUE TO SMOKE?

Most smokers are well aware of the dangers and risks associated with smoking, e.g. lung cancer, CHD, bronchitis and emphysema, and many are aware of the more recently documented health risks of smoking, e.g. complications to pregnancy, circulatory diseases, premature menopause and ageing. But they still smoke. Often they protect themselves by denial:

• 'it won't happen to me'
• 'I can give up any time'
• 'I will stop in 5 years'.

Part of the problem can be that many serious ill effects of smoking do not manifest themselves until later. Smokers who feel healthy now, do not believe any damage has or will be done and cannot actually see the damage being done to their lungs or arteries. It is also true that not every smoker will get a fatal disease, but a 50:50 chance of dying from smoking-related disease is a high risk. Knowing the facts then is not enough—there are some very powerful facts that keep people smoking.

Drug dependence

The main reason for not giving up even when a smoker wants to is the addictive nature of nicotine.

Nicotine reaches the brain approximately 7 seconds after the first puff on a cigarette and an average of 10 inhalations is taken on each cigarette—a very high frequency of 'shots' makes smoking a very over-learned behaviour.

Most people smoke to obtain nicotine—a smoker will often subconsciously increase puffs on a low-nicotine cigarette to keep the level maintained.

The withdrawal symptoms of nicotine can be serious, e.g. cravings, irritation, sleep disturbance and anxiety. These symptoms are the main reason for relapse.

Enjoyment

Many smokers enjoy the taste and ritual handling of the cigarettes. They may reward themselves with a smoke and it is an important part of their lifestyle.

Cigarettes also have a social function and can act as ice-breakers, be used as time fillers and to deal with boredom.

However, most people smoke not for enjoyment, but because they feel miserable if they do not smoke.

Relaxation

Smokers learn to use cigarettes as a means of relieving stress and believe that cigarettes 'calm the nerves'.

In fact nicotine is a powerful stimulant and what actually happens is that withdrawal symptoms emerge when a smoker has not smoked for a while. The next cigarette alleviates these symptoms and the smoker feels better and 'relaxed'.

Concentration

Some smokers smoke to aid their concentration but this is more a result of habit and association. The smoker has a cigarette to help him or her concentrate (and to ward off withdrawal restlessness) and therefore feels more concentrated.

A smoker learns to make good use of the cigarette and regulates the nicotine as required.

Health beliefs

Smokers are very good at denial or adopting a fatalistic approach to the consequences of smoking:

• 'I could get knocked down by a car tomorrow'; 'I'm going to die anyway.'
Out of 1000 young male smokers, 1 will be murdered, 6 will be killed on the roads and 250 will be killed by tobacco (Peto 1980).
• 'My uncle is 92 and smoked 40 a day.'
40% of smokers do not collect their pension and die before retirement, compared with only 15% of non-smokers. The most recent study has found that one in two smokers die from smoking and lose on average 23 years of life (Doll et al 1994).

Weight control

Fear of gaining weight is a very powerful obstacle to quitting, particularly amongst young women who are under constant social pressure to be thin.

Nicotine delays the stomach emptying and speeds up the action of the colon. The smoker feels replete for longer. Smoking at the end of a meal also defines the end of that meal. On giving up, the stomach changes and empties faster, causing many quitters to eat more.

Mood control

Smokers feel that cigarettes control their temper and moods. Smoking calms them down and prevents them from being irritable and bad tempered. Conversely, they can feel cheered up and revived when they have a cigarette.

Fear of failure

The fear of failure is probably the single biggest obstacle to stopping smoking. But research shows that the more often people try to stop the more likely they are to succeed eventually (Barnes et al 1985). By planning the attempt to quit, the smoker is more likely to succeed.

Components of smoking behaviour

Smoking is not a simple process but a complex behaviour which may be summarized as a blend of three components:

1. physical/chemical addiction
2. learned behaviour becoming an automatic habit
3. psychological/emotional dependence.

Physical/chemical addiction

When the nicotine falls below an established level the smoker feels the desire to smoke. The need to smoke to maintain the level of nicotine in the blood is an addiction.

The plasma nicotine level falls rapidly so a cigarette is usually needed every hour to maintain the smoker's preferred level—most smokers smoke 15–20/day.

Learned behaviour becomes an automatic habit

Smoking is a behaviour acquired with social reinforcement, usually peer pressure as a teenager.

Inhaling tobacco smoke is initially repugnant, but each puff gradually increases the physical tolerance and smoking becomes easier. The nicotine addiction is gradually built up until the actual act of smoking produces enough reinforcement without social pressure. Smoking then becomes associated with different everyday activities, e.g. smoking and drinking coffee, smoking and driving, and smoking after a meal.

These links are established over many years in some cases and can be difficult to break; they usually become so automatic as to be subconscious. Most smokers would not be able to identify every cigarette smoked during the day, only the significant ones, e.g. first thing in the morning, one after lunch, etc.

Psychological/emotional dependence

Smokers use cigarettes to cope with stress, and to combat negative feelings of anxiety, frustration and anger.

Smokers may experience exaggerated emotions when trying to quit because they have previously used cigarettes to subdue these feelings. Some smokers feel on quitting that they have lost something—a friend, or a prop.

WHY DO SMOKERS STOP SMOKING?

Just as people start to smoke and continue to smoke for different reasons, the decision to stop is a very personal one and may be the result of a number of different factors. Most of the quitters you will have contact with in your work will fall into the first two categories below.

Awareness of health risks

Although the majority of smokers are aware of the health risks of smoking, such as lung cancer and heart disease, a smoker may acquire new information or become aware of a risk to his or her own health, e.g. a pregnant women reads about the complications caused in pregnancy by smoking, or a smoker with a persistent cough realizes that smoking makes it worse.

Doctor's advice

Advice from a GP or practice nurse can be a powerful motivator for a smoker to quit smoking. For instance, a patient with CHD disease may be told about the link between smoking and his/her heart disease and advised to stop smoking to improve prognosis and recovery.

Financial considerations

Increases in the price of cigarettes, or greater demands on finances can mean the cost of smoking can become more apparent to a smoker. The savings made by stopping smoking can be a significant reward for a quitter to maintain motivation to stay stopped.

Family

Encouragement from the family, particularly young children, can be a powerful reason to stop smoking. Becoming a parent or a grandparent for the first time can also be a factor.

Restrictions and social pressure

Smoking is becoming more and more restricted in public places, workplaces and social settings and a smoker may feel antisocial and decide to stop.

HOW DO SMOKERS STOP AND HOW CAN YOU HELP THEM?

There are two models that can be used to understand why smokers quit and how they can be helped. These are known as the Health Belief Model and the Prochaska & Diclemente model and are discussed in greater depth in Chapter 8.

Health Belief Model

This model (Becker 1974) helps to explain what determines whether or not people follow treatment regimens or take any necessary preventive action.

This theory can be used to understand whether a smoker will try to quit and how he or she might go about doing so.

Behaviour is seen as determined by:

- the value placed on achieving a goal, in this case stopping smoking
- a belief in the likelihood that a particular action will achieve that goal, e.g. smokers may be convinced that attending a hypnotherapist or following the advice in a quitter's pack will help them stop.

Whether an individual takes action depends on the following factors:

- perceived susceptibility or vulnerability to disease/illness—'Will I suffer ill health from smoking?'
- perceived severity of the results of contracting the disease—'How ill will I be?'
- perceived benefit of taking the preventive action—'Will quitting now make any difference to my health?'
- perceived cost of taking the action—the time and money invested—'Do the benefits outweigh the costs?'
- health motivation level—the extent to which the individual is generally interested or concerned with health; this can depend on a number of factors—age, sex, social class, circumstances, etc.
- cue to action—the stimulant or trigger required for the individual to take action, e.g. pregnancy, increased price, work policy.

Smokers may fail to take action to stop smoking because of their beliefs at any of a number of points. For example, a smoker may smoke less than 20 cigarettes a day and mistakenly believe this to be a safe level, or a smoker may recognize the personal seriousness of the risk of smoking but believe that the effort of giving up outweighs the benefits of quitting.

It is therefore important to explore the smokers' beliefs about smoking and health, and discuss their motivations, before giving any information about quitting.

The Cycle of Change Model

According to this model (Prochaska & Diclemente 1983), quitting is not a single simple act but a process involving change at a number of levels until there is a final behavioural change and the smoker stops smoking (see Fig. 5.2). The move through the cycle can take weeks, months or even years and may be repeated more than once before the smoker stops for good.

Before you can give any help to the smoker, you need to know where the smoker is in the cycle to determine the appropriate approach to take. For example:

• A smoker may believe smoking is not harming him and even feel better when he has a cigarette. This is the 'contented smoker' stage and a change in attitude is needed. The smoker's positive beliefs about smoking need to be explored and challenged with discussion and relevant corrective information.

• A smoker may know the risks of smoking and can feel the ill effects on his

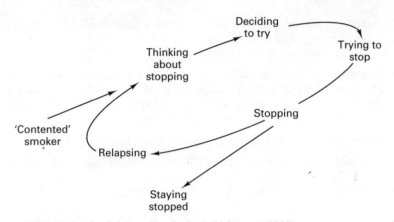

Figure 5.2 The cycle of change (Prochaska & Diclemente 1983).

health. This smoker has passed the 'contented' stage but now needs to be convinced about the personal benefits of stopping. This will encourage a move into the 'intention to stop' stage.

• A smoker has made the decision to stop. A quit day should be fixed and the smoker will then need some advice on what preparations to make, what to do on the day and what to expect afterwards.

The health professional's role—practical aspects of intervention

Among the range of professionals who offer help to smokers trying to quit, health professionals have the highest credibility—to the extent that if GPs simply instruct smokers to stop smoking during routine consultations this can result in a 5% quit rate among practice patients (Russell et al 1979). There is little formal documentation of nurses' interventions although Macleod Clark et al (1990) have shown that most cessation work, particularly more intensive counselling and sustained follow-up, is actually undertaken by nurses.

Patients expect health professionals to ask about their smoking, and can interpret professional silence as tacit condoning of smoking. Nurses and other health care staff are therefore in a unique position to help their patients stop, by virtue of their skills, their 'expert' status, patient expectations and the context in which their patient contacts take place.

Target patient groups

Most patient contact occasions provide opportunities to intervene on smoking. Consider the various patient groups you might meet, and how smoking might be an issue for some of the less obvious ones:

• young children—may be living in a smoky atmosphere, aggravating respiratory problems
• teenagers—may be experimenting with smoking or already presenting with smoking-related symptoms; by age 16, around 25% are likely to be regular smokers

- pregnant women
- parents—may be smoking around the house, aggravating children's health problems as well as their own and increasing the likelihood that their children will grow up to be smokers; there is an added household safety risk when young children have access to smokers' materials
- adults with smoking-related conditions (heart, respiratory or circulatory disease, ulcers, gum diseases, cancers)
- adults in general—around 30% are likely to be smokers, more in areas of deprivation where smoking prevalence can be well over 50%.

The care of CHD patients provides an even more potentially fruitful context for stop-smoking interventions. These patients have had dramatic personal proof of the health consequences of smoking, and the challenge to their carers is to enable them to accept and learn from the experience.

The professional's role in a stop-smoking intervention

The aim of a stop-smoking intervention with patients from any group is to encourage and enable the patients to make health-enhancing behaviour changes for themselves. This may involve work on motivation, skill-building, confidence building—it will certainly demand the best of communication skills. The role of enabler is a subtle one—it does not involve treating or teaching patients in a traditional sense, but working with them to help them identify solutions and strategies for themselves. It can be hard for professionals to take on this role, which can feel like handing over responsibility or expertise, but this is exactly what must be done for a successful intervention—it is the smokers who give up smoking, not their counsellors.

Just as there is no single reason why people start to smoke or want to stop, there is no single best way to give up or to intervene. Barth's 1994 review of the literature outlines the main range of interventions and discusses their relative effectiveness. He concludes that priority should be given to maximizing opportunistic advice-giving by health professionals, and to the development of smoking-cessation protocols for health care settings. The review also confirms that in terms of cost-effectiveness and acceptability, the most appropriate intervention strategy for health professionals to use is a combination of opportunistic and planned one-to-one advice, or 'minimal intervention'.

What is minimal intervention?

A minimal intervention involves effective and efficient use of health professionals' time to equip patients with the knowledge and motivation they need to make health-enhancing behaviour change later. Drawing on Prochaska & Diclemente's cyclic model of behaviour change (see Fig. 5.2), minimal intervention aims to move a patient towards behaviour change one stage at a time. In the context of smoking cessation, a minimal intervention will not necessarily result in instant successful quitting, but it will help the patient move towards it through understanding his or her own smoking behaviour and devising a relevant action plan. The evaluation implication for health professionals should be reassuring—the professional is not expected to produce a successful quitter in one go every time!

In a minimal intervention, responsibility for successful behaviour change remains with the patient, as does control of the process. This approach is highly acceptable to smoking patients, who need to make their own decision to quit, in their own time, to have the best chance of success. Moreover, the approach is highly cost-effective. Good quality minimal intervention with a high number of patients results in far more ex-smokers than the equivalent amount of time spent in more intense interventions with smaller groups of patients, e.g. in stop-smoking clinics.

Macleod Clark's research with coronary patients suggests that there is a best time to intervene to maximize the chance of successful quitting—ideally after their first coronary event. This may be because of the type of smoker involved: it is possible that smokers who go on smoking even after the onset of related disease are a particularly 'hard-core' group. This would be even more likely to be true of patients who are still smoking after more than one coronary event.

The same research suggests that interventions should be considered with recent ex-smokers too: coronary patients seem to be slightly more likely to relapse later than other ex-smokers who, if they stay abstinent for a year, usually stay smoke-free for good. It is therefore worth asking all coronary patients if they have ever been smokers, and reinforcing cessation among ex-smokers.

Having established that minimal interventions are recommended in most situations, it must be acknowledged that some patients will need more sustained interventions.

The main group of such patients will be the 'contented smokers': those who, for whatever reason, do not associate their smoking with health damage, or long-term relapsed quitters who have resigned themselves permanently to smoking. Using Becker's theory, explained earlier in this chapter, exploration of a patient's health beliefs will reveal whether any of these situations applies.

Another group of patients who might need a longer intervention are people with low self-efficacy—patients who do not feel that they have the skills to give up smoking, and who seek the support of other people to help them do it. Again, exploration of the patient's health beliefs about the perceived costs of giving up smoking should reveal this.

A final group who might need more sustained support are people who have absolutely no other source of personal or social support. People who come from households or social groups with a high smoking prevalence and low interest in quitting might come into this category. In these circumstances it is not uncommon for other smokers to undermine an attempt to quit, making it extremely difficult for a potential quitter to succeed. While some population sectors may be particularly prone to this problem, e.g. some deprived communities with high unemployment, the issue of family and social support should always be explored.

Motivational interview techniques for smoking cessation

The core skill of motivational interviewing is active listening—the use of open questioning, reflecting patient responses and picking up on cues. It can be helpful to plan an intervention like this in the same way as one would plan for other health promotion or educational interventions—by identifying aims, objectives, methods and desired outcomes, which will in turn help suggest appropriate evaluation methods. The aims and objectives in such an intervention plan might therefore read:

* *Aim:* to increase the patient's motivation to make a behaviour change.
* *Specific objectives:*
   —to identify the patient's position in the cycle of change
   —to establish the patient's health beliefs about quitting smoking
   —to enable the patient to progress to the 'deciding to stop' stage.
* *Desired outcome:* patient will name a quit date.

The method to use in pursuit of these objectives is one which will involve the patient in doing most of the talking and all of the decision-making. Remembering that most smokers wish that they could stop, even if they do not readily express this desire, 10–15 minutes should be enough if the subject is raised appropriately to allow the conversation to progress quickly to the nitty-gritty of quitting.

A conversation outline might be as follows:

Raise the subject: ask the patient whether he or she smokes, or has recently stopped. Depending on the patient's smoking status, either:

• Congratulate all non-smokers on their status—reinforcement of this positive behaviour encourages them and can act as an example to others, as patients tend to tell everyone when they meet approval! Record non-smoking status in notes: writing things down emphasizes their importance. You may wish to consider asking if the patient spends much time in smoky atmospheres as this can be particularly health-damaging for patients with other cardiovascular risk factors.

• Congratulate all ex-smokers on their achievement, explore any anticipated problems with staying stopped. As with non-smokers, explore the patient's exposure to passive smoking. Again, record ex-smoker status in notes.

• Ask all smokers how they feel about their smoking—this should be the opening strategy which will give you a very rapid insight into the patient's position in the cycle of change, and allow you to start an exploration of health beliefs about smoking and quitting. It is not really very useful to ask detailed questions about how long patients have been smoking, or how much they smoke: all this does is give you a few more facts, when the important one is that they smoke at all. It can also be risky to get into conversations about the number of cigarettes smoked—patients can interpret this as implying there is a safe or acceptable level of smoking.

After raising the subject: ask one or two open questions, for example:

- 'How do you feel about your smoking?'
- 'How do you see it relating to your heart condition?'
- 'What might be putting you off having a go at quitting?'

You will be able to position the patient within the cycle of change, and you should have gained a few insights into useful avenues to explore with the patient.

How the conversation proceeds depends on the patient's starting point, as follows.

'Contented smoker' patients

There should be very few of these, and it need not be assumed that contented smokers are necessarily hard-core, determined-to-continue smokers. It may just be that they don't know enough about smoking and how to stop. However, there is a possibility that remaining smokers amongst cardiac patients may well be hard-core smokers, denying the risks of smoking and refusing to accept the need to stop. You will know this from responses to your initial open questions.

For these smokers, your minimal intervention will be aimed at simply moving them into thinking about stopping: a more intensive intervention will be required to move them further if indeed they agree to proceed.

Hard-core smokers in denial will need to be encouraged to accept the scientific evidence about smoking and the benefits of quitting. Common reactions from this group will be reliance on the example of the immortal smoker, or quoting facts about every other risk factor, i.e. ignorance of relative risk. The health professional's role in these cases is:

- to correct misinformation—it can be useful to have simple, relevant fact sheets or booklets to hand for back-up, and make it absolutely clear that the evidence on smoking is conclusive
- to give clear advice that the patient should stop smoking as soon as possible, personalizing the danger of continuing and the benefit of stopping
- to warn the patient of follow-up enquiry, but leave the patient with information on where and how to get help.

The contented smoker who simply has not thought about quitting smoking before is of course easier to deal with, and many can quickly be moved on to the 'deciding to quit' stage. A few more open questions to explore health beliefs and establish that denial is not a problem, should indicate that it is more likely to be a case of ignorance of the benefits of quitting, or concern about the perceived 'costs' of quitting, e.g. fear of failure, anxiety or weight gain, or lack of social support.

Again in this case, it can be helpful to have simple relevant patient education literature to hand for reference. If patients express an interest in thinking about giving up smoking, it may be appropriate to arrange a special follow-up appointment, but if not, make a point of raising the subject again at the next routine visit. Make it clear that your unequivocal advice is to stop smoking as soon as possible, and leave the patient with information on where and how to get help.

'Thinking about stopping' patients

Most patients who smoke will already have progressed at least to this stage, which you will be able to tell from their responses to your subject-raising questions.

- 'I know I should stop . . .'
- 'It's a stupid habit . . .'
- 'I've only myself to blame . . .'
- 'The damage is done now . . .'

These patients have started to think negatively about their smoking, so it is the professional's role to reinforce that thought process, correct any misinformation and encourage them to believe that quitting would be both beneficial and possible. Use open questions to explore beliefs about quitting, for example:

- 'Can you think of any ways in which quitting smoking might do you good?'
- 'Is anything putting you off having a go at quitting?'
- 'How confident would you feel about having a go at quitting?'
- 'Have you ever had a look at any of the booklets available to help people stop smoking?'

These will help the patient to talk through concerns and identify positive beliefs or actions to build on.

Having helped the patient to establish that quitting would be personally beneficial, the professional's role is to encourage the patient to name a quit day, thereby moving on to the next stage in the cycle.

'Deciding to stop' patients

These patients will need reinforcement of their positive decision and beliefs, together with clear guidance on how to go about quitting. The procedure can be described as seven steps, which are summarized in a patient hand-out in Box 5.1.

Step 1: Name a quit day. A named day is essential, as is the intention to quit completely on that day rather than start cutting down. Cutting down is only useful as part of the preparations towards a named quit day. The patient should allow at least 1 week to prepare properly, and choose a day which will be relatively free from other major stresses. Many people like to choose a significant day like New Year, a birthday or No-Smoking Day, but this does not really matter as long as the day becomes a target quit day.

Step 2: Consider the benefits of stopping versus the costs. The patient should think through all his or her personal reasons for quitting—the expected gains—and identify any reasons why smoking should continue. Honesty about both is important as many smokers still cling to underlying positive beliefs about smoking, and unless these are dealt with openly they can sabotage a quit attempt.

Step 3: Keep a cigarette diary for a day or two. The aim of this is to enable the

---

Box 5.1 How to become a non-smoker in seven simple steps

---

1. Name a quit day, a few days or weeks away, and use the in-between days to prepare for quitting.
2. Make a list of your reasons for quitting, and any reasons you might have for continuing to smoke. Make sure that you really want to quit this time.
3. Keep a cigarette survey sheet for a day or two to analyse your smoking pattern.
4. Work out what you will do in different smoking situations:
   —what distractions or substitutes will you have around for when the cravings come?
   —do you need to practice a relaxation exercise?
   —what will you say if someone offers you a cigarette?
   —will you need to arrange to be able to talk to a friend in any desperate moments?
   Write down your plans somewhere handy, and keep looking back at your reasons to quit for motivation.
5. The night before your quit day, have your last cigarette, but make sure you don't enjoy it—smoke an old stale one, or smoke out in the rain—just make sure it isn't a happy memory. Then get rid of all your smoking equipment—ashtrays, lighters and any spare cigarettes.
6. On quit day—think positive! You've made your plans for coping, so put them into action. Make a note of any particularly difficult moments during the day, and rethink your plans if you need to.
   Drink lots of water or fruit juice (try to avoid caffeine) and have some low-calorie nibbles on hand. At the end of your first day, reward yourself, even if no-one else does! Spend your cigarette money on a treat and enjoy it—you deserve it.
7. Later days—repeat Step 6 as long as you need to. Go back to your list if your will-power flags, and keep rewarding yourself for every smoke-free day. Don't panic about the odd lapse—simply review your plans for the difficult moments and change them if necessary.
   Start calling yourself a non-smoker—YOU ARE!

---

smoker to understand his or her own smoking patterns. By recording each cigarette and the circumstances in which it is smoked, the smoker will be able to identify those cigarettes which are smoked out of addiction, and those which are prompted more by habit. Each type can then be tackled separately.

Step 4: Develop coping strategies. The patient needs to think about ways to deal with the different smoking situations identified in the diary—coping strategies like relaxation exercises for stressful moments, refusal techniques for dealing with unexpected offers, distractions or substitutes like low-calorie snacks or glasses of water to deal with nicotine cravings. The health professional should have a stock of these tips, which are listed in most self-help literature, but the important thing is for smokers to decide on the ones they feel will work for them.

Step 5: The night before the quit day. The patient should have a final cigarette and then dispose of all smoking materials. It can be helpful to make sure that the last cigarette is not a positive experience which the smoker may later remember with fondness. A hurried, stale cigarette in uncomfortable surroundings can act like aversion therapy. Most smokers then find it helpful to get rid of all ashtrays, lighters and cigarettes, but some say they prefer the reassurance of keeping a packet of cigarettes to hand in case of desperation.

Step 6: The quit day. Coping plans are put into action. Ideally the day will be a relatively stress-free one, when the smoker will have access to exercise opportunities, fresh fruit and cool drinks, and any social support needed. However, some smokers prefer to make the day as normal as possible, to get used to facing real-life situations and stresses without cigarettes. Some kind of personal treat will be important to celebrate a first day off smoking—often, smokers don't get this kind of positive feed-back from other people or themselves but it can really boost motivation.

Step 7: The maintenance step. Repeating the coping strategies identified at Step 6 until a new set of health-enhancing behaviours is learned, reviewing progress and rethinking any relapse situations. Relapses should be seen as isolated incidents rather than failures—they usually occur in unforeseen or extra-stressful situations, or in off-guard moments (particularly in social settings and when alcohol is involved).

'Staying stopped' patients

This group of patients will include recent quitters, who may need continued reassurance and reinforcement in the early weeks (most relapses occur within the first 3 months), and longer-term ex-smokers. Most quitters who abstain for a full year end up as permanent ex-smokers, but relapse sometimes happens after very long intervals. For example, women who stop smoking during pregnancy sometimes go back to smoking when their children start school.

Very late relapse is also encountered among some CHD patients, who may feel that the danger of a further attack has passed. It is therefore always worth reinforcing the continuing benefits of permanent cessation for all ex-smoker patients.

'Relapser' patients

This patient group can be treated in a similar way to patients who are 'contented smokers' or 'thinking about stopping', as appropriate, with the modification that the previous experience of quitting should be drawn on. It may be that the previous quit experience was a bad one, leaving the smoker with negative health beliefs that can be explored and modified. Or the quit process itself was satisfactory but sabotaged by a relapse incident, in which case there is considerable scope to build on positive experience.

In summary, the motivational interview approach to smoking cessation interventions involves the health professional in helping smokers to understand and control their own quit-smoking process.

The communication skills involved are open questioning, active listening and relevant information-giving.

The expression of continuing interest by a health professional can enhance motivation and boost patient quit rates.

Common questions and answers

Smokers will express concerns, doubts and objections to your advice throughout the process of change. They may just be expressing doubt to seek reassurance, or be testing you to find an excuse to reject your advice. However, there are ways to respond to this without needing to be an expert on every aspect of smoking. Here are some of the most common questions raised by smokers, with suggested approaches to answering them.

'There's no point in giving up smoking—I'm already ill, too old, . . .'

There are very few patients for whom stop-smoking advice is really inappropriate, and it is unlikely that you will come across them in normal care circumstances. Even if a patient's existing health problem is irreversible, there will be health benefits of some kind to everyone: easier breathing, less strain on the heart, fresher-tasting mouth, improved circulation, better wound healing, etc.

Care should be taken with CHD patients, though, to acknowledge and avoid aggravating other potential risk factors like excessive weight gain, additional anxiety, and increased use of other drugs like caffeine and alcohol.

All smokers will benefit financially, and even if there is nothing at all the patient would like to do with the substantial cash savings, including charitable donation, there is the comfort of not swelling the tobacco industry's profits. You might also appeal to patients' sense of responsibility—reducing other people's exposure to passive smoking, reducing the number of bad examples children see, etc.

'What's the point—everyone else in the house smokes'

The example of other smokers is a big problem for people giving up smoking. It is a fair point that exposure to passive smoking is health-damaging, although it is not as bad as active smoking. However, a successful quitter can become an example of good practice, possibly inspiring other smokers to have a go too. Ideally, other smokers in the household should be approached to consider quitting with the patient, or at least to avoid undermining the patient's attempt.

Convalescence is a good time to address the problem of passive smoking in the home, say by restricting smoking to certain rooms or times in the house.

'But it's the only thing that calms me down'

While many people use tobacco to relieve stress, nicotine is a stimulant. A discussion of alternative ways to relax, or better still to tackle the source of stress can help. Non-smokers get stressed too, and have similar but less harmful responses. The point of dealing with stress in this way is not so much that the response is a real relief, simply that in most cases the 'ritual' provides a distraction from the stressful situation. Making a cup of coffee, eating a bar of chocolate, or having a cigarette is no more than an excuse for a 5-minute break, which is what relieves the stress. Much better stress-relievers are those which involve bodily relaxation—a short walk, a breathing or muscle-control exercise, a warm bath or lie down, etc.

'I gave up smoking before and put on 2 stones'

This is a particularly common fear among women, and is also an important concern for CHD patients, who must avoid excessive weight gain. We can eliminate the myth that cigarettes are a weight-control method. The only way to gain weight when quitting is to consume more calories than the body uses. The only way to control weight is to adjust that balance. When people gain weight on quitting smoking, it is because they are replacing cigarettes with food. The patient should avoid calorie-laden snack items, or compensate by increasing levels of activity.

The average long-term weight gain is only 2–3 lb, which in most cases will have no health consequences. Small weight gains can easily be dealt with at a later date, after the smoker is safely off cigarettes. For most patients it would take a weight gain of 3 stones to cancel out the health benefit to the heart of quitting smoking.

'I've tried everything—hypnosis, groups—nothing works'

There is no magic treatment to make smokers stop. All the therapies, pharmaceutical or otherwise, are no more than aids to cessation—the real work has to be done by the smokers themselves. A smoker who attributes success or failure to a therapy does not understand the quitting process, so an explanation of the different components of smoking can help.

'What about the patches?'

Properly used, patches can increase the likelihood of successful quitting among nicotine-addicted patients who are motivated and supported to quit. However, there are several patient groups who should not use nicotine-based products, CHD patients and pregnant women being the main ones. The patches are not licensed for supply to these groups, and these patients should be advised about other ways to cope with nicotine withdrawal symptoms.

Creating the climate for cessation

The whole-practice approach

Even the best smoking cessation and prevention programmes need to be set in a supportive context if they are to succeed. Education programmes commonly fail when their recipients do not have their lessons reinforced by experience. In the smoking cessation context, quitters often relapse in the face of unrestricted smoking by their peers and workmates.

It is therefore essential to pay attention to the context in which any smoking cessation intervention is delivered. In the health care setting, this can pose less of a problem, as most facilities are already completely smoke-free. If this is not the case, a policy should be introduced as soon as possible.

Interventions have the best chance of success when they are understood, accepted and reinforced by everyone associated with the environment in which the intervention is taking place. In a hospital or primary care setting, it is important to ensure that all staff sectors are involved. This applies particularly to reception and auxiliary staff who by virtue of their less formal contact with patients often have a crucial communication role. Any smoking action plan should therefore acknowledge and clarify all staff groups' roles. Areas to consider in planning a comprehensive approach to smoking include:

- Rules about staff, patient and visitor smoking on the premises:
  —what are they?
  —how will staff, patients and visitors know what they are?
  —who will enforce the rules and how will breaches be dealt with?
- Intervention procedures:
  —how will smokers be identified on registration with the practice and subsequently?
  —what arrangements will be made for proactive opportunistic or systematic interventions?
  —will any particular patient groups be targeted (e.g. symptomatic patients, pregnant women, parents of infants)?
  —what arrangements will be made to cater for smokers who make spontaneous requests for help (and to encourage them to do so)?
  —what records will be kept to document, evaluate and review interventions?
- Promotion of non-smoking as the norm:
  —what patient education materials, e.g. leaflets and posters, will be displayed?
  —how will tobacco promotional material be avoided, e.g. consider whether waiting-room magazines etc. have tobacco advertisements in them?
  —how will staff and patient interest be maintained, e.g. participation in national and local no-smoking campaigns?

The development of a comprehensive approach to smoking in a health care setting need not be arduous, but it is a process which will demand careful communication and wide representation. It can be helpful to include an intervention procedure so that smokers are not 'missed'—sample protocols for hospital and primary care settings are given in Boxes 5.2 and 5.3.

When developing intervention procedures, it is important to be aware of different client groups and their specific needs, e.g. CHD patients will need to be approached very differently from teenage patients or pregnant women. Consider too whether you have any literacy or cultural issues to consider among different patient groups.

The secret of success in the design and implementation of comprehensive programmes is responsibility: named individuals should have responsibility for overall coordination and specific aspects of the programme, but everyone involved should understand and accept their personal role. Care should be taken over colleagues who smoke: they have a useful contribution to make both in being seen to abide by the rules on smoking and by using their experience as smokers to work sympathetically with patients.

Box 5.2 Suggested smoking cessation protocol for hospital settings

---

General environment
- Smoking should be banned completely or restricted to separately-ventilated, designated areas which are not used for any other purpose.
- Supplies of suitable stop-smoking literature and posters should be maintained on each ward.

Proactive intervention
- A named coordinator should be identified on each ward—normally the ward sister/charge nurse.
- Sufficient staff members on each ward should be adequately trained to deliver a simple stop-smoking intervention.

Suggested admission, care and discharge procedure
- Admission:
  —record each patient's smoking status on admission document
  —remind patient about hospital rules on smoking
  —liaise with coordinator to arrange separate counselling session for all suitable patients.
- Delivery of advice:
  —introduce subject by reminding patient why the hospital has a policy on smoking
  —invite patient to consider stopping smoking, or to discuss concerns about difficulty coping with restrictions on smoking while in hospital
  —talk patient through short-term coping strategies
  —remind patient about personal benefits of stopping for good
  —discuss strategies for ensuring visitors' support
  —invite patient to discuss the subject again if required
  —leave patient with self-help pack
  —record intervention in patient notes.
- Discharge—where notes show that stop-smoking advice has been given:
  —congratulate patient on time off smoking
  —remind patient where to get more help with staying stopped
  —refer to intervention on GP discharge letter
  —tell patient that the primary health care team will be asked to continue working on stopping smoking
  —ensure patient has self-help pack on departure.

A further secret of success is 'lightness of touch'. While the smoking issue is an extremely serious one, the approach taken needs to be light-hearted rather than doom-laden scare tactics. While fear-arousing messages can act as motivators to some smokers, they must be balanced with the message that quitting smoking is both beneficial and possible. Patients must be confident that you are there to support, not criticize, when they come forward for help.

Finally, measure, record and celebrate success. If realistic programme goals are set, it should be possible to document considerable achievement in tackling patient smoking. Bearing in mind that minimal interventions are not immediately concerned with long-term cessation as an outcome, success should be measured in terms of moving patients round the cycle of change:

Box 5.3 Suggested smoking cessation protocol for primary care settings

General environment
- Smoking should be banned completely or restricted to separately-ventilated, designated areas which are not used for any other purpose.
- Supplies of suitable stop-smoking literature and posters should be maintained and displayed routinely.
- Waiting room materials should be free of tobacco advertising.

Proactive intervention
- A named coordinator should be identified—normally a practice nurse.
- All practice staff should be briefed on the practice's policy on smoking, and trained to deliver interventions appropriate to their normal role.
- Patient record systems should incorporate reference to smoking status and interventions undertaken.
- Practice information leaflets should make reference to the main points of the smoking policy, including availability of cessation advice.

Suggested opportunistic intervention procedure
- Ensure that all case notes have prominent mark of patient's smoking status.
- Routinely ask all patients if smoking status has changed.
- Point out any relationships between smoking and patient's presenting condition.
- Offer self-help information on quitting, or a planned appointment to discuss smoking at a later date.

---

moving a contented smoker to thinking about stopping is a successful outcome! An attempt to quit which ends in relapse is still a successful outcome, as most smokers need a few attempts before they quit for good.

The health care professional needs to analyse the large-scale task of helping patients stop into all its component parts, from setting up a system to identify patients to removing tobacco advertisements from the waiting room. Evaluate success in terms of the extent to which you have completed your own tasks—each one is a contribution to the big picture.

■ KEY POINTS

- Smoking is the chief cause of avoidable premature death and ill health in the world. 111 000 people die each year from smoking-related disease in the UK alone.

- One in four of these deaths is from CHD, and cigarette smoking is responsible for at least 20% of all deaths from CHD.

- In 1992, 29% of men and 28% of women over 16 smoked in the UK.

- Tobacco smoke contains a cocktail of over 4000 chemicals, 60 of which are known or suspected carcinogens. Carbon monoxide and nicotine are thought to be important causes of CHD in smokers. Evidence shows that passive smoking also causes CHD.

- There are significant benefits of quitting. Immediately after quitting the body clears itself of poisons. Nicotine levels reduce by half within 8 hours, and 24–48 hours after quitting, carbon monoxide is down to the level of a non-smoker.

- Within 1 year of quitting the excess risk of CHD from smoking reduces by half. After 15 years the risk is down to about the same as in someone who has never smoked. For an individual who has heart disease or who has had a heart attack, the risk of premature death or another attack reduces by up to 50% or more.

- People usually start to smoke in adolescence as a result of peer pressure, rebellion, or out of curiosity.

- Smokers continue to smoke for a number of reasons including enjoyment, relaxation, concentration, health beliefs and mood control. The main reason for continuing to smoke is dependence on nicotine, a very powerful drug.

- The three main components of smoking are physical and chemical addiction, habit, and psychological dependence. All three need to be addressed and tackled in an attempt to quit.

- Health professionals have high credibility with smokers and can be effective in helping them to stop for good.

- Most patient contacts provide an opportunity to intervene on smoking. The most effective intervention strategy for health professionals is minimal intervention.

- Minimal intervention aims to equip patients with the knowledge and motivation they need to change behaviour, one stage at a time.

- Motivational interviewing should be used in giving smoking cessation advice, involving open questioning and active listening, and the patient doing the decision-making. Advice and information given should be relevant to what the patient says.

- The whole practice can be involved in creating the climate for cessation. Rules about staff, patient and visitor smoking should be in place. Smokers should be identified on registration, and procedures outlined for interventions. Non-smoking should be promoted as the norm throughout the practice.

PRACTICAL EXERCISE

Eliminate all tobacco advertising from the waiting room

Something that often slips through the net in a health service setting is tobacco advertising in waiting room literature and magazines. To emphasize the no-smoking norm, it is important that this is eliminated.

What you can do:

- Nominate yourself as the coordinator to audit current literature and check all new magazines etc. that come in.
- Go through all the magazines in the waiting room and tear out all tobacco advertisements.
- If the practice subscribes to magazines that routinely contain tobacco

advertising, cancel the subscription and take out a new one for a magazine that does not carry tobacco advertisements.
- Any new literature in the waiting room should be screened for advertisements. Make a note of any magazines that routinely carry tobacco advertisements and take extra care when checking these—or do not hold them in the waiting room at all.
- Explain your advertising policy in your practice leaflet.

REFERENCES

Barnes G E, Vulcano B A, Greaves L 1985 Characteristics affecting successful outcome in the cessation of smoking. International Journal of Addictions 20(9): 1429–1434

Barth A 1994 Smoking: a review of effective interventions. Anglia and Oxford Regional Health Authority, Oxford

Becker M H 1974 The health belief model and personal health behaviour. Health Education Monographs 2: 324–508

Doll R, Hill A 1950 Smoking and carcinoma of the lung. British Medical Journal 2: 739–748

Doll R, Peto R, Wheatley K, Gray R, Sutherland I 1994 Mortality in relation to smoking: 40 years' observations on male British doctors. British Medical Journal 309: 901–911

Environmental Protection Agency 1992 Respiratory health effects of passive smoking: lung cancer and other disorders. Office of Health and Environmental Assessment, Washington DC

Glantz S A, Parmley W W 1995 Passive smoking and heart disease. Journal of the American Medical Association 273(13): 1047–1058

Health Education Authority (HEA) 1993 The smoking epidemic: a prescription for change. HEA, London

International Agency for Research on Cancer (IARC) 1986 IARC monographs on the evaluation of the carcinogenic risk of chemicals to humans. Volume 38: IARC, Lyon

Independent Scientific Committee on Smoking and Health (ISCSH) 1988 Fourth report of the Independent Scientific Committee on Smoking and Health. (Chairman Sir Peter Froggatt) HMSO, London

Macleod Clark J M, Haverty S, Kendall S 1990 Helping people to stop smoking: a study of the nurse's role. Journal of Advanced Nursing 16: 357–363

Office of Population Censuses and Surveys (OPCS) 1991 Deaths by cause. HMSO, London

Office of Population Censuses and Surveys (OPCS) 1992 Cigarette smoking (in Great Britain) 1972–90. HMSO, London

Office of Population Censuses and Surveys (OPCS) 1994 General household survey. HMSO, London

Peto R 1980 Editorial. Health Education Journal 39: 45–46

Prochaska J O, Diclemente C C 1983 Stages and processes of self-change of smoking: towards the integrative model of change. Journal of Consulting and Clinical Psychology 51(3): 390–395

Royal College of Physicians 1983 Health or smoking. Pitman, London

Russell M, Wilson C, Taylor C, Baker C 1979 Effect of general practitioners' advice against smoking. British Medical Journal 2: 231–235

US Department of Health and Human Services 1986 The health consequences of involuntary smoking: a report of the Surgeon General. DHHS Publication No. (PHS) 87-8398, Washington

US Department of Health and Human Services 1989 Reducing the health consequences of smoking: 25 years of progress. A report of the Surgeon General. DHHS Publication No. (CDC) 89-8411, Washington

US Department of Health and Human Services 1990 The health benefits of smoking cessation. A report of the Surgeon General. DHHS Publication No. (CDC) 90-8416, Atlanta GA: Office on Smoking and Health

Wald N, Nicolaides-Bauman A 1991 UK smoking statistics, 2nd edn. Oxford University Press, London

Wells A J 1994 Passive smoking as a cause of heart disease. Journal of American College of Cardiology 24: 546–554

World Health Organization (WHO) 1991 Epidemiology: tobacco attributable mortality, global estimates and projections. Tobacco Alert, WHO, Geneva

FURTHER READING

Barth A 1994 Smoking: a review of effective interventions. Anglia and Oxford Regional Health Authority, Oxford

Ford B J 1994 Smokescreen: a guide to the personal risks and global effects of the cigarette habit. Halcyon Press, Australia

A readable and up-to-date book covering the history and the personal and global costs of smoking. Substantial information on smoking-related disease plus a comprehensive chapter on smoking and cardiovascular disease.

Glynn T J, Manley M W 1992 How to help your patients stop smoking: a national cancer institute manual for physicians. National Cancer Institute, US Department of Health and Human Services

An American guide to simple and brief interventions with smokers that all members of the health team can undertake. Includes sample tear-out materials.

Royal College of Physicians 1992 Smoking and the young. Royal College of Physicians, London

Very good for facts and figures and covers the psychology of smoking in some depth.

Lifestyle management: diet

Nicola S. Gilbert   Bruce A. Griffin

6

■ CONTENTS

INTRODUCTION

Hyperlipidaemia, obesity, diabetes mellitus (DM) and hypertension are recognized as major risk factors for CHD. Dietary modification has an important role to play in the management of these risk factors. It is not uncommon for individuals to present with one or more of these conditions. Therefore dietary management must be planned on an individual basis and will vary from person to person. Many people will be referred to a state registered dietitian (SRD) for personalized dietary advice.

SRDs are nutrition specialists who possess the unique skills to translate nutritional science into practical dietary messages. Their role is to ensure that the health messages received by both individuals and the general public are consistent and based on sound scientific principles. An increasing number of SRDs now work as part of a primary health care team counselling individuals on therapeutic diets. Others are employed as nutrition facilitators where their main remit is to provide training for practice nurses and other health professionals on dietary management. However, as the 'health care team' evolves both in the primary and secondary health care setting, many health care professionals have a greater responsibility for dietary management as an integral part of patient care in the following ways:

- in the initial screening and assessment
- identifying those who need referral to an SRD
- motivating and encouraging change
- giving first-line dietary advice
- providing continued support.

Dietary management is important in modifying the following well-documented CHD risk factors:

- hyperlipidaemia
- obesity
- diabetes mellitus
- hypertension.

This chapter will focus on the guidelines and rationale associated with the management of hyperlipidaemia and obesity; the specific dietary recommendations for the management of diabetes mellitus and hypertension will be covered only briefly. However, all the key principles of dietary management that will be discussed apply in the management of all of the above risk factors.

HYPERLIPIDAEMIA

Therapeutic definition of dyslipidaemia

A therapeutic definition of dyslipidaemia in the context of dietary guidelines for CHD prevention can be considered in accordance with a plan devised by the WHO Expert Committee for population and individual strategies for the primary and secondary prevention of CHD respectively. The rationale for this division lies in the variable nature (genetic and environmental) and extent of CHD risk factors present in the two categories, the recognition of which should facilitate the choice of appropriate dietary treatments. Thus, guidelines for dietary management for secondary CHD prevention may be inappropriate for the prevention of CHD in the general population.

In a clinical setting a phenotypic classification of dyslipidaemia is required in order to identify the principal targets for dietary intervention. In the most simplified form, this classification would consist of the three categories defined by the European Atherosclerosis Society Task Force (1992), namely:

- hypercholesterolaemia
- combined (mixed) hyperlipidaemia
- hypertriglyceridaemia.

This system of nomenclature defines broad categories that are useful for identifying the principal dietary target(s). However, within these categories there are a number of discrete metabolic disorders each of which may require specialized dietary treatments.

What are dietary lipids?

Triglycerides or triacylglycerols represent the edible fats in our diet. These consist of a backbone of glycerol to which are attached three fatty acids. The melting point of different dietary triglycerides and thus their 'hardness' increases with the chain length of their constituent fatty acids (number of carbon atoms) and number of double bonds (degree of saturation). Therefore, triglycerides containing saturated fatty acids (SFAs) with no double bonds are harder than those containing polyunsaturated fatty acids (PUFAs).

Cholesterol is a sterol that is essential for the synthesis of cell membranes, steroid hormones and vitamin D. Gurr (1993) provides more detailed information on the definition, metabolism and composition of dietary fats and cholesterol in foods.

Principles of a lipid (cholesterol) lowering diet: fat quantity versus quality

The first and probably most important principle of any lipid-lowering diet is a reduction in dietary fat to the recommended value of 35% of total energy intake (DoH 1994). The basic aim of this principle is to achieve a reduction in the intake of calories derived from fat by replacing energy-rich triglycerides with nutrients of a lower energy content such as complex carbohydrates. This dietary measure, in combination with increased physical activity, is an attempt to correct the chronic imbalance between high energy consumption and low energy expenditure that frequently leads to an increase in body weight and obesity. The latter is recognized as an independent risk factor for CHD (BMI > 30) and is strongly linked to conditions associated with increased CHD risk such as diabetes mellitus, hypertension and hyperlipidaemia.

The replacement of fat with complex carbohydrates should produce the desired effect of lowering total plasma cholesterol and LDL-cholesterol. However, carbohydrates in their refined form (containing high levels of sucrose) may also increase plasma triglycerides and lower HDL-cholesterol and would thus be unsuitable for treating hypertriglyceridaemic states. To avoid these unfavourable changes whilst maintaining the reduction in cholesterol, saturated fatty acids (SFAs) should be replaced in part with unsaturated fatty acids, monounsaturated fatty acids (MUFAs) and poly-unsaturated fatty acids (PUFAs). Diets that include a high intake of PUFAs can have adverse effects for reasons that will be discussed below.

It is important to realize that the amount of SFAs in our diet greatly exceeds that of dietary cholesterol, and as such, it is the former rather than the latter which exerts a major impact on plasma cholesterol (plasma cholesterol is increased by only about 0.5 mmol/l per 100 mg dietary cholesterol). While dietary PUFAs (n-6) are able to increase the rate at which cholesterol is excreted from the body and reduce the production of LDL-cholesterol, much of their influence in lowering plasma cholesterol is likely to be mediated through the 'permissive' effects of replacing SFAs.

Scientific basis for current recommendations for the consumption of dietary n-3 and n-6 PUFA

In considering the role of dietary unsaturated fatty acids (see Table 6.1) in CHD prevention it is only possible to provide a brief summary of recent developments in this expanding area of nutritional research. More detailed and definitive information on the nutritional and physiological significance of dietary unsaturated acids and recommended intakes can be found in the report of the British Nutrition Foundation's Task Force (1992).

The substitution of SFAs with n-6 PUFA (linoleic acid) from oils derived from corn, sunflower, safflower and soya is unequivocally associated with decreases in the concentration of total plasma cholesterol and LDL-cholesterol. However, current guidelines suggest that intake should be restricted to between 10 and 13% of energy intake. Levels that exceed this may lower HDL-cholesterol and increase the risk of gallstones by increasing the lithogenicity of bile. Current intake in the population of n-6 PUFA is estimated at 6% of energy intake. The recent COMA report cautioned against increased intake since the safety of levels above 6% of energy intake 'remains untested' (DoH 1994).

In contrast to the guidelines for n-6 PUFA, the government recommend doubling the intake of n-3 PUFA, which at present is estimated to be 1% of our energy intake. This figure translates into an increase of 0.1 g/day (from 0.1 g/day to 0.2 g/day) or the equivalent of eating two meals of oily fish per week. The basis for this recommendation is suggested to lie in the anti-thrombotic potential of n-3 PUFAs rather than their potent action in lowering serum triglycerides.

Diets enriched with moderate levels of n-3 PUFA significantly attenuate both the magnitude and duration of postprandial lipaemia following a fat-

Table 6.1 Dietary unsaturated fatty acids

Fatty acid	Class*	Example	Source	Principal lipid effect
Polyunsaturated (PUFA)	n-(6)	Linoleic acid	Vegetable oils	Serum/LDL-cholesterol ↓
	n-(3)	EPA, DHA	Fish oils	Serum triglycerides ↓
Monounsaturated (MUFA)	n-(9)	Oleic acid	Olive oil	LDL oxidation ↓

* n = number of carbon atoms-(position of double bond)
Key: EPA = ecosapentaenoic acid; DHA = docoshexaenoic acid

containing meal and have been shown to reduce fasting triglyceride levels by up to 60%. There is evidence to suggest that the origin of these effects may lie in the ability of n-3 PUFAs to increase the insulin-sensitivity of certain tissues. As already mentioned, much of the benefit associated with n-3 PUFAs may lie in their anti-thrombotic properties. In general, SFAs increase thrombotic tendency whereas PUFAs, especially the n-3 series, have the opposite effect.

The lipid-lowering properties of dietary n-3 PUFAs make them a potent tool for the treatment of hypertriglyceridaemia or combined hyperlipidaemia. In the latter case, a dietary supplement could be given in combination with drugs designed to lower plasma LDL-cholesterol such as the HMGCoA reductase inhibitors (Contacos et al 1993; see Ch. 10).

Oxidation hypothesis of atherosclerosis and role of dietary PUFA

An important factor that mitigates against a policy of increasing the consumption of dietary PUFAs concerns their susceptibility to oxidation within lipoproteins and cell membranes. The enrichment of diets with PUFAs results in an increase in the levels of the same fatty acids within the lipids of circulating lipoproteins. Before cholesterol can accumulate in the artery wall, the LDL-cholesterol particles must first be oxidized. Oxidized LDL can no longer bind to its native LDL receptor but instead binds to scavenger receptors on the surface of inflammatory cells, such as macrophages, in the artery wall. The general consensus of the effects of dietary PUFAs on this process is that highly polyunsaturated n-3 PUFAs increase the susceptibility of LDL to oxidation. The full impact of this effect on CHD risk is at present unknown.

Monounsaturated fatty acids (MUFAs)

Historically, MUFAs have often been considered to be neutral with respect to their influence on lipoprotein levels and as such offer a valuable alternative to complex carbohydrate and PUFAs as substitutes for SFAs. More recently, MUFAs have attracted considerable attention because of the observation of a significantly lower incidence of CHD in Mediterranean countries. In some of these countries consumption of MUFAs, in the form of olive oil (24% total energy), is nearly double that of northern European countries. The lower CHD incidence may be as a result of the protective effects of MUFAs against LDL oxidation. In addition to this property, the first press or 'virgin' olive oil contains a number of phenolic compounds derived from the skin of the olive that are thought to also have beneficial properties as antioxidants.

Dietary *trans* fatty acids and CHD risk

The prefixes *trans* and *cis* are chemical terms which describe the configuration or shape of a molecule. SFAs have straight chains and as a result pack tightly into membranes and lipoproteins. Conversely, PUFAs and MUFAs in the *cis* configuration have bends or 'kinks' in their chains which give them greater flexibility in membranes and lipoproteins. PUFAs and MUFAs in the *trans* configuration lack these kinks and tend to behave like SFAs.

The hardening of vegetable oils in the manufacture of margarines and related products (biscuits and pastries) by the widely adopted practice of partial hydrogenation results in the removal of double bonds and re-configuration of many of the *cis* fatty acids into *trans* acids. *Trans* fatty acids are also present in dairy produce as by-products of the ruminant's gut bacteria. In the light of evidence from a number of cross-sectional and prospective studies (Stender et al 1995), it has been suggested that *trans* fatty acids may have greater responsibility for the link between dietary fat and CHD than SFAs. This largely stems from the fact that high intakes of *trans* fatty acids have been associated with increases in the concentration of LDL-cholesterol, decreases in HDL-cholesterol, and an elevation in the concentration of a particle related to LDL called Lp (a), and CHD mortality. While the intake of *trans* fatty acids in the UK is estimated to be about 2% of total energy, the actual figure may be significantly greater than this and approaching that estimated for the USA (5–7% total energy). It has been recommended that levels of intake should not exceed 2% of energy consumption and strategies should be devised for reducing intake, e.g. modification of food manufacturing processes.

The effects of dietary fibre (non-starch polysaccharides) and alcohol

Non-starch polysaccharides (NSP) are the major components of the plant cell wall and include cellulose and non-celluloses (pectins in fruit and vegetables, glucans in oats and barley, and gums in food additives). Cellulose, which is insoluble, has an indirect effect in lowering plasma cholesterol when taken as a replacement for saturated fat in the diet. The non-celluloses which are, in the main, soluble compounds, produce a more pronounced lowering of plasma cholesterol through the binding of bile acids in the small intestine and interruption of the enterohepatic circulation. The soluble NSP thus act in a similar way to sequestrant resins such as cholestyramine and colestipol (see Ch. 10). However, despite the reported effects of soluble NSP, the health benefits associated with a high-fibre diet may not be due to the NSP alone, but to some other dietary constituent (DoH 1994).

Alcohol

A strong inverse relationship exists between the moderate consumption of alcohol (< 2–3 units/day (16 g ethanol) or 14 units/week for females; 21 units/week for males) and the incidence of CHD. The potential for alcohol to confer protection against CHD may be mediated through its HDL-cholesterol-raising properties and ability to reduce thrombotic tendency. In addition to these effects, red wine contains natural antioxidant compounds (polyphenols) which may further contribute to cardioprotection. Nonetheless, it is well established that levels of alcohol consumption above the recommended values are associated with increased CHD morbidity and mortality and for this reason current guidelines do not recommend alcohol as a means of reducing CHD risk.

Role of antioxidant micronutrients

As previously described, the oxidation hypothesis of atherosclerosis is based on the premise that LDL must be oxidatively modified before it can deposit its cholesterol in the artery wall. The oxygen free-radicals responsible for generating the oxidative stress that damages lipids in membranes and lipoproteins may be regarded as reactive fragments of molecules produced as by-products of metabolic reactions. To combat damage caused by free-radical attack, the body has evolved antioxidant defence mechanisms. These take the form of enzyme systems located within cells, and aqueous and lipid-soluble antioxidant micronutrients present in cell membranes and circulating lipoproteins. Examples of the principal antioxidant micronutrients (vitamins) include ascorbic acid (vitamin C), α-tocopherol (an active form of vitamin E) and β-carotenoids (derived from vitamin A).

Epidemiological studies have supported the 'oxidation' hypothesis in showing that low plasma levels of essential antioxidants are associated with increased CHD risk. The studies also suggest that antioxidants from dietary sources should, at least in theory, be able to provide protection against this increased risk if plasma levels of the principal antioxidants can be made to exceed 'threshold' values (Gey 1993). The word 'threshold' in this context means optimum levels for the prevention of free-radical-mediated damage to lipids and other biological molecules. The dietary intake required to exceed these optimum levels is above recommended daily amounts (RDA). RDA are calculated to produce plasma levels that are sufficient to prevent symptoms of vitamin deficiency (Table 6.2) but not free-radical damage.

Evidence for the preventive efficacy of optimal antioxidant levels in terms of CHD prevention, although not comprehensive, is believed by many to be sufficient to warrant modification of current dietary recommendations. The target levels indicated in Table 6.2 are regarded as being 'safe' and should be achieved by the consumption of a diet rich in vegetables, fruits, nuts and seeds, with saturated oils being replaced by less saturated oils.

Current research into the antioxidant potency of a number of other compounds such as carotenoids other than β-carotene (e.g. lycopene) and a group of substances known as the phenolic flavenoids (e.g. catechins) present in red wine and tea may reveal an important supplementary role for these compounds in conferring protection against CHD.

Table 6.2 Recommended dietary intake of antioxidant vitamins necessary to achieve optimum antioxidant status in plasma (Gey 1993)

Vitamin	Recommended daily intake	Threshold plasma level (μmol/l)
C	60–250 mg (1–4 × RDA*)	40–50
E	60–100 IU (4–6 × RDA)	28–30
A	1 mg (= RDA)	2.2–2.8
(β-carotene)	6–15 mg	0.4–0.5

* Recommended daily amount

Summary of current recommendations

- Reduce total energy intake if overweight to achieve ideal body weight.
- Reduce total fat intake to ≤ 35% total energy intake.
- Increase proportion of energy from complex carbohydrates.
- Modify the type of fat by increasing unsaturated : saturated fatty acids balance.
- *Trans* fatty acids to contribute ≤ 2% of energy intake.
- Increase intake of soluble fibres.
- Optimal intake of dietary antioxidants.

OBESITY

Overweight individuals have a twofold increase in the risk of developing CHD (HEA 1990).

Most overweight individuals can be detected visually; however, Quetelet (1869) was the first person to observe that among adults of normal build but different heights, weight was roughly proportional to height squared. The ratio of these quantities was named the body mass index (BMI) and is now the most useful way of classifying obesity in a clinical setting, requiring minimal equipment or expertise.

$$BMI = \frac{weight\ (kg)}{height\ (m)^2}$$

It is essential to note that BMI is only applicable to *adult* men and women. It is not satisfactory for children, adolescents or the elderly in whom the proportion of lean body mass (LBM) is changing.

Garrow (1981) proposed a classification of obesity based on calculation of the body mass index (Table 6.3).

Increasing BMI has a positive relationship with dyslipidaemia and blood pressure and subsequently an increased risk of CHD. As BMI increases above 25, risk of all-cause mortality increases (WHO 1990). Recent work on obesity (Garrow 1991) shows that the primary metabolic defect is reduced insulin sensitivity. Susceptibility to arterial disease shows a parallel increase with glucose intolerance, one route by which obesity predisposes to CHD. Glucose intolerance is also highly correlated with hypertension.

Android obesity, i.e. a central distribution of excess adipose tissue, is associated with metabolic changes that confer greater risk of CHD than

Table 6.3 Grades of obesity (Garrow 1981)

Grade	BMI	
0	< 20	Underweight
1	20–24.9	Normal weight
2	25–29.9	Overweight
3	30–39.9	Moderately obese
4	> 40	Severely obese

peripherally distributed fat, gynoid obesity (Larsson et al 1984, Donohue et al 1987). Males and females with a waist : hip ratio (WHR) of > 1.0 and 0.8 respectively are considered most at risk. As BMI takes no account of body fat distribution, the combined measurements of BMI and WHR are more likely to identify overweight individuals most at risk of CHD than use of BMI alone, and are simple, cheap and reliable techniques suitable for use in clinical settings.

Prevalence of obesity

In the UK the incidence of obesity and consequently the risk of CHD is increasing. Surveys show that between 1984 and 1990, obesity within the population has increased from 32 to 36% in females and 40 to 45% in males (Knight 1984, Gregory et al 1990). In a survey conducted in 1993, 16% of females and 13% of males were identified as obese (BMI > 30) (Health Survey for England 1995). These figures highlight clearly a need for cost-effective treatment of obesity and preventive strategies to avoid individuals becoming overweight.

Management of obesity

Genetic, hormonal, metabolic and social factors play an aetiological role in the development of obesity but fundamentally an imbalance between energy intake and energy expenditure is the pathophysiological disturbance which results in increased body fat deposition (Garrow 1981).

The aim of any weight loss programme is to achieve and maintain a target weight. Active treatment should be geared to those people with grades 2 and 3 classified obesity who are most at risk of serious medical and psychological problems and who should be able to achieve a healthy weight. It is also recommended that those in grade 1 are treated, particularly those with a high central fat deposition, if they are young or have additional medical complications and risk factors, to prevent their progression to grade 2 or 3 (Thomas 1994).

Any treatment of obesity will only be successful if an energy deficit is created by reducing energy intake and/or increasing energy expenditure, which leads to loss of body fat whilst meeting all other nutrient requirements. The optimal rate of weight loss is between 0.5 and 1 kg per week. This can be managed by inducing an energy deficit of between 3500 and 7000 kcal in a week, as 1 kg of adipose tissue stores approximately 7000 kcal.

Ideally, a safe weight loss programme is one that will maintain muscle and organ protein stores, i.e. lean body mass (LBM), while selectively promoting loss of body fat. This should maintain an appropriate resting metabolic rate (RMR) and deliver the essential nutrients necessary for the conversion of stored fat to energy. Fluid, electrolyte and pH balance are maintained and, through diet and behavioural modifications, long-term body composition is improved.

In practice, treatment of obesity is often difficult and there is a vast array of diet aids, slimming programmes and publications readily available to the general public. Many rely on gimmicks and fail to address the complex issues which lead to weight gain and as such may be associated with adverse effects (Lissner et al 1991).

Conventional diet therapy

Most weight loss programmes based upon dietary manipulation alone advise a daily energy deficit of between 500 and 1000 kcal as a safe and acceptable target. A more rapid rate of loss is undesirable due to accompanying breakdown of LBM. Everybody has a different requirement for energy which will vary from day to day, largely depending upon activity levels. As a guide, the average man and woman attempting to lose weight will require a diet plan providing a daily intake of about 1500 kcal and 1200 kcal respectively to achieve the recommended rate of weight loss.

Alternative diet therapies

'Very low calorie diets' (VLCDs) popular in the 1970s and 1980s involve the use of meal replacement formulas and bars to provide < 1000 kcal, and sometimes as little as 400 kcal, daily. They can be easily obtained by the general public as they are not controlled by medical prescription. They often achieve an initially fast weight loss but at the expense of LBM and accompanying fluid losses. Side effects include fatigue, nausea, dizziness, constipation, muscle cramps and depression. The first VLCDs were not nutritionally adequate and combined with loose medical supervision resulted in a number of deaths. Current VLCDs are presumed safe although concern regarding preservation of LBM still exists.

'Yo-yo dieting' or weight cycling frequently occurs when normal eating practices resume after a period of dieting. This in part may be due to a fall in the RMR through loss of LBM and also the failure to educate the individual on healthy eating practices for life. VLCDs should only ever be used under medical supervision for extreme obesity where life is threatened. They are not suitable for use by those with other medical complications or anyone who merely has a desire to be thinner. They carry the risk of both physical and psychological side effects, and therefore cannot be regarded as promoting healthy lifestyle changes (Sanders & Bazalgette 1994).

Other weight loss programmes include:

- surgical interventions, e.g. gastroplasty, gastric bypass
- procedural interventions, e.g. gastric balloon, waist cord, jaw wiring, liposuction
- pharmacotherapy, e.g. appetite suppressants, thermogenic agents, bulking agents.

These programmes have been used in isolation or in combination with diet and/or exercise, and have produced weight loss in the short term. Generally, weight is regained when treatment stops due to lack of education and motivation to achieve and maintain healthy lifestyle habits.

Diet and exercise prescription

Diet and exercise regimens are becoming increasingly popular as a dual approach to treating obesity. Many GPs are now able to refer suitable clients to a locally registered programme for exercise prescription.

While it is easy, at least in theory, to reduce energy intake by 500 kcal by controlling food intake, it has been shown that it is more difficult to increase energy output by increasing physical activity (Passmore & Eastwood 1993). For example, 30 minutes of steady breast-stroke swimming will expend little more than 250 kcal.

However, even if exercise contributes to only a little negative energy balance, it benefits by promoting physical fitness (see Ch. 7). Beneficial effects observed from closely monitored combined diet and exercise programmes include:

- loss of body fat (particularly centrally deposited fat) whilst maintaining LBM
- maintenance of desirable body weight
- prevention of 'yo-yo dieting'
- reduced hypertension
- increased insulin sensitivity
- improved self-esteem.

Therefore for the overweight individual a combined approach to weight loss and maintenance shows encouraging results that are likely to confer significant benefits in reducing the risk of CHD.

DIABETES MELLITUS

CHD is the major cause of mortality in individuals with maturity onset diabetes mellitus. Many are overweight and have concomitant dyslipid-aemia and hypertension. These are also potential long-term complications for people with insulin-dependent diabetes mellitus (IDDM).

The dietary management of diabetes aims to minimize the risk of both micro- and macrovascular complications as well as maintaining normo-glycaemia and optimal nutrition. Nutritional recommendations are outlined in Box 6.1.

HYPERTENSION

The benefits of treating moderately severe hypertension are generally agreed (Editorial 1984). Lifestyle changes are important first-line interventions and should continue, in combination with pharmacological therapies when required, to achieve optimal blood pressure levels. Weight reduction and sodium restriction are the cornerstone of non-pharmacological therapy but the dietary intakes of calcium and potassium have also been implicated. This subject is covered in greater detail in Chapter 4.

Dietary recommendations

1. All overweight hypertensive individuals should comply with a sensible reducing diet to attain a healthy body weight.
2. Minimize the use of salt in cooking and at the table and the consumption of highly salted foods to restrict salt intake.

> **Box 6.1** Summary of nutritional recommendations for the 1990s for people with diabetes mellitus (Nutrition Sub-committee, British Diabetic Association 1991)
>
> - Energy: at a level which attains a BMI in the region of 22
> - Carbohydrate: 50–55% of total energy intake; added sucrose or fructose < 25 g/day
> - Dietary fibre: > 30 g/day
> - Total fat: 30–35% of total energy intake
>   —SFAs < 10%
>   —MUFAs 10–15%
>   —PUFAs < 10%
> - Protein: 10–15% total energy
> - Salt: < 6 g/day and < 3 g/day if hypertensive
> - Avoid 'diabetic foods'

3. Eat a well-balanced diet including adequate amounts of fresh fruit and vegetables.
4. Achieve an optimal daily calcium intake (COMA 1991).

Practical suggestions to meet these dietary goals will be discussed in detail later in this chapter.

Primary prevention/population approach

Surveys of the UK population suggest that few people comply with lifestyle recommendations to decrease the risk of CHD. Only 12% of males and 11% of females are free from the four major risk factors associated with CHD; namely, smoking, lack of physical activity, hypertension and hypercholesterolaemia (Allied Dunbar 1992, Breeze 1994).

Obesity, physical inactivity and poor nutrition are risk factors in their own right and also through their adverse effects on blood pressure, plasma lipid levels and plasma antioxidant levels.

SERUM TRIGLYCERIDES: AN EMERGING CHD RISK FACTOR IN THE GENERAL POPULATION

A raised level of serum cholesterol is now thought to provide an inadequate scientific explanation for the relationship between diet, lipids and CHD in free-living populations, within which serum cholesterol levels are actually a poor discriminator of CHD risk. While measures of serum cholesterol continue to be of value in the management of patients with clinically defined hyperlipidaemias and CHD, their value in a population approach to the prevention of CHD is limited. It is becoming increasingly apparent that a major proportion of the variability in increased CHD risk in healthy asymptomatic populations can be ascribed to an inappropriately high energy intake in the form of fat, which causes body tissues such as adipose tissue and skeletal muscle to become resistant to the normal action of hormones such as insulin (see polymetabolic syndrome below). This defect manifests itself not through raised levels of serum cholesterol but as a collection of metabolically related abnormalities in lipoproteins that are the product of insulin resistance. These include:

- moderately raised fasting triglycerides (> 1.7 mmol/l)
- low HDL-cholesterol (< 1.0 mmol/l)
- predominance of small, dense LDL particles
- intolerance to dietary fat after a fat-containing meal (enhanced postprandial lipaemia)
- increased triglyceride-rich lipoproteins (chylomicron/VLDL remnants).

This collection of abnormalities is known as the atherogenic lipoprotein phenotype (ALP) and forms part of a common condition known as the poly-metabolic syndrome or Syndrome X or Reaven's syndrome. It is likely to be very common in northern Europe with a population frequency of about 25% in adult males and postmenopausal women and is associated with a three- to fourfold increase in the relative risk of CHD in otherwise normal people.

The relevance of this relatively new high-risk syndrome in a chapter devoted to dietary lifestyle management is that the ALP is particularly responsive to dietary modification, despite being largely determined by genetic factors.

The basic principals of the lipid-lowering diet still apply, especially regarding the need to reduce energy intake as fat calories, although the attention given to the monitoring of plasma cholesterol level is reduced, with greater emphasis on the management of triglyceride levels.

Recent assessment of UK dietary intakes show that both men and women derive about 40% of their energy from fat, with saturated fatty acids contributing 17% (Gregory et al 1990). Trends since 1980 indicate that dietary fat intakes are not declining and the quality of fat is not changing despite persistent advice following the NACNE (1983) and COMA (DoH 1984) reports which increased awareness in the mid-1980s.

'THE HEALTH OF THE NATION'

The need for a population strategy to reduce the risk of CHD has been addressed by the Government in the 'Health of the Nation' white paper released in 1992.

Part of the strategy to minimize the risk of CHD is to prevent and reduce obesity and improve diet and nutrition amongst the population. The following targets have been set to be achieved by 2005:

- to reduce the average percentage of food energy derived by the population from saturated fatty acids by at least 35% (from 17% in 1990 to no more than 11%)
- to reduce the average percentage of food energy derived by the population from total fat by at least 12% (from about 40% in 1990 to no more than 35%)
- to reduce the percentage of men and women aged 16–64 who are obese by at least 25% for men and 33% for women (from 8% for men and 12% for women in 1986–87 to no more than 6% and 8% respectively).

In addition, a further risk factor target—to reduce the mean systolic blood pressure in the adult population by 5 mmHg—will require a nutritional contribution from reduction in sodium intake as well as alcohol and obesity.

To meet these targets, effective health promotion strategies need to be employed. The white paper makes it clear that the necessary changes will not be brought about by regulation and direction but are to be reached by education, encouragement and persuasion, and by practical action to enable people to change their diets. Many programmes already exist both nationally and locally, e.g. Change of Heart, Look After Your Heart and the Kilkenny Health Project, in response to dietary recommendations of the NACNE (1983) and COMA (DoH 1984) reports.

Recently, a nutrition task force formed with representatives from the British Government departments, the NHS, industry and the Health Education Authority (HEA). The task force aimed to identify opportunities for health promotion, educate and offer advice to implement healthy eating campaigns and policies to enable the general public to make informed healthy eating choices more easily.

Programmes are to attempt to change lifestyle practices by bringing about a change in behaviour, not merely a change in knowledge. State registered dietitians together with nurses and other health care professionals have an important role in initiating and coordinating projects to promote healthy eating in the local community. They need to be able to translate the nutritional guidelines into consistent dietary messages which the general public understand, thereby enabling them subsequently to make healthy choices easily.

RECOMMENDED DIETARY GUIDELINES

The NACNE (1983) and COMA (DHSS 1984, DoH 1994) reports clearly outline nutritional requirements for health. In 1994, the British Government published a document, *Eight Guidelines For A Healthy Diet*, reinforcing these recommendations in a booklet suitable for use by the general public which offers simple suggestions to implement the guidelines stated below:

1. Enjoy your food.
2. Eat a variety of different foods.
3. Eat the right amount to be a healthy weight.
4. Eat plenty of foods rich in starch and fibre.
5. Don't eat too much fat.
6. Don't eat sugary foods too often.
7. Look after the vitamins and minerals in your food.
8. If you drink, keep within sensible limits.

Further guidance on practical means of making healthy diet choices has been outlined in *The Balance of Good Health*, a national food guide produced by the Health Education Authority (1994) in partnership with the Department of Health and Ministry of Agriculture, Fisheries and Food (MAFF) after extensive consumer research. It aims to give individuals consistent and practical advice about healthy eating, making it more easy to understand by using a visual display of food types and portion sizes for a healthy well-balanced diet.

It is based on the five commonly accepted food groups which are:

- bread, other cereals and potatoes
- fruit and vegetables
- milk and dairy foods
- meat, fish and alternatives
- fatty and sugary foods.

Its key message is to consume a variety of foods in the proportion shown by the different areas occupied by each of the food groups in the visual display. It is not necessary to achieve the balance shown at every meal, or even every day, although this may be the most sensible and practical approach. Balance can be achieved over a period of a week or two.

The guide encourages people to eat more portions of fruit and vegetables than most currently do (five or more portions a day is recommended), and it also suggests that they eat increased amounts of bread, other cereals and potatoes. Specific information about portion sizes is not included as people have different needs which are difficult to quantify.

It is anticipated that everyone will be able to use the national food guide to make balanced food choices whether at home planning meals or writing a shopping list, or in a supermarket or restaurant. However, *The Balance of Good Health* is also an excellent teaching tool for use by all health professionals involved in promoting healthy eating practices to groups and individuals.

FOOD LABELLING

With an expanding market for new product ranges and greater varieties of food items, especially pre-packed and convenience foods, it is becoming increasingly difficult for the consumer to identify healthy food choices. Many manufacturers guide consumers by highlighting healthier options with nutritional claims such as 'low fat' or 'lower in fat' but these can be misleading, e.g. a bag of 'low fat' crisps contains less fat than the usual variety but is still a high-fat snack, and many of these products may prove to be more expensive than nutritionally similar, cheaper options.

Nutritional information on food labels gives the purchaser an opportunity to compare the nutritional content of products, learn about food composition and make informed choices when selecting foods.

According to the Food Labelling Regulations of 1984, almost all foods sold to the 'ultimate consumer' or to a catering establishment must be labelled with the weight of the food item and a list of ingredients which must appear in descending order of weight. Nutrition labelling recommendations followed publication of the COMA report (DHSS 1984) as a way of providing product information to enable people to select foods wisely.

There has been much debate over the content and presentation of the nutritional information, resulting in some confusion with many differing formats in circulation. So that trade within the European Community is not impaired, rules on nutrition labelling were agreed by EC members in 1990, and this has brought about reasonable consistency both nationally and within Europe.

In summary, they state that whenever nutrition labelling is given, the information must consist of either Group I or Group II:

- Group I—energy values and the amounts of protein, carbohydrate and fat
- Group II—energy values and the amounts of protein, carbohydrate, sugars, fat, saturates, 'fibre' and sodium.

Additional nutrients may also be listed. Nutrition labelling is to remain voluntary unless a specific claim is made for any of the nutrients in Group II (see above) in which case there must be nutrition labelling to support the claim.

Teaching clients to read food labels is a useful way of guiding sensible food choices. An example of a food label is given in Box 6.2.

Using the information on food labels

Hint one

Read the list on the label, which gives the ingredients in descending order of weight.

If fat is in the top three or listed several times by various names then the food is probably high in fat. This will also apply to sugar.

Fat may be hidden under the following aliases: vegetable fat, vegetable oil, animal fat, shortening, lard, cream, butter, margarine.

In the product in Box 6.2 sugar is present in many forms, e.g. honey, glucose syrup, sugar cane and apricots.

Hint two

Reading the nutrition labelling gives a more accurate guide to the composition of foods. You can calculate the percentage energy from fat, carbohydrate or protein from the nutrition information.

To calculate the fat to energy ratio:

Multiply the number of grams of fat in a serving by 9, divide by the total energy in kilocalories in the same serving and multiply by 100. (Alternatively, multiply the number of grams of fat in a serving by 37, divide by the total energy in kilojoules and multiply by 100.)

Box 6.2 Information on the label of a fruity chewy cereal bar

Ingredients list
Dried apricots, Rolled oats, Oat flour, Honey, Vegetable oil, Glucose syrup, Raw sugar cane, Cornflour, Sea salt

Nutrition information (per 30-gram serving)

Energy	150 kcal/630 kJ
Protein	2 g
Carbohydrate	24 g
Fat	5 g

For example, in a serving providing 150 kcal and containing 5 g fat:

$$\text{Fat to energy ratio} = \frac{5 \times 9}{150} \times 100$$
$$= 30\%$$

Foods with < 30% fat should be chosen most frequently.

This method can also be used to assess the energy contribution from carbohydrate and protein where 1 g of either nutrient provides approximately 4 kcal (17 kJ).

IMPLEMENTING DIETARY CHANGE

Preparing your client for change

Before giving any dietary advice you will need to establish whether your client is prepared to make any lifestyle changes. An initial consultation to assess motivation is an effective use of time.

If your client is ready and eager to make changes then a routine dietary assessment, the setting of realistic goals and constructive dietary advice can follow. However, it is widely recognized that even highly motivated individuals such as those with risk factors will continue to require support and guidance to succeed.

Motivation often wanes as clients feel cheated because immediate benefits are not observed. At this stage it will be necessary to remotivate to prevent your client giving up.

For those clients identified as having risk factors and not yet prepared to make changes, giving detailed dietary advice at this stage is likely to alienate them even further. It is better to have an informal session explaining simple ways to achieve a healthier lifestyle and potential short-term benefits relevant to that individual, e.g. being able to fit into favourite clothes or go for a long walk without being out of breath. It is important to stress that a healthy lifestyle is a balanced one achieved by realistic and gradual change. Many people are discouraged from attempting change if they feel it means having to give up everything they enjoy in life.

Assessing dietary habits

Before attempting to offer any constructive dietary advice it is essential to know what your clients eat and why they choose to eat particular foods. Only then can you offer useful tips and suggestions that will help your clients to adapt their diet.

You will also need to consider the many factors which influence food choices. Recognition of the factors affecting an individual's eating habits will enable the provision of personal and motivating dietary advice. For example, if cost is a major concern, then advice on cheap healthy meals is required; but it would not be appropriate for the business man needing ideas for healthy options for eating out.

Methods of dietary assessment

The main methods include:

- 24-hour recall
- food (record) diary or questionnaire
- 7-day weighed food inventory
- diet history.

24-hour recall

Advantages:
- A quick method of obtaining information on dietary intake.
- No commitment other than memory is required from the client.

Disadvantages:
- Tends to be inaccurate as people generally have great difficulty in recalling the previous day's intake.
- The previous day may not be typical.
- There is known to be variation between week days and weekend days.

Main uses. The main use of the 24-hour recall is in clinic or home situations where an assessment of nutritional intake is needed on which to base advice.

Daily food record or questionnaire

Advantages:
- Gives a reasonable overall idea of types of food eaten and frequency of intake.
- Establishes meal pattern and possible lifestyle factors, e.g. number of meals out.
- Gives a reasonable estimate of nutritional intake and adequacy of diet.

Disadvantages:
- No idea of portion sizes.
- Difficulties in assessing accurate energy intake.
- Time-consuming for client, which may be reflected in inaccurate records.
- Method may not appeal to all social groups.

Main uses:
1. To give a general idea of diet in an area or within a population group.
2. Assessment of frequency of certain food items consumed upon which simple advice can be based.

7-day weighed food inventory

Advantages:
- Accurate nutritional assessment of foods documented.

Disadvantages:
- Time-consuming requiring a high degree of motivation from the client.
- Under-reporting of food intake.
- Alteration of usual food intake.

Main uses. In research and population surveys of nutritional intakes.

Diet history

Dietitians routinely use diet histories to gain a subjective assessment of a person's eating habits. A diet history gives a limited knowledge about a person's eating style and habits but is simple and quick to perform, especially if one simply wishes to gain an insight into the regularity of meals, snacking habits, cooking methods and favourite food choices. Knowledge of these factors will give a rough appreciation of energy and fat intake and consumption of fruit and vegetables.

Steps in taking a diet history. The length of the session will vary according to the information you wish to obtain and your client's attention span.

Stage one:
- Establish what is consumed on a 'typical' day.
- Determine meal and snack pattern, foods usually chosen, approximate quantities consumed, work and exercise routine.

Stage two:
- Establish the weekly pattern.
- Consider weekend differences, meals out, extra snacks, alcohol.

Stage three:
- Fill in any other relevant details, e.g. shopping and cooking arrangements, cooking techniques, frequency of any specific foods consumed.

Stage four:
- Clarify and cross-check. Food models and photographs are particularly useful in clarifying types of foods and quantities consumed.

Assessing diet histories. After taking a diet history you should be able to:

1. Give an overall assessment of the client's eating pattern and habits.
2. Assess what changes need to be made.
3. Prioritize the changes and agree short- and long-term goals with your client.

Giving dietary advice

For most people, changing lifelong habits is a gradual process requiring frequent sessions for further advice, new ideas and continuing support. Providing too much advice initially will often lead to confusion and distract from the individual's immediate priorities.

Use of a simple action plan (Box 6.3) clearly identifies immediate targets. Targets set should be agreed as realistic and achievable within a specified time span, and regularly reviewed.

The decision on how much information is offered and the number of sessions in which it is given will vary with each client and the priorities of the health professional. Usually it is preferable to hold frequent appointments, i.e. monthly, until the client has achieved the agreed short-term targets and is confident to be monitored less often.

Dietary advice should be practical and appropriate to the individual's medical condition, lifestyle, financial status and food preferences.

Box 6.3 Examples of agreed dietary targets

Date	Change	Achieved
2 Feb.	Eat breakfast each morning before work	
1 Mar.	Use semi-skimmed instead of full-fat milk	
7 Mar.	Eat three pieces of fruit daily	
14 Mar.	Try cooking a new 'healthy' recipe each week	
28 Mar.	Go for a brisk walk before dinner every day	

The list is endless!

Once a target has become a regular habit, it can be ticked off and a new target set. This will help to develop a healthy lifestyle without too many drastic changes at once.

Practical dietary advice

In dealing with individuals or groups, whether overweight or hyperlipid-aemic or at a slimming club, you need to be able to offer constructive advice that is practical and can easily be followed.

Although medical and social conditions and therefore requirements will vary from person to person the dietary issues relevant in reducing risk of CHD can be summarized as follows:

1. Eat a variety of foods.
2. Reduce fats and oils.
3. Increase complex carbohydrates.
4. Eat more fruit and vegetables.
5. Increase fibre intake.
6. Reduce sugar intake.
7. Reduce salt intake.
8. Drink sensible amount of alcohol.

There are a number of 'healthy eating' brochures and leaflets available from the MAFF, the HEA, large supermarket chains and your local community dietitians, which are a useful source of additional practical information.

It is important to note that not all individuals will need or be able to make these changes but most will require practical hints and tips to guide gradual change.

Practical hints for healthier eating

Eat a variety of foods. Use *The Balance of Good Health* to advise on the variety and proportion foods to eat daily.

Hints to encourage food variety:
- Try new foods and recipes.
- Make the most of foods in season.
- Explore all types of a food, e.g. different types of bread—bagels, French, granary, rye, crusty rolls.
- Have a number of small portions of different foods at a meal.

Reducing fats and oils. Fat is an essential component of the diet, a concentrated energy source that makes meals tasty, palatable, satisfying and rich in texture, and the sole source of essential fatty acids and fat-soluble vitamins in the diet.

Recent surveys in the UK show that most of the fat in the diet comes from meat and meat products, spreading fats and oils, dairy products and cakes and biscuits. Therefore, most people should be able to reduce their fat intakes by eating less of these products and making use of low-fat alternatives.

Hints to reduce fat in the diet:
- Protein and dairy foods:
  - —Choose lean cuts of meat and chicken and fresh fish or seafood
  - —Choose tinned fish not canned in oil or drain off the oil.
  - —Trim all fat and skin from meat and chicken, preferably before cooking.
  - —Choose low-fat varieties of processed meats, avoiding high-fat sausage and luncheon meat products.
  - —Whether meat, chicken or fish, serve a small portion as an accompaniment to a high-carbohydrate food.
  - —Make use of low-fat dairy products, e.g. skimmed milk, cottage cheese, yoghurt, fromage frais.
  - —Cheese is the highest-fat dairy food; even the low-fat hard cheeses are still high in fat and therefore you still need to limit the serving. Grating cheese or using a cheese slicer to cut cheese thinly helps. Avoid adding additional cheese to dishes such as spaghetti bolognese.
- Added fats and oils:
  - —Learn to use cooking methods which require little fat. Grill, bake, microwave, steam, stir fry or 'dry fry' in a non-stick pan.
  - —Enjoy fresh bread, crackers, scones with only a small scrape of spread or better still 'continental style' without any at all.
  - —Use salad dressings and sauces which are fat-free or low in fat, e.g. herb, vinegar and yoghurt dressings. Avoid butter- or cream-based sauces and sour cream; make use of low-fat yoghurt and fromage frais.
- Snack foods and takeaways:
  - —Keep away from crisps, chips and nuts. Enjoy lower-fat snacks such as pop corn, raw vegetables, crackers and toasted pitta bread which are all-low fat alternatives and easy to prepare.
  - —Most takeaways are high in fat. Choose only occasionally and select lower-fat options such as chicken or grilled burgers and follow with fresh fruit. Try to avoid deep-fried, battered or pastry items.
- Processed foods:
  - —Learn to read the labels and select those which are lower in fat. There are lower-fat alternatives for many foods, e.g. scones and bagels instead of croissants (see below).
  - —You can make your own 'healthy' recipes by reducing the amount of fats and oils and other high-fat ingredients.
  - —Enjoy a small amount of sweets, chocolate, pastries and cakes as a treat occasionally.

Modifying the type of fat in the diet:
• Eat fish more often, replacing meat with tuna, mackerel or sardines in traditional dishes such as spaghetti bolognese or shepherds pie.
• Use less meat in dishes by adding beans and pulses to stews, chilli con carne and casseroles.
• Use unsaturated spreading fats and oils in cooking and dressings, e.g. sunflower, safflower, rapeseed, olive and peanut oils.
• Cut back on biscuits and cakes.

Increasing unrefined carbohydrates. Traditionally, rich sources of carbohydrate have been classified in terms of simple (sugars) or complex (starches). Sugars contain few other nutrients except energy (calories) and have little satiety value. In contrast, complex sources are usually filling foods and good sources of a variety of vitamins and minerals as well as fibre.

The Balance of Good Health clearly reflects current dietary guidelines to consume complex carbohydrates as the major energy source.

A common mistake is to assume that carbohydrate-rich foods are high in calories (energy) and are therefore fattening foods. They only become fattening if they are eaten with additional oil or spreads, e.g. chips, garlic bread, doughnuts, etc. An excessive intake of complex carbohydrate foods is unlikely as they are bulky and promote early satiety.

Clients should be encouraged to turn typical eating habits inside out. Carbohydrate foods should become the base of all meals and snacks. Advice must be constructive to encourage people to change attitudes and become creative with rice, pasta, bread, and potatoes that have traditionally been considered as an accompaniment or afterthought in our meal planning. An added incentive to make these changes is that meals are generally cheaper.

Increasing the complex carbohydrate in the diet:
• Plan each meal around a carbohydrate food, making it the centre of attention and adding the rest of the meal around it, e.g. add filling to a sandwich, sauce to pasta, topping to jacket potato or rice. Alternatively, take half your usual protein portion and fill up with a generous serving of starchy foods and vegetables.
• Choose breakfast cereals that are low in sugar and high in fibre. These are also ideal as snacks at any time during the day. Be careful with toasted mueslis and similar cereals which are high in fat and sugar.
• Eat plenty of all types of fruit, be it fresh, canned, stewed or baked.
• Enjoy all different types of bread and rolls.
• Replace rich cakes and puddings with scones, muffins or crumpets, particularly wholemeal varieties.
• Experiment with root vegetables; add extra parsnips, carrots, swede, turnip, and try out pumpkin and squash, which are all filling and cheap foods.
• Be adventurous with cooking, try out new recipes and make cereals, grains, pulses and vegetables the focus of the meal.

Ideas for replacing high-fat carbohydrate foods with a lower-fat carbohydrate alternative are given in Table 6.4.

Table 6.4 Low-fat carbohydrate replacements for high-fat carbohydrate foods

High-fat carbohydrate food	Alternative
Lasagne	Pasta with a small amount of meat/beans and tomato sauce
Pasta with rich creamy sauce	As above
Croissant	Bagel or bread roll
Pizza with everything	Thick-crust pizza with seafood or vegetables and less cheese
French fries	Jacket potato
Doughnut	Scone, crumpet or teacake
Toasted ham/cheese sandwich	Toasted banana or baked bean sandwich— thick-sliced bread and scrape of spread
Chocolate bar	Plain muesli bar—low-fat brands

Increasing consumption of fruit and vegetables. Controversy exists over the protective role of antioxidant supplements, but evidence supports health benefits from a high daily intake of fruit and vegetables. In addition, all fruit and vegetables are low-fat, high-fibre foods, promoting satiety, and therefore ideal food choices for people attempting to lose weight. Many of the suggestions discussed earlier will promote an increased intake of fruit and vegetables.

• Aim to eat five portions or more of any fruit and vegetable each day.
• Eat all types of fruit; fresh, tinned, dried, stewed and baked.
• Eat fruit as a healthy, filling snack.
• Eat fruit as part of a main course, e.g. in stir fries or curries, or add to salads for variety and colour.
• Be adventurous with desserts; enjoy fresh whole fruits or fruit salads or baked fruits with low-fat yoghurts and fromage frais.
• Use seasonal fruits or tinned fruits for crumbles and summer pudding.
• Select fruit-based desserts for dinner parties or when eating out, instead of rich creamy cakes and desserts.
• Serve at least two vegetables in addition to potatoes at meal times.
• Serve a side-salad with all meals and especially with pizza, lasagne and other dishes which are frequently eaten without vegetables.
• Experiment with vegetarian dishes.
• Try stuffed vegetables, e.g. marrow, courgettes, peppers, tomatoes, as the main part of a meal.
• Try out stir-fries based on oriental vegetables as a quick and easy meal.
• Don't be put off by the price of fresh vegetables. Choose those in season, which tend to be cheaper, and make use of tinned and frozen vegetables, which are just as good nutritionally.
• Add vegetables to casseroles and composite dishes, e.g. shepherds pie, chilli con carne.
• Choose fruit- and vegetable-based starters as fillers to meals at home or when eating out, e.g. grapefruit, melon, corn on the cob, crudités.

Increasing dietary fibre (non-starch polysaccharides). Because the definition of dietary fibre has been misinterpreted, the COMA panel have attempted to standardize the measurement and components of fibre by adopting the term 'non-starch polysaccharides' (NSP). The term 'fibre' will frequently be used in public communications but health professionals should be encouraged to use the more accurate term of NSP.

Many of the suggestions listed above will promote an increase in both water-soluble and insoluble NSP.

Additional hints for a healthy fibre intake:
• Select whole grain breads and breakfast cereals, wholemeal pastas and brown rice.
• Cook with wholemeal flour or a mixture of white and wholemeal.
• By choosing foods naturally high in fibre you will not need to add additional bran which can impair absorption of other nutrients.
• Increase intake of soluble fibres by:
  —enjoying more fruit and vegetables and eating the skins and seeds where appropriate
  —experimenting with beans and pulses in cooking
  —including oat-based cereals and foods.

Reducing sugar intake. Sugar is the popular name for sucrose, the most commonly occurring simple sugar in the western diet and the most refined of all carbohydrate foods with all other nutrients removed during processing. Sugar and related substances appear in many forms in the diet, e.g. honey, molasses, maltodextrins, glucose, corn syrup, fructose, and all provide energy (calories) and little else.

It is now recognized that sugar is not the direct cause of disease apart from its contribution to tooth decay. It is more by association that sugar is related to health problems. Sugar is a compact and delicious form of calories, especially in the form of sugar-coated fats such as chocolate, cake and ice-cream. This combination of high calories and fat, lacking fibre, vitamins and minerals, is where the potential for overuse and subsequent health disadvantages lie.

Ways to consume less sugar:
• Gradually reduce the amount of sugar added to drinks and breakfast cereals.
• Select 'unsweetened' and 'no added sugar' brands.
• Use less sugar in traditional recipes or replace it with an artificial sweetener.
• Make use of low-kilocalorie artificial sweeteners but where possible get used to a less-sweet taste. Be careful as not all sweeteners are low in calories.
• Choose processed foods with less sugar by learning to read labels and recognizing sugar by its other names.

Reducing salt intake. Salt in the diet is provided as sodium chloride but only the sodium component is a health concern due to its regulatory effect on blood pressure and volume, and fluid balance.

Sodium is found naturally in many foods but recent dietary habits have distorted sodium intake through the addition of large amounts of salt to meals and snack foods. Other sources of dietary sodium include monosodium glutamate (MSG), sodium bicarbonate and effervescent vitamin C tablets.

Hints to use salt wisely:
• In general there is no need to add salt either at the table or in cooking.
• Use salty sauces and flavourings sparingly, e.g. soy sauce, stock cubes, yeast extracts.
• Experiment with herbs, spices, lemon juice, garlic and other salt-free flavourings.
• Reduce your intake of salty snack foods, processed foods and takeaways, which are often high in fat and calories too.
• Learn to read labels to check the salt content of processed foods; look for new varieties with reduced salt or low-sodium content.
• Make this campaign a gradual process as your taste adapts to a lower salt intake.

Drinking alcohol sensibly. Drinking alcohol in moderation and within the recommended limits is not considered detrimental to health. As discussed earlier, any suggested benefits from regular alcohol consumption are controversial and therefore most people should be encouraged to keep to sensible limits and drink no more than 1–2 units daily with 2–3 alcohol-free days every week.

All alcoholic beverages are high in calories and drinking often promotes a carefree attitude towards eating a sensible diet. People who are trying to lose weight or attempting to alter dietary habits should minimize their alcohol intake. For many this may be difficult, as alcohol is a major source of relaxation and social focus, and much encouragement is needed to succeed.

It is worth noting that any attempt to restrict dietary energy intake can be reversed very quickly with a few drinks in the pub.

Tips for sensible drinking:
• If you choose to drink alcohol, enjoy one or two on an occasion and avoid binges.
• Organize social events which do not involve drinking, e.g. tenpin bowling, cinema, ice-skating.
• Use tricks to make the alcohol go further. Drink low-alcohol beers, mix your wine with water to make a spritzer, make shandies with a low-calorie lemonade and use a large low-calorie mixer to dilute a measure of spirit. Try out many of the new non-alcoholic beverages and alternate with an alcoholic one.
• Only drink in company.
• Offer to drive to the pub as an excuse not to drink at all.
• If you need to restrict your energy intake, treat alcohol as a luxury. There are far more nutritious and tasty ways to consume calories.

The cost of eating healthily

Poverty and diet
There is much evidence to show that a healthy diet costs more than a less-

healthy diet. Some healthier options are cheaper, e.g. skimmed milk and low-fat spreads tend to be less expensive than their full-fat counterparts, but wholemeal bread is more expensive than white bread.

The effects of poverty on diet are more far-reaching than simply adapting the amount and choice of foods bought. Cooking and storage facilities are both limited, whilst access to supermarkets to buy cheaper foods may mean expensive bus or taxi fares.

High earners spend considerably less of their available income on food and are able to travel to supermarkets, buy in bulk and enjoy a greater choice of foodstuffs obtainable at a lower cost. Lower-income shoppers on the other hand may avoid supermarkets due to the temptations on offer being difficult to resist, resulting in overspending on essential items and not just luxuries.

For many, health considerations may not be a priority; the provision of cheap, filling food being of far greater importance. Emotional and social issues manifesting as low self-esteem, depression and feelings of despair may in turn lead to smoking or drinking or eating 'junk' foods. It is rather simplistic to expect these clients to substitute their sweets, chocolates or biscuits for 'healthier' options. A 'client-centred' approach is needed, where clients are able to discuss their needs and wants and practical individual advice is offered.

Practical shopping tips
- Make a shopping list of essential items and avoid buying extras.
- Look for the supermarket's own-label lines which are usually cheaper than leading brand names.
- Stock up on special offers.
- Cheaper fruit and vegetables are available at local markets rather than supermarkets.
- Fruits and vegetables in season will be cheaper than less-available varieties.
- Buy in bulk and store foods if possible.
- Do not attempt to replace usual food choices with more expensive 'low-fat', 'low-sugar' and 'reduced-salt' alternatives but focus purchases on cheaper filling items such as pasta, potatoes, rice, bread, beans and pulses.

Reduce costs in other ways by cutting down on transport costs and fuel bills, for example:

- Cook meals which require using only one or two hobs, such as spaghetti bolognese or stew and rice.
- Boil only the amount of water you need in a kettle.
- Boil vegetables in only a small amount of water.
- A toaster uses less electricity than a grill so is a better choice for toasting bread, crumpets, etc.
- Use the oven to the full, e.g. serve jacket potatoes with any oven-cooked dish, and braise vegetable in water in the oven.
- Share a car or taxi with friends to reduce transport costs.

With care, planning and a willingness to try new recipes, healthy eating need not be more expensive. By following *The Balance of Good Health*, expensive items such as meat, cheese and dairy products will be eaten in smaller quantities and replaced with cheaper staple items such as cereals, bread and potatoes and legumes.

Convenience foods

Convenience foods can contribute to a healthy diet and, whilst there are many high-fat and salty varieties sold, they do not have to be unhealthy. There are many nutritious, economical convenience foods available.

Tins and packets. The supermarket's own label is usually the cheapest. Healthy options include:

- all varieties of tinned beans and pulses
- tinned soups
- tinned vegetables, particularly tomatoes and sweet corn
- tinned fruit, preferably in juice rather than syrup
- instant mashed potato—rich in vitamin C
- tinned fish, e.g. mackerel, pilchards, sardines, preferably canned in brine or sauce
- dried milk powder or UHT low-fat liquid milk
- wholemeal or rye crackers.

Frozen foods. Examples of healthy options are:

- all types of frozen vegetables
- fish fingers and frozen fish portions, with or without sauce
- packs of chicken and other lean-meat portions and minced meat
- pizza, which can be served with additional salad or vegetables
- special, prepared dishes, e.g. sweet and sour chicken, shepherds' pie, which can be served with additional vegetables.

■ **KEY POINTS**

- Diet plays an important role in a variety of disease processes.
- Plasma lipid levels may be influenced by dietary changes and current recommendations by national bodies suggest specific dietary strategies to lower plasma lipid levels and in turn reduce CHD risk.
- The composition of dietary fats as well as their quantity must be taken into account in assessing any diet.
- Modern dietary guidelines emphasize the importance of increased fruit and vegetable intake. This provides increased dietary fibre as well as potentially important antioxidant vitamins.
- Obesity is the result of an imbalance between energy intake and expenditure.
- BMI is a useful tool in assessing levels of obesity in adults.
- A variety of weight loss programmes exist and all approved programmes should be gradual and, where appropriate, should be performed under supervision.

• Food labelling provides useful nutritional information but requires guidance in interpretation.

• Dietary advice should be tailored to the individual and should be based on detailed dietary assessment, which may be performed in different ways.

Case Study 6.1

Mrs X is 48 years old, 175 cm tall and weighs 85 kg. She is married and lives with her husband, two teenage sons and a daughter. She does not smoke, rarely drinks, takes little exercise and works in an office 3 days a week. She has a family history of CHD and a recent fasting lipid profile showed a normal blood cholesterol but slightly raised triglycerides of 3.5 mmol/l. Her GP has suggested she attempt to lose weight.

You take the following diet history at her first appointment.

Diet history
Breakfast
Muesli or porridge with full-fat milk, 1 slice of toast with margarine, tea without sugar

Mid-morning
Doughnut on 5 days/week; coffee with full-fat milk daily

Lunch
Sandwich with 2 slices of bread, margarine, cheese or peanut butter
Yoghurt or chocolate biscuit

Afternoon
Tea with full-fat milk and digestive biscuits every weekday

Evening meal
Meat or fish, roasted or grilled on 6 days/week
Mashed potatoes with milk and margarine on 4 days/week, roast on 1 day/week and chips on 1 day/week
1 small portion of vegetables
Tinned fruit (in natural juice) and low-fat custard

Evening
Handful of peanuts or crisps on 2–3 days/week
Cheese and crackers on 4 days/week

Weekends
Similar to weekdays but eats out every other week at Chinese or Indian restaurants
Sunday: Roast dinner at lunch time with roast potatoes and Yorkshire pudding, vegetables and gravy, fruit pie or trifle with custard
Sandwiches and cake at tea time

Questions
Using the information you have been given answer the following:
1. What is her BMI?
2. What is the desired weight loss?

3. What points would you need to clarify from her diet history?
4. What initial targets would you set?
5. What advice would you give?
6. What do you consider her biggest hurdles?
7. At what stage would you consider referring Mrs X to an SRD?

Answers
1. BMI = weight (kg)/height (m^2) = 28.
2. A desirable weight loss is between 1 and 2 kg per week. Mrs X will be aiming to reach < 76 kg to achieve a BMI < 25.
3. Points to clarify from the diet history include:
   —timing of meals and snacks
   —type of muesli; is it sugar coated?
   —preferred type of bread
   —spreads used, i.e. butter or margarine or low-fat spread?
   —sugar in coffee?
   —whether additional fat is used when cooking; clarify cooking techniques
   —rough guide to portion sizes of foods, i.e. biscuits, meat, potatoes
   —were any snacks eaten that were not mentioned?
   —general likes and dislikes
   —general information to help you to give advice, i.e. cooking and food storage facilities available
   —is the family likely to be supportive?
   —whether there are any physical activities she is particularly interested in
   —where she usually does her shopping
4. Initial targets will vary according to her motivation and your knowledge of Mrs X and her family. The following are very simple and should be easy to follow:
   —aim for a regular meal pattern
   —avoid snacking but choose low-energy snacks if hungry, e.g. fruit, yoghurt
   —include daily physical activity.
5. Advice must be simple and practical and fit in with her job and family, for example:
   —shopping tips
   —suggested meal patterns
   —low-fat cooking techniques and recipe ideas
   —suitable snacks
   —ways to get more exercise.
6. The biggest hurdles will be continuous motivation, and time to plan for healthy diet and exercise whilst bringing up a teenage family with different dietary needs.
7. Mrs X should be monitored regularly. She should be referred to an SRD:
   —if there is no significant weight loss after 2–3 months, or indeed if there is weight gain
   —if an initial weight loss cannot be sustained or if motivation is poor
   —if other risk factors or complications arise.

PRACTICAL EXERCISE

When shopping for food examine the food labels on different products. Compare and contrast the nutritional values of prepackaged convenience foods with more basic food items. On the basis of this experience, consider how best to guide your patients in putting dietary guidelines into practice.

REFERENCES

Allied Dunbar, Sports Council and Health Education Authority 1992 Allied Dunbar national fitness survey. Belmont Press, England

Breeze E 1994 Health survey for England 1992. HMSO, London

British Nutrition Foundation Task Force 1992 Unsaturated fatty acids: nutritional and physiological significance. Chapman & Hall for the British Nutrition Foundation, London

Contacos C, Barter P J, Sullivan D R 1993 Effect of pravastatin and ω-3 fatty acids on plasma lipids and lipoproteins in patients with combined hyperlipidaemia. Arteriosclerosis and Thrombosis: 13: 1755–1762

Department of Health 1991 Dietary reference values for food, energy and nutrients for the United Kingdom. Report on Health and Social Subjects 41. HMSO, London

Department of Health (DoH) 1992 The health of the nation: a strategy for health in England. HMSO, London

Department of Health (DoH) 1994 Diet and risk. Report of the Committee on Medical Aspects of Food Policy (COMA). HMSO, London

Department of Health and Social Security (DHSS) 1984 Diet and cardiovascular disease. Report on Health and Social Subjects No. 28 (COMA Report). HMSO, London

Donahue R P, Abbott R D, Bloom E, Reed D M, Yano K 1987 Central obesity and coronary heart disease in men. Lancet 1: 821–824

Editorial 1984 Diet and hypertension. Lancet ii: 671–673

European Atherosclerosis Society Task Force 1992 Prevention of coronary heart disease: scientific background and new clinical guidelines. Recommendations of the European Atherosclerosis Society prepared by the International Task Force for the Prevention of Coronary Heart Disease. Nutrition, Metabolism and Cardiovascular Diseases 2: 113–156

Food Labelling Regulations 1984 SI 1305. HMSO, London

Garrow J S 1981 Treat obesity seriously: a clinical manual. Churchill Livingstone, Edinburgh

Garrow J S 1983 Indices of adiposity. Nutrition Abstracts and Reviews 53: 697–707

Garrow J S 1991 The health of the nation: the BMJ view. Latimer Trend, London

Gey K F 1993 Prospects for the prevention of free radical disease, regarding cancer and cardiovascular disease. British Medical Bulletin 49: 679–699

Gregory J, Foster K, Tyler H, Wiseman M 1990 The dietary and nutritional survey of British adults. HMSO, London

Gurr M 1993 Fats. In: Garrow J S, James W P T (eds) Davidson's human nutrition and dietetics, 9th edn. Churchill Livingstone, Edinburgh, pp 77–103

Health Education Authority (HEA) 1990 Health update 1: coronary heart disease. HEA, London

Health Education Authority (HEA) 1994 The balance of good health. HEA, London

Knight I 1984 The heights and weights of adults in Great Britain. HMSO, London

Larsson B, Svardsudd K, Weln L, Bjornturp P, Tubblin G 1984 Abdominal adipose tissue distribution, obesity and risk of cardiovascular disease and death: a 13 year follow up of participants in the study of men born in 1913. British Medical Journal 288: 1401–1404

Lissner L, Odell P M, D'Aigostino R., Stokes J, Kregar B E, Belanger A J, Brownell K D 1991 Variability of body weight and health outcomes in the Framingham population. New England Journal of Medicine 324: 1839–1844

National Advisory Committee on Nutritional Education (NACNE) 1983 Proposals for nutritional guidelines for health education in Britain. Health Education Council, London

Nutrition Sub-committee, British Diabetic Association 1991 Dietary recommendations for people with diabetes: an update for the 1990s. Journal of Human Nutrition and Dietetics 4: 393–412

Office of Population Censuses and Surveys (OPCS) 1995 The health survey for England 1993. HMSO, London

Stender S, Dyeberg J, Holme R G, Ovesen L, Sandstrom B 1995 The influence of *trans* fatty acids on health: a report from the Danish Nutrition Council. Clinical Science 88: 375–392

Thomas B 1994 Manual of dietetic practice. Blackwell Scientific Publications, London

Vesby B 1995 Nutrition, lipids and diabetes mellitus. Current Opinion in Lipidology 6: 3–7

Waddon T A, Bartlett S, Letizia K A, Foster G D, Stunkard A J, Conill A 1992 Relationship of dieting history to resting metabolic rate, body composition, eating behaviour, and subsequent weight loss. American Journal of Clinical Nutrition 56: 203–208

Westerterp K R, Meijer G, Janssen E M E, Saris W H M 1992 Long term effect of physical activity on energy balance and body composition. British Journal of Nutrition 68: 21–30

World Health Organization (WHO) 1990 Study group on diet, nutrition and prevention of non-communicable diseases. Diet, nutrition and the prevention of chronic diseases: report of a WHO study group. Technical Report Series; 797. WHO, Geneva

FURTHER READING

Ewles L, Simnet I 1992 Promoting health: a practical guide. Scutari Press, London

Health Education Authority (HEA) 1991 Diet, nutrition and 'healthy eating' in low income groups. HEA, London

Kanfer F H, Goldstein A P 1986 Helping people change. Pergamon Press, Oxford

Leeds A, Judd P, Lewis B 1990 Nutrition matters for practice nurses. John Libbey, London

Marllatt A, George W 1984 Relapse prevention: introduction and overview of the model. British Journal of Addiction 79: 261–275

Marshall J, Heugham A 1992 Eat for life diet. Vermilion, London

Sanders T, Bazalgette P 1994 You don't have to diet! Bantam Press, London

Resources
Health Education Authority:

—'Enjoy healthy eating' booklet.
—A guide to healthy eating.
—The balance of good health.

Information for educators and communicators
National Dairy Council:

—Making sense of food.
   A practical booklet on healthy eating supported by a recipe leaflet.
—Make a meal of it.
—The meal ticket.
   A video and support material on healthy eating.

Lifestyle management: exercise

Gillian E. Armstrong

7

■ CONTENTS

INTRODUCTION

Exercise is known to influence almost all of the coronary heart disease (CHD) risk factors. In this chapter, the physiological basis for the potential benefits of different types of exercise are reviewed.

Barriers and promoters to the uptake of regular exercise as an integral part of day-to-day life are discussed.

The rationale for exercise prescriptions amongst different patient groups is appraised. A summary and suggestions for further reading are provided.

PHYSIOLOGY OF EXERCISE

All human movement and muscular contraction requires energy, the immediate source of which is ATP (adenosine triphosphate). As the muscles contract, their stores of ATP are quickly depleted. In order for the muscles to continue working, additional ATP is needed.

The method by which the muscles resynthesize ATP depends upon the intensity and duration of the activity. Activities that require sudden bursts of effort, such as jumping and sprinting, need a large production of energy over a short period of time, whereas other activities such as walking call for continued energy production for an extended period of time.

Anaerobic and aerobic energy systems

Anaerobically means without the need for oxygen. An anaerobic energy system provides a very short but fast supply of ATP, sufficient for only short bursts of activity.

Aerobic means in the presence of oxygen. Such an energy system can provide ATP for prolonged periods of time. The aerobic system is the one that the body uses most often for everyday life. Aerobic exercise training improves a person's stamina and endurance.

Maximum oxygen uptake (VO₂max)

At rest, the body uses 3.5 millilitres of oxygen per kilogram of body weight per minute (3.5 ml/kg/min). During activity, the additional muscular activity results in greater oxygen consumption.

The maximal oxygen uptake (VO_2max) is a physiological measure of the greatest amount of oxygen that the body is capable of delivering to the working muscles. VO_2max therefore depends upon the efficiency of the cardiorespiratory system. The higher a person's VO_2max, then the fitter that person is.

The average VO_2max for a middle-aged sedentary adult is 35 ml/kg/min. A patient with moderately severe heart failure may only have a VO_2max of 15 ml/kg/min. On the other hand, a middle distance runner's VO_2max may be 60 ml/kg/min.

Direct measurement of oxygen uptake requires sophisticated equipment to measure expired respiratory gases while the subject is exercising at a maximal level. However, values for VO_2max can be extrapolated from the length of time a subject manages on a graded exercise test.

In the USA it is usual to document aerobic capacity in metabolic equivalents (METs) rather than in ml/kg/min. METs are multiples of the oxygen consumption at rest. 1 MET corresponds to a VO_2max of 3.5 ml/kg/min, and 6 METs corresponds to a VO_2max of 21 ml/kg/min. Conversely, MET scores can be calculated from a known VO_2max by dividing by 3.5. For example, a VO_2max of 35 ml/kg/min equates with a maximum MET value of 10.

Anaerobic threshold

During exercise testing, as the workload increases, there comes a point, where the resynthesis of ATP cannot be met by aerobic mechanisms alone. At this stage, there is a significant increase in anaerobic metabolism, heralded by a disproportionate rise in blood lactate levels and in ventilation. This point is known as the anaerobic threshold. As lactic acid accumulates within the muscles, the ensuing fatigue means that the exercise cannot continue for more than a few minutes.

Thus, while the VO_2max gives a measure of a person's peak functional capacity, it is the anaerobic threshold which provides a better indication of submaximal exercise capacity. Hayward et al (1995) conclude that the anaerobic threshold gives greater information about the level of activity a patient will comfortably manage during daily life.

In health, the anaerobic threshold usually occurs at around 70% of the VO_2max. However, in cases where O_2 delivery is compromised (e.g. in heart failure) it occurs at a much lower percentage of the VO_2max. If, for example, we look at two individuals with the same VO_2max, it is the one whose anaerobic threshold occurs at a lower percentage of his or her VO_2max who has the greater limitations during day-to-day life.

Exercise training results not only in improvement in a person's VO_2max, but greater stamina as measured by an improved ratio of anaerobic threshold/predicted VO_2max.

Cardiovascular and respiratory responses to acute exercise

Cardiovascular responses

Aerobic metabolism can only take place for as long as there is sufficient oxygen available to the muscles to fully meet their oxygen demands during exercise. The cardiovascular responses to exercise are:

- an increase in cardiac output
- a redistribution of blood flow to the active muscles.

Increase in cardiac output from rest. The amount of blood ejected from the left ventricle each minute is called the *cardiac output*. This is the product of *heart rate* and *stroke volume*.

During exercise, cardiac output rises as a result of increases in heart rate and stroke volume. Figure 7.1 shows how this is achieved.

From the figure it can be seen that only the heart rate increases in direct proportion to oxygen consumption. This is because as the exercise becomes harder and the heart rate is higher, then the length of diastole shortens. This reduces ventricular filling time and therefore stroke volume reaches a plateau.

Fitter people have a lower resting pulse. Not only that but they are then able to perform their day-to-day activities at a lower percentage of their maximum heart rate (see Fig. 7.2). The fitter myocardium results in a larger stroke volume with every beat. This means that the same cardiac output is achieved with a lower heart rate.

The heart muscle receives its blood supply during diastole. As the heart rate increases, the period of diastole shortens and the time for coronary perfusion is therefore reduced. For cardiac patients, exercise training could make the difference between disabling angina and no angina during activities of daily life.

Selective distribution of blood flow to the active muscles. The regulation of blood flow is achieved by both local metabolic and centrally mediated autonomic changes.

At rest, only 15–20% of the total cardiac output is distributed to the muscles, with the majority going to the brain and abdominal viscera. During exercise, blood is shunted away from the gut, liver and kidneys, so that as much as 85% of the total cardiac output is directed to the exercising

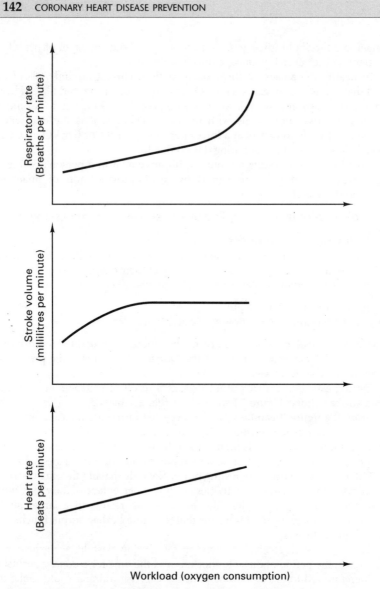

Figure 7.1 The effects of increasing levels of exercise on respiratory rate, stroke volume and heart rate.

muscles. Oxygen is then only delivered to those areas where it is principally needed.

Respiratory responses

As well as the cardiovascular changes, in order to match increased oxygen consumption, both the rate and depth of breathing increase. During light to moderate exercise, there is a linear relationship between ventilation and

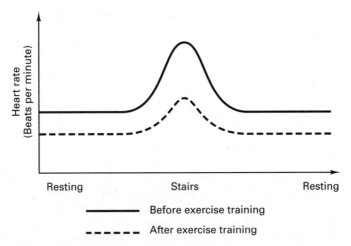

Figure 7.2 The effects of exercise training on heart rate.

workload. During vigorous exercise there will come a point when the cardiovascular system is working to capacity. Metabolism then switches to anaerobic pathways. With the onset of anaerobic metabolism, blood levels of lactic acid rise stimulating a disproportionate rise in ventilation. See Figure 7.1.

The effect of different types of muscular activity on the cardiovascular response

Muscles work in either of two ways. The type of muscle work used depends upon the specific task being performed.

Isotonic exercise

Isotonic exercise involves the rhythmical movement of the arms, trunk and legs against a low resistance. This type of muscular activity greatly increases the demand for oxygen in the blood and is often referred to as 'aerobic exercise'. Examples include brisk walking, jogging, cycling, swimming and keep fit classes.

During isotonic exercise, the blood vessels within the exercising muscles vasodilate as a result of the action of local metabolites on the vascular smooth muscle, whereas vasoconstriction occurs in the inactive muscles. The combined effect is to cause a greater amount of blood to flow through the active muscles where it is needed most.

When the exercise involves a sufficiently large muscle mass, the net effect is a lowering of peripheral vascular resistance and reduction in afterload. Since:

arterial blood pressure = cardiac output × peripheral vascular resistance

systolic blood pressure then rises only moderately, despite large increase in the cardiac output.

If, on the other hand, the exercise involves smaller muscle groups (e.g. during arm exercises), then there is relatively more vasoconstriction (within the inactive leg muscles) and therefore peripheral vascular resistance and systolic blood pressure are relatively greater. Blood pressure is therefore higher during isotonic upper body exercise than during isotonic leg exercise.

One final difference between isotonic arm and leg exercise is in the contribution made by the heart's stroke volume during the activity. Isotonic exercise of the upper body involves a smaller muscle mass, resulting in a lower rate of venous return and therefore a smaller stroke volume. This means that at the same percentage of VO_2max, the heart rate is higher during isotonic arm exercise than during isotonic leg exercise.

Since myocardial O_2 consumption is greater when the heart is working against a pressure load rather than a volume load, the combination of a higher blood pressure (BP) and heart rate (HR) during arm exercise, led to fears about myocardial ischaemia and ventricular arrhythmias if the arms were raised above the head for long periods of time. According to Balady (1993) these fears are unfounded because the increased diastolic blood pressure during arm exercise augments diastolic coronary perfusion.

Isometric exercise

Isometric muscle work means that the muscles are contracting without any movement of the joints. For example, lifting and carrying a heavy object requires a lot of isometric muscular work around the neck, shoulders and trunk.

When the muscles are in a constant state of tension, the arterial vessels are compressed thereby greatly reducing blood flow through the muscle. As a result, isometric exercise is primarily anaerobic and therefore cannot be sustained for long periods of time without muscle fatigue.

Cardiovascularly, if an exercise or activity requires a lot of isometric or static muscle work, then arterial BP (systolic and diastolic) increases markedly in a *pressor response*. The magnitude of this response is dependent upon the muscle mass involved in the activity and how hard these muscles are having to work.

Wall motion abnormalities in the myocardium may be aggravated by isometric exercise. Patients with dilated ventricles should be actively discouraged from isometric activities because of the excessive level of myocardial pressure work associated with them.

To make matters worse, during isometric activities, there is a tendency for people to hold their breath and strain. This is referred to as a *Valsalva manoeuvre*, the immediate effect of which is a substantial rise in BP, and a reduction in venous return. This could result in serious arrhythmias and ischaemia, particularly in patients with poor left ventricular (LV) function.

EXERCISE AND CORONARY HEART DISEASE

When screening for coronary heart disease (CHD), many health professionals fail to consider inactivity as a major risk factor. As a result, health promotion programmes concentrate on other aspects of lifestyle change (smoking cessation, diet, etc.). However, studies have shown that physical inactivity increases the risk of a first heart attack by a factor of 2.4 (Powell et al 1987).

Exercise is thought to reduce the risks of developing CHD by a variety of different mechanisms, summarized in Box 7.1. Fitness cannot be stored. Athleticism in youth is not protective against CHD later in life (Brill 1989, Morris et al 1990). The protective effects of exercise therefore relate only to current exercise habits.

Recent research has focused on the influence of exercise in modifying the thrombotic process. Connelly (1992) and Elwood (1993) found fibrinogen concentrations and blood viscosity were lowest amongst physically active men. Data from the latter study showed that the crucial factor was an individual's total amount of exercise time rather than the intensity at which he or she exercised.

Primary prevention of coronary heart disease

Box 7.1 Protective effects of regular exercise (Morris & Froelicher 1993, Connolly 1992, Elwood 1993)

Haemodynamic alterations
- Decrease in resting heart rate
- Decrease in heart rate and systolic blood pressure during subsequent activity
- Reduced myocardial oxygen demands at rest and during exercise
- Increase in left ventricular end diastolic volume
- Increased maximal oxygen uptake

Morphological alterations—cardiac muscle*
- Increase in myocardial mass/increase in ejection fraction
- Increase in coronary artery size
- Increase in myocardial capillary-to-fibre ratio—better perfusion
- Increase in collateral development

Musculoskeletal alterations
- Increase in oxygen extraction and utilization of skeletal muscles
- Increased efficiency of skeletal muscles during activity
- Increase in bone density—decreased risk of osteoporosis

Metabolic alterations
- Increased level of HDL cholsterol
- Decreased level of triglycerides
- Favourable alterations in insulin and glucagon responses
- Lower levels of adrenaline released in response to any stress
- Enhanced fibrinolytic system and reduced platelet aggregation

*Only with a high-intensity exercise programme, which may not be appropriate for all cardiac patients.

Several large epidemiological studies show that regular exercise gives primary protection against CHD. The Multiple Risk Factor Intervention Trial (Leon et al 1987) clearly showed that the protective effects of regular exercise extend even to those classified as being at high risk of developing CHD. Researchers found that amongst high-risk, but asymptomatic, middle-aged American men, the most active group had a 20% lower risk of CHD.

Blair (1989) in one of the few studies involving women, established that a similar relationship existed for women. More recent work on CHD in women done by Lavie (1995) has reaffirmed the need to encourage women to attend cardiac rehabilitation, since at baseline, they have lower exercise capacity and quality of life measures. Therefore the improvements (physiological and psychological) seen after such a programme, may be of greater clinical benefit to women than men.

Paffenbarger et al (1986) found that the risk of CHD in more active males was about 40% below that of their less active colleagues. They were also able to show that the protection against heart disease was lost when their subjects stopped exercising. Conversely, previously inactive subjects who then took up exercise acquired a lowered risk of CHD, thus confirming that the protective effects of exercise are present only for as long as the person continues to exercise.

A prospective study by Morris et al (1990) on healthy male executive grade civil servants showed that those who reported regular moderately intense exercise (e.g. swimming, jogging, tennis, etc.) had, after 10 years, rates of CHD three times lower than their sedentary colleagues.

Despite all of the known benefits of exercise in reducing the risks of early morbidity and mortality through CHD, sadly the levels of physical activity within the population as a whole, remain low. This is reflected in the Allied Dunbar National Fitness Survey of England and Wales (1992) which reported that 76% of men and 68% of women were below their desired activity level for their age group.

Secondary prevention of coronary heart disease

A report by a British Heart Foundation working group (1990) concludes that the relative risks of physical inactivity may be greater than commonly accepted and approach similar levels of risk attributed to smoking, hypertension and hypercholesterolaemia.

Greenland & Chu (1988) found that exercise training resulted in an average increase in exercise capacity of 15–25% over and above that which could be attributable to the normal process of recovery.

As well as reducing myocardial oxygen demands at rest, after training all activities of daily living can be performed at a lower heart rate and systolic BP (Leon et al 1990). This means that an individual can then continue with a desired activity without developing symptoms such as breathlessness or angina.

Myocardial infarction (MI)

Meta-analysis of 22 randomized clinical trials of exercise training in patients postmyocardial infarction revealed a 22% reduction in cardiovascular morbidity amongst exercisers and a 25% reduction in sudden death rates. However, despite the significant impact on mortality, there is little evidence to suggest that exercise reduces the risks of non-fatal reinfarction (O'Connor et al 1989, Oldridge et al 1988).

The benefits of exercise training to patients who have had large anterior Q wave infarcts has been questioned by some researchers. Judgutt et al (1988; cited in Pollock & Schmidt 1995) found that patients with left ventricular asynergy of greater than 18% developed more cardiac shape distortion, expansion and thinning; and their ejection fractions and functional capacity worsened after training. However, a more recent study by Giannuzzi et al (1992; cited in Pollock & Schmidt 1995) randomized patients 6 weeks after a Q wave infarct (ejection fraction above 25%) into either moderate intensity exercise training or a control group. As expected, exercise capacity only improved in the exercise group. They found, however, that in both groups, patients with poor left ventricular function (ejection fraction of less than 40%) exhibited adverse ventricular remodelling over time, and that exercise training did not appear to influence the process.

Angina

It is widely believed that the increase in physical work capacity seen in cardiac patients following exercise training, is primarily the result of peripheral adaptations (improved efficiency of the active skeletal muscles), rather than a consequence of improved myocardial efficiency. Skeletal muscles that are able to extract and utilize oxygen more effectively place less demands on the cardiovascular system. There is, however, some evidence to support the idea that improved myocardial blood supply and ventricular function after training is also achieved. Raffo et al (1980), in a prospective randomized control trial, found that in patients with angina (no previous history of MI) exercise training resulted in an increased HR/ST threshold. The HR/ST threshold refers to the heart rate at the point in the exercise test at which the patient develops ST segment depression, indicative of myocardial ischaemia. If the HR/ST threshold is raised, then myocardial ischaemia is no longer evident until a higher heart rate is reached. This they concluded could only be the result of enhanced myocardial oxygen delivery caused by the growth of new collaterals, an increase in the capacity of existing collaterals or by biochemical changes within the myocardium.

Todd et al (1991) undertook a similar study and, by using thallium scans, found that exercise training produced better coronary perfusion and on average a 34% reduction in ischaemia.

In both studies, patients were carefully selected and had a reasonably good exercise tolerance prior to training. This meant that they were able to safely participate in a high-intensity exercise programme. It is important to note that this sort of training programme is only appropriate for carefully screened and selected cardiac patients. If prescribed indiscriminately, vigorous exercise could precipitate a major coronary event (see 'Exercise safety', p. 161).

Fletcher (1986) assessed the effectiveness of inpatient education for patients who had undergone percutaneous transluminal coronary angioplasty (PTCA). He found that their short hospital stay (mean 4.9 days) precluded thorough patient and family education on risk factor modification. The rehabilitation team found that often patients were under the impression that their coronary artery disease had been cured and, because of the apparent simplicity of the angioplasty procedure, were not stimulated to reduce their risk factor profile.

This study reinforces the need for outpatient cardiac rehabilitation for all patients with coronary heart disease, and not just those who have had an infarct or bypass surgery.

Coronary artery bypass grafting (CABG)

Hanson et al (1985) concluded that an early (first 4 months postoperatively), moderate-intensity daily home exercise programme (walking or cycle ergometry) was as effective as a traditional medically supervised exercise programme in bringing about improvements in CABG patients' exercise capacity. Froelicher et al (1985) found that exercise training initiated as late as 2 years after surgery was effective in increasing patients' exercise capacity. Patients undertook moderate-intensity aerobic training for 45 minutes, three times a week for a 1-year period. Patients with signs and symptoms of unsuccessful revascularization were also included. In fact, these patients showed the greatest improvement in exercise capacity after training (21% increase compared with 13%). This study confirms that exercise training improves exercise capacity above and beyond that which could be reasonably attributed to the natural process of recovery and resumption of usual activities of daily living.

Heart failure

Patients with chronic stable heart failure show a reduced exercise capacity as a result of physical deconditioning. Low-intensity exercise training not only results in desirable changes in muscle strength, it delays the onset of anaerobic metabolism in skeletal muscle, reverses the impairment of peripheral vasodilatation and improves blood flow to exercising muscles (Uren & Lipkin 1992). Soler-Soler & Permanger-Miralda (1994) in a discussion paper on the role of lifestyle modifications, highlight the deleterious effects of 'rest' for patients with heart failure. They state that the time may be here for routinely prescribing formal exercise training to patients with compensated heart failure. Obviously, closer monitoring would be required and the exercise intensity would need to be strictly controlled, since even apparently small increments in intensity could result in the patient exercising too vigorously.

PRESCRIBING THE CORRECT EXERCISE

Not all cardiac patients have access to a physiotherapist for specialist advice, exercise prescription and training. Indeed, Lipkin (1991) concludes that formal exercise training (i.e. in a hospital setting) is probably not justified for all cardiac patients. It is therefore essential that other health care professionals can offer their patients advice and encouragement on exercising. Many factors need to be taken into consideration. Simply telling someone to take more exercise is not sufficient. The exercise prescription should specify:

- the type of exercise
- the intensity of exercise
- the frequency of exercise
- the duration of exercise.

Type of exercise

When recommending the type of exercise a person should do to improve his or her fitness and stamina, the following factors need to be considered:

1. The activity should involve isotonic rhythmic movement of as large a number of different muscle groups as possible. This then utilizes aerobic pathways and places a demand on the oxygen transport system.
2. The activity should be of sufficient intensity to cause the heart and respiratory rate to rise.
3. The activity should be one that the person is capable of continuing for 10–30 minutes at a time.
4. The activity should require minimal skill levels to reduce the person's likelihood of injury.
5. The participant should find the activity enjoyable. This makes the exercise programme easier to comply with.
6. If special facilities/equipment are needed, then these should be readily accessible and affordable.

Walking (outdoor and treadmill)

Walking is a natural form of exercise for all ages and is an excellent introduction to exercise for sedentary and unfit individuals. Walking is primarily an aerobic exercise of the lower limbs, although as the pace increases the upper limbs are used more.

Walking paces vary from a leisurely stroll to power walking. In order to be of benefit, walking needs to be of a pace sufficient to place a demand on the cardiovascular system causing a rise in heart rate.

The results of the Allied Dunbar Fitness Survey (1992) indicate that because of the poor exercise levels amongst the population as a whole, brisk walking for half an hour each day is sufficient for desirable changes to take place in the fitness of over two-thirds of the population. Morris et al (1990) found that the quantity of walking a person did was not associated with any decline in cardiac events, i.e. those who walked over 1 hour a day had the same incidence of coronary events as those who did no walking. Fast walkers, however, had particularly low rates of CHD. This confirmed the importance of performing exercise of sufficient intensity.

Most patients tend to overestimate their walking speed. Outdoor walking is self-paced and is therefore subject to individual perceptions and motivation. Ideally, a pedometer should be recommended for feedback and encouragement.

The main drawback to outdoor walking is, of course, the weather. Cardiac patients should be told to avoid prolonged periods of exercising outdoors when it is very cold or windy, since this is more likely to precipitate angina.

Treadmill walking is a suitable alternative, although it necessitates equipment only usually found in sports centres and hospitals. Visual displays of distance covered, time and even calories burned, provide powerful motivation.

Unlike outdoor walking, the main advantage of treadmill walking is that, once programmed, the walking speed is set by the machine, therefore the exercise intensity can be much more accurately controlled.

For those unaccustomed to the treadmill, an inefficient gait increases energy expenditure. Likewise, gripping too tightly on the handrail causes undesirable isometric work. During walking, the likelihood of injury is very low in comparison to other modes of exercise.

Jogging

Jogging provides a much higher intensity form of aerobic exercise and is therefore only suitable for those under 50 years of age with an already very good exercise capacity. Jogging is a high-impact activity making musculo-skeletal injuries much more likely. Proper footwear is essential. Joggers should be advised to avoid cement and asphalt surfaces, but keep to shock-absorbing surfaces like running tracks. Grass is a reasonable alternative provided the surface is not too rough or uneven. When recommending jogging as an exercise, it is usual to advise that after a warm-up, short periods of jogging should be interspersed with equal periods of walking (conversational jogging). This allows less fit individuals to keep their exercise intensity from becoming maximal, a situation which is more likely to result in cardiovascular complications.

Mini-trampoline rebounding

Commercially available mini-trampolines can be a good alternative to jogging for those with minor lower limb orthopaedic problems since they reduce the shock transmitted through the joints. This type of exercise is not suitable for people with poor balance, unless the trampoline incorporates a handrail.

Stair-climbing/step-ups

Exercise should be an integral part of everyday life, yet if given the choice between using the stairs or using an escalator, few opt to use the stairs.

Blamey et al (1995) found that 'Stay Healthy, Save Time—Use the Stairs' posters strategically placed in an underground station, resulted in significantly greater stair usage. Provided that it is done slowly at a level well within the person's capabilities, stair-climbing is an aerobic activity. However, for patients with weak thigh muscles or congestive heart failure, the activity may be anaerobic. If this is the case, then patients will complain that it feels very strenuous and makes them very breathless. For less fit individuals it is usually better to make use of the step at the foot of the stairs, to step up and down from. This will allow a relatively constant effort to be maintained for the duration of the exercise, as opposed to strenuous effort when ascending several steps followed by much easier effort when descending.

Repetitive stepping may exacerbate arthritic problems in hips, knees and ankles.

Cycling

Cycling works the large muscle groups of the legs in a steady aerobic manner. Cycling, like walking, is an easy activity to maintain at a steady level for the duration of the activity, an important consideration where precise control of exercise intensity is indicated. Cycling is an excellent form of non-weight-bearing exercise and is suitable for a wide range of fitness levels since the intensity can be altered by adjusting the pedalling speed or the terrain. The saddle height should be set so that the knee is only slightly bent at the downstroke; this ensures that the muscles work through a large range of movement, thus increasing the efficacy of the exercise.

In 1995, the British Government signalled a welcome shift in its transport policy, pledging more money to improve the facilities for inner city cyclists. At present only about 2.5% of all journeys are done by bicycle. Bhopal & Unwin (1995) state that 62% of all car trips are under 5 km in distance, and could quite easily be done by bicycle. Exercise bicycles are popular pieces of equipment bought for using at home. Unfortunately, most of these people give up once the novelty has worn off and the boredom has set in. Watching a favourite television programme while exercising can be good distraction therapy.

Exercise bicycles were once the cornerstone of many of the early cardiac rehabilitation programmes. However, cycling is a skill which uses muscles in a way not frequently used in day-to-day life. *Training specificity* refers to the adaptations that occur in response to exercise. Adaptations occur only in the muscles being exercised. Since most of the improvements that occur after moderate-intensity training come about as a result of peripheral adaptations in the muscles rather than enhanced cardiac function, exercise training which uses a single modality such as cycling is unlikely to improve upper body endurance, something which is necessary for many activities of daily living.

Rowing machines

The advantage of a rowing machine over other modes of exercise is that it combines the use of upper and lower limb muscle work. This makes the oxygen costs greater when compared with cycling. Most rowing machines also allow the participant to use legs only or arms only, making them useful for those with disabilities. They are generally not suitable for those with knee problems. Work rate can be adjusted by altering the resistance or increasing the velocity of each stroke. The equipment is of course expensive, which makes it inaccessible to some.

Swimming

Swimming incorporates upper and lower limb aerobic muscle work and as such can be a good form of exercise for those having already completed an exercise-based cardiac rehabilitation programme. For those who are unable or find it difficult to participate in weight-bearing exercise because of ortho-paedic limitations or obesity, the buoyancy of the water greatly reduces joint loading. The hydrostatic pressure of the water coupled with the horizontal position of the body, also enhances venous return. Many elderly people do not go swimming because they are frightened of slipping on wet floors and falling.

The wide variation in skill levels with swimming makes it a difficult mode of exercise for which to quantify individual training intensity accurately. For example, poor swimmers may not be able to attain an effective training stimulus because they are continually stopping. Similarly, highly skilled swimmers may find swimming is too easy, making it difficult to get enough cardiovascular exercise.

The temperature of the pool is a particularly important consideration. In a cold pool, to prevent excessive heat loss, a widespread peripheral vaso-constriction occurs with a resultant rise in arterial blood pressure. There is also an increase in the heart and respiratory rates. For cardiac patients this could precipitate ischaemic symptoms.

Rope skipping
Skipping is a high-impact, high-intensity exercise which also requires significant coordination, and as such is not recommended for cardiac patients. It is possible to use skipping as one of the exercises in a supervised cardiac rehabilitation circuit programme, providing it is reserved for those with good exercise tolerance at least 12 weeks post-event.

Callisthenics
Callisthenics is the name given to light mobilizing exercises of the upper and lower limbs designed to promote general fitness. Callisthenics are most often used in the inpatient setting for stable, uncomplicated cardiac patients, since the exercises represent a low demand on the cardiovascular system (somewhere in the region of 2–3 METs). When planning the exercises, the therapist should alternate between leg and arm work to prevent local muscle fatigue.

The term callisthenics should not be confused with 'Callanetics'. Callanetics are small repetitive end-of-range movements, localized to individual muscle groups and designed to improve muscle tone. These exercises contain a large isometric element and as such are less suitable for cardiac patients, particularly hypertensives.

Dancing
The aerobic benefits of dancing will vary considerably depending on the type of dance and the tempo of the music. Dancing is usually very sociable and enjoyable and as such may not be looked upon as 'exercise'. This makes it a good activity for those who think that exercise is the preserve of the fit and sporty.

Aerobic/keep fit exercise classes
Provided that the class is well structured and kept to low-impact moves, exercise classes can be very enjoyable. Participants should be encouraged to continually monitor themselves and work at their own pace. One of the disadvantages of exercise classes is that most participants try to keep up with

the pace set by the instructor, rather than pacing themselves. Prolonged bouts of exercise with the arms above the head will increase the work of the cardiovascular system, so it is wise initially to encourage participants to modify the exercise, by keeping their arms below chest height. Exercise classes can be very daunting for beginners who they think they are not coordinated. A good instructor can offset this by building up sequences of movements from two or three basic steps, rather than simultaneously changing arms and legs.

The importance of rehabilitation in a community setting has been emphasized by Bertie et al (1992) and Thompson (1994). Many of the hospital cardiac rehabilitation programmes will have a community link, with exercise classes in church halls or community centres. These should be staffed by chartered physiotherapists or qualified fitness instructors. Participants usually require medical confirmation of their suitability. A useful video for those uncertain of how to structure an exercise class has been produced by the YMCA (details at end of chapter, p. 170).

Exercise videos for home use

Cardiac patients should be guided to a low-impact/low-intensity version of aerobic exercise, which includes a distinct warm-up and cool-down. Patients should not be expected to exercise unsupervised at home until they have been taught the various components (frequency/intensity/duration) of an exercise prescription and how these factors interrelate. It is worthwhile reinforcing this point at all times. The type of exercise chosen should be well within the person's current capabilities. Exercises can always be modified so that if, for example, the person is getting breathless while performing arm exercises with the hands above the head, then he or she should be told to do a similar move but with the arms out in front.

With so many exercise videos on the market, the choice is bewildering. Most still aim at the already fit and healthy, 'lipstick and leotard' set, making them difficult to recommend to typical cardiac patients. For this reason, some cardiac rehabilitation programmes have produced their own videos, with much more satisfactory results.

Racquet games

By nature, racquet sports are highly variable in their intensity. If the participants are of a low skill level, then they could spend most of their time walking slowly or hanging about waiting for others. On the other hand, if the opponents are not equally matched in terms of skills, then the game may be far too demanding for one of them. Games like squash require bursts of energy. Sprinting for a ball is primarily anaerobic in nature and will be of no benefit to the cardiovascular system. In fact it is more likely to strain the cardiovascular system than train it. Instead of playing to get fit, advise people to get fit beforehand.

Canadian Airforce 5BX and XBX physical fitness programme

Despite the fact that several researchers have successfully used this programme with cardiac patients, it is not one that the author recommends. The plan consists of five different exercises which should be completed in 11 minutes. Although the principles of graduated progression are emphasized, the authors of the programme claim that an additional warm-up is unnecessary. Exercise duration is kept fixed and progression is made by increasing the intensity. High-intensity, short-duration exercise is not suitable for symptomatic individuals. In addition, the exercises themselves, if performed in the manner described, could result in musculoskeletal/back injury (e.g. sit up with legs straight and feet hooked under a chair).

Competitive exercise

Highly competitive exercise should be discouraged, since participants will be much less able to self-monitor and regulate their levels of exertion. If people feel that their team is relying upon them, they will not slow down even if they develop symptoms such as palpitations, breathlessness or chest pain.

Weight training

So far, aerobic exercise has been emphasized. However, most household, recreational and occupational activities require equal, if not greater, upper body strength than cardiovascular fitness. Increasing evidence now points to the value of light upper body resistance training to complement an aerobic training programme for cardiac patients. It is important to point out that these strengthening programmes emphasize isotonic muscle work using high repetitions of light weights. Pure isometric muscle work should be minimized (Butler et al 1992, Balady 1993). A small study by Ghilarducci et al (1989) found that strengthening exercises with much heavier weights (80% of the patient's maximum voluntary contraction) caused no signs or symptoms of myocardial ischaemia, or abnormal heart rate or blood pressure responses. The 10 patients studied were all stable, aerobically trained cardiac patients, with a mean age of 57 years.

Readers are referred to the guidelines laid down by the American Association of Cardiovascular and Pulmonary Rehabilitation (1995) before recommending this type of exercise to patients with heart disease.

■ KEY POINTS ON RESISTANCE TRAINING FOR CARDIAC PATIENTS (AACVPR, 1995)

- Low-level resistance training should be individualized.
- Resistance training should require no greater cardiovascular demands or perceived exertion ratings than aerobic exercise.
- Use of ECG and BP monitoring is recommended in a supervised setting.
- Surgical and MI patients should wait at least 6 weeks before beginning low-level resistance training.
- Patients with congestive heart failure, uncontrolled arrhythmias, severe valvular disease, uncontrolled hypertension > 160/100 and aerobic capacity < 3 METs should be excluded.

Exercise intensity

For convenience, exercise intensities can be classified as follows:

* *Light intensity*—easily within an individual's current exercise capacity, placing very little demand on the oxygen transport system
* *Moderate intensity*—within an individual's current exercise capacity, but causing an increase in respiratory and pulse rates
* *Vigorous intensity*—intense enough to represent a substantial challenge to a person's cardiorespiratory system (ACSM 1991).

The aim of an exercise programme should be to gradually expose the individual to an amount or level of exercise sufficient to bring about a cardiovascular training effect. This level is known as the training threshold. If the exercise intensity is too low, i.e. it is below the threshold, then no improvements in aerobic capacity will take place. The threshold of exercise for cardiovascular protection has been calculated to be about 630 kJ/day (Haskell 1985).

The American College of Sports Medicine (Leon et al 1990) conclude that in order to attain the health-related benefits of exercise, a person need only engage in moderate physical activity; vigorous levels of exercise are associated with increased risk of injury and sudden death. This is particularly encouraging for previously sedentary individuals or for those at risk of or with established coronary heart disease. In general, the less fit an individual is, then the lower the exercise intensity should be. The importance of a proper warm-up and cool-down period cannot be overemphasized.

Warm-up

The warm-up is the preparatory phase of an exercise session and has an important role in reducing the risks of musculoskeletal injury and cardio-vascular complications. In its simplest form, a warm-up would involve performing the prescribed exercise at a much lower intensity (e.g. slow walking, pedalling without any resistance, etc.).

A typical warm-up lasts 10–15 minutes (dependent on the intensity of the exercise to follow) and should include the following elements:

* limbering up and mobilizing exercises of the main joints
* low-intensity aerobic exercise to allow the cardiovascular system to accommodate the increased demands being placed upon it
* static stretching exercises.

One of the major purposes of the warm-up is to prepare the cardiovascular system for the physical exertion ahead. If individuals attempt strenuous exercise without having warmed up, then their heart rate will rise rapidly in response to the sudden increase in demand. This in turn causes a sudden and large increase in the myocardial oxygen demands, predisposing the individual to arrhythmias and/or ischaemia.

A warm-up allows more time for the selective redistribution of the body's cardiac output (see p. 141). Without this, the muscles are forced to work anaerobically, leading to a build-up of lactic acid. This then causes the muscles to fatigue at a workload or level that they might otherwise have been capable of sustaining.

As the name suggests, a warm-up slowly elevates the temperature of the body as a whole and in particular the temperature of the muscles. This increase in temperature reduces the viscosity of the muscles so that they contract more efficiently. Warm muscles, ligaments and tendons are able to lengthen more readily when stretched. This greatly reduces the likelihood of sprained muscles and other musculoskeletal injuries.

Cool-down

When the training portion of the exercise session ends, it is important not to stop abruptly but to gradually reduce the level of activity before stopping. A cool-down is therefore described as the period of lower-intensity exercise at the end of an exercise session. The structure of a cool-down is essentially the reverse of the warm-up. There are several reasons why a cool-down is important.

1. During exercise, venous blood is assisted in its return to the heart by the action of the skeletal muscles wrapped around the veins. If a person suddenly stops exercising (particularly if the body is in an upright posture), then without the muscle pump to maintain venous return, blood begins to pool in the extremities. This can lead to post-exercise hypotension, resulting in fainting or the unpleasant symptoms of light-headedness and dizziness.

2. Even though the exercise is over, the active skeletal muscles still need a large supply of oxygenated blood to replenish their energy reserves. If the heart's stroke volume is less because of the smaller venous return, then the heart rate has to remain elevated in order to maintain the cardiac output (cardiac output = stroke volume × heart rate). This means that myocardial oxygen consumption continues to rise even though the person has stopped exercising.

3. Maintaining an adequate blood flow to the skeletal muscles into the recovery period enhances the removal of the waste products of metabolism (e.g. lactic acid) which may have accumulated during exercise. These waste products have been blamed for much of the muscle soreness that develops following exercise.

Controlling the exercise intensity

Various methods can be used to prescribe and monitor exercise intensity. Clinically, amongst the most useful are:

- heart rate
- patient-perceived exertion
- breathlessness
- METs.

Target heart rate. As previously stated, there is a linear relationship between heart rate and oxygen consumption. To increase cardiac fitness, aerobic exercise needs to be of an intensity that raises the heart rate (HR) to between

50 and 70% of its maximum. The lower and upper limits of the target heart rate can be calculated as follows:

Lower limit of target HR = HRmax × 0.5
Upper limit of target HR = HRmax × 0.8

The maximum heart rate (HRmax) is the heart rate at which maximal oxygen uptake is achieved. If the patient has recently undergone a graded maximal exercise test, then the peak heart rate on exercise should be used to calculate the training heart rate. Where no recent exercise test has been done, an estimated HRmax can be made simply on the basis of the person's age (estimated HRmax = 220 − age in years).

Another method of calculating the target heart rate is by the Karvonen formula (Hal 1993):

Lower limit of target HR = 0.5 × (HRmax − HRrest) + HRrest
Upper limit of target HR = 0.8 × (HRmax − HRrest) + HRrest

Whatever method is used, patients need to be taught how to take their own pulses. Usually the radial artery is easy to palpate. The beats are counted over a 15-second period, then multiplied by four, to give a measure of the heart rate.

When individuals first embark on an exercise programme, they will have little idea of what level of exercise corresponds to their training heart rate. This means that heart rate measurements should be taken frequently if exercise intensity is to be reliably regulated.

■ KEY POINTS WHEN USING HEART RATE AS THE SOLE METHOD FOR CONTROLLING EXERCISE INTENSITY:

• Bear in mind, that an individual's signs and symptoms are overriding factors when prescribing the intensity of an exercise. For example, patients with COAD may be unable to maintain the exercise intensity calculated using only the heart rate guidelines, because they become short of breath.

• Commonly prescribed cardiac drugs considerably lower a patient's maximum heart rate (Pollock & Schmidt 1995), for example patients on beta-blocking medications.

• Patients with an irregular pulse need to count for an entire minute.

• Patients have to interrupt their exercise session to find and check their pulse.

• If the heart rate is fast, this makes it difficult to count every beat.

• Patients with poor perfusion to their fingers will have difficulty finding a strong radial pulse.

• Patients can become obsessive about counting their pulse during activities, possibly increasing anxiety amongst certain individuals.

Patient-perceived exertion. In the 1970s, Gunner Borg discovered that subjective perception of effort or exertion could be used to predict heart rate during a graded exercise test. He developed a visual analogue scale from 6

Box 7.2 Rating of perceived exertion (RPE) scale			
6		13	Somewhat hard
7	Very, very light	14	
8		15	Hard
9	Very light	16	
10		17	Very hard
11	Fairly light	18	
12		19	Very, very hard
		20	

to 20 used to describe the intensity of effort being put into an activity (see Box 7.2). This has been tested extensively using both normal individuals and cardiac patients. A rating of perceived exertion (RPE) of 12–13 has been found to be highly correlated to 60% HRmax, while an RPE of 16 corresponds to 85% HRmax (Birk & Birk 1987). Consequently, most individuals will achieve a training effect by exercising at a 'somewhat hard' level.

At the onset of an exercise programme, individuals can be instructed to exercise at a specified heart rate and to self-monitor the RPE at that intensity (ACSM 1991). Once they have learned to recognize the feeling that arises when the exercise intensity is at the right level then there is no need for them to stop exercising in order to check their pulse. RPE can be successfully used by patients who have difficulty checking their own pulse accurately, in patients taking beta-blockers and after heart and heart lung transplant. It should be remembered, however, that a small percentage of individuals cannot use the scale with any accuracy and instead tend to select unrealistic RPE scores (Hall 1993).

Breathlessness. 'Sing—Talk—Gasp' (Hall 1993). This is probably the simplest yet most effective means of teaching exercise participants the skills of self-monitoring. If they are able to sing as they exercise, then the intensity should be increased. If they do not have enough breath to sing, yet are still able to talk in sentences as they exercise, then they are achieving the correct intensity. If they are unable to talk in sentences and are gasping for breath, they are working at too high an intensity and need to decrease the pace at which they are exercising.

METs or metabolic equivalents. MET is the unit of measurement used to describe the oxygen costs of an activity. 1 MET equals the oxygen costs of resting metabolism.

1 MET = VO_2 at rest = 3.5 ml/kg/min

MET values for common leisure activities are listed in Table 7.1. Once a person's peak MET is known, then a mode of exercise equivalent to approximately 65% of that can be selected. A person's peak MET is usually reported in the exercise tolerance test results.

For example, a person with a maximum MET of 5, should choose an activity from the tables that corresponds to an MET of around 3. This would include activities such as walking (3 m.p.h.), leisurely cycling and ballroom dancing.

Table 7.1 Estimated energy requirements of selected activities (Fletcher et al 1990)

Activity	METs	Activity	METs
Light intensity		Mowing the lawn	
Baking	2.0	(power mower)	3.0
Billiards	2.4	Playing drums	3.8
Bookbinding	2.2	Sailing	3.0
Canoeing (leisurely)	2.5	Swimming (slowly)	4.5
Conducting an orchestra	2.2	Walking (3 m.p.h.)	3.3
Ballroom dancing	2.9	Walking (4 m.p.h.)	4.5
Golf (with cart)	2.5		
Horseback riding (walking)	2.3	**Vigorous intensity**	
Playing a musical instrument:		Badminton	5.5
accordion	1.8	Chopping wood	4.9
cello	2.3	Climbing hills (no load)	6.9
flute	2.0	Climbing hills (with 5-kg load)	7.4
horn	1.7	Cycling (moderately)	5.7
piano	2.3	Dancing (aerobic or ballet)	6.0
trumpet	1.8	Dancing (ballroom or square)	5.5
violin	2.6	Field hockey	7.7
woodwind	1.8	Ice skating	5.5
Volleyball (non-competitive)	2.9	Jogging (10-minute mile)	10.2
Walking (2 m.p.h.)	2.5	Karate or judo	6.5
Writing	1.7	Roller-skating	6.5
		Rope-skipping	12.0
Moderate intensity		Skiing (water or downhill)	6.8
Callisthenics (no weights)	4.0	Squash	12.1
Croquet	3.0	Surfing	6.0
Cycling (leisurely)	3.5	Swimming (fast)	7.0
Gardening (no lifting)	4.4	Tennis (doubles)	6.0
Golf (without cart)	4.9		

NB These activities can often be done at variable intensities, assume that the intensity in each case is not excessive and that the courses are flat (no hills) unless otherwise specified.

If on the other hand a person's MET was 10, then he or she should select from activities corresponding to 6–7 METs (e.g. badminton, water-skiing and fast swimming).

Disadvantages of the MET system are that it does not make any allowance for environmental factors or differing skill levels.

Exercise duration

The conditioning period (exclusive of a warm-up and a cool-down) may vary in length from 10–30 minutes. As a general rule, the greater the intensity of the conditioning period, the shorter the duration needed to bring about a training effect and vice versa. High-intensity, short-duration exercise is not desirable except for fit individuals with no known pathology.

Sedentary individuals and those with known pathologies should be guided towards lower-intensity, longer-duration exercise. To begin with, they will be unable to exercise for long (e.g. 10 min) at the desired intensity. The emphasis should then be on increasing the exercise duration as opposed to increasing the exercise intensity. In other words, as fitness improves, the duration of the conditioning part of the exercise should be increased in 5-minute increments, with the duration of the warm-up and cool-down remaining constant.

An exercise session which lasts longer than 30 minutes (excluding warm-up and cool-down) is more likely to provoke musculoskeletal overuse injury. DeBusk (1990) found that patients who exercised for three 10-minute sessions a day, in lieu of the more usual single session of 30 minutes, showed similar improvements in their fitness. This confirms that a day's exercise can, if need be, be broken up into multiple shorter bouts in order to fit in with the individual's lifestyle.

Exercise frequency

The frequency of exercise should reflect the needs, interests and functional capacity of the participants. Very unfit individuals will benefit most from short-duration, very frequent exercise (i.e. several times a day). Whereas the optimal frequency of exercise for those on a maintenance programme might be alternate days, three times a week.

Continuous versus interval training methods

As the name suggests, during continuous exercise, after a warm-up, the level of exercise is maintained at a steady intensity for the duration of the training period. The session is completed by a cool-down period before stopping. During interval training, there is the usual warm-up and cool-down, but the training period is interspersed with short rest periods. The main advantage of interval training is that it allows those with a low exercise tolerance to exercise for longer at their prescribed intensity.

Exercise progression

Progression should be made by adjusting the frequency and the duration. It is usual to build up tolerance by increasing the frequency of the exercise sessions, then the duration. For safety reasons, the exercise intensity should remain constant. Table 7.2 shows the recommended exercise prescription for differing patient populations. If the exercise intensity is controlled using the METs system already discussed, then as the person's fitness improves, the same exercise may no longer be equivalent to a 'moderate' intensity.

For example, people with a functional capacity of 5 METs would initially select an activity equal to around 3 METs, e.g. walking at 3 m.p.h. As they became fitter, their functional capacity would improve, say to 7 METs. If, however, they continued to choose walking at 3 m.p.h. as their training method, then instead of exercising at 60% of their maximum, they would then only be exercising at 40% of their functional capacity. If, however, exercise intensity is guided by heart rate or perceived exertion levels, then individuals would be automatically adjusting the amount of exercise they were doing in order to stay within their training zone.

Table 7.2 Suggested guidelines for exercise prescription—unsupervised exercise

	Frequency	Intensity		Time (minutes)
		%HRmax	RPE	
Healthy, active adults	2–4/week	75–85%	14–16	30–40
Healthy, sedentary adults	3–5/week	65–80%	12–14	20–30
Asymptomatic adults with two or more risk factors	3–5/week	60–75%	12–13	20–30
Chronic stable angina pectoris	Twice daily	10 beats below ischaemic threshold	10–11	5–10
Within first 2 months after uncomplicated MI or CABG	Once daily	40–55%	10–11	15–20
2 months following uncomplicated MI or CABG	4–6/week	60–75%	12–13	20–30

Walking programme. Box 7.3 provides an example of a walking programme which a patient could use on discharge from hospital following an uncomplicated MI or cardiac surgery. Progress depends upon the individual; as a rule patients should not move on to the next stage of the programme until they are consistently (i.e. on four separate occasions) finding the exercise too easy.

Exercise safety

Injuries (both musculoskeletal and cardiovascular) resulting from exercise are generally avoidable. Exercise participants must be made aware of, and

Box 7.3 A walking programme	
Stage 1.	Walk 0.25 miles twice each day (takes 10 min if walking at 1.5 m.p.h.).
Stage 2.	Walk 0.5 miles each day (aim to do in 15 min).
Stage 3.	Walk 0.75 miles each day (aim to do in 20 min).
Stage 4.	Walk 1 mile each day or 2 miles three to four times a week (walk at 3 m.p.h.).
Stage 5.	Walk 1.25 miles each day or 2.5 miles three to four times a week—with 10 minutes in the middle spent walking briskly.
Stage 6.	Walk 1.5 miles each day or 3 miles three to four times a week—with two 10-minute periods of brisk walking.
Stage 7.	Walk 1.75 miles each day or 3.5 miles three to four times a week—with the majority of the time spent walking briskly.

understand the risks associated with non-compliance with their individual exercise prescription. Patients needlessly place themselves at increased risk because they are under the mistaken belief that exercising harder and for longer will speed up their recovery—the so-called 'no pain–no gain' myth.

Orthopaedic problems may be either chronic overuse injuries such as shin splints, caused by repetitive trauma, or acute injuries such as sprained ligaments caused by sudden excessive overloading of the soft tissues. Most are the result of inadequate warm-up, unaccustomed vigorous exercise or poor technique.

Cardiovascular complications (myocardial ischaemia, ventricular fibrillation, etc.) usually result from a person's failure to pay heed to warning symptoms such as feeling unwell, dizziness, chest pain and breathlessness. Isometric exercise or activities which involve a large isometric component, should be discouraged for the reasons previously discussed. Participants should not exercise within 2 hours of eating a meal, otherwise blood flow is diverted away from the gut and the digestive process is hindered. Cardiac patients should be advised on how to gradually warm up prior to exercise and then how to cool down prior to stopping, thus reducing the risk of serious cardiovascular complications. They should be encouraged to report any change in their typical cardiac symptoms (e.g. increasing frequency of angina during activities of daily living or failure of quick-acting nitrates to relieve angina once it has developed) and should be reminded not to exercise if they have forgotten to take their usual medications. Exercise testing should be used to screen out high-risk individuals. Such individuals usually require further medical or surgical intervention and should therefore be guided to a low-intensity, low-duration, high-frequency exercise plan.

During an exercise test, specific indicators of a poor clinical status are:

- decrease in systolic blood pressure during exercise testing or failure of systolic blood pressure to rise despite increasing workload
- exercise test terminated at a low workload because of myocardial ischaemia (> 2 mm ST depression)
- appearance of serious ventricular arrhythmias.

Other clinical markers of poor cardiovascular function include a myocardial infarction complicated by congestive heart failure, cardiogenic shock and/or complex ventricular arrhythmias, multiple myocardial infarctions, impaired ventricular function (i.e. ejection fraction < 25%), angiographic evidence of significant (> 75%) occlusions in the left main or left anterior descending coronary arteries and an unpredictable pattern of angina.

Contraindications to exercise

Contraindications to exercise listed by the ACSM include:

- uncontrolled hypertension
- moderate to severe aortic stenosis
- acute systemic illness or fever
- uncontrolled atrial or ventricular arrhythmias
- resting sinus tachycardia > 120 b.p.m.

- uncontrolled congestive heart failure
- third degree AV heart block
- active pericarditis or myocarditis
- recent embolism
- thrombophlebitis
- uncontrolled diabetes.

METHODS OF MEASURING EXERCISE TOLERANCE

An accurate knowledge of a person's aerobic exercise capacity is needed in order to give appropriate exercise advice. This can be obtained subjectively by using a questionnaire such as those shown in Boxes 7.4 and 7.5.

The New York Heart Association's functional classification, although often used clinically, is not sensitive enough to show small but significant changes in a person's aerobic capacity. This is because there are only four broad categories:

Class I   No symptoms with ordinary physical activity
Class II   Symptoms with ordinary physical activity
Class III Symptoms with less than ordinary physical activity
Class IV   Symptoms at rest.

Box 7.4 Duke activity scale index (DASI) (Hlaty et al 1989)

Can you?

1. Take care of yourself, i.e. eating, dressing, bathing or using the toilet.	2.75
2. Walk indoors, such as around your house.	1.75
3. Walk a block or two on level ground.	2.75
4. Climb a flight of stairs or walk up a slope.	5.50
5. Run a short distance.	8.00
6. Do light work around the house—dusting, washing dishes.	2.70
7. Do moderate work around the house—vacuuming, sweeping floors, carrying in groceries.	3.50
8. Do heavy work around the house—scrubbing floors, lifting/moving furniture.	8.00
9. Do yard work—raking leaves, weeding, pushing a power mower.	4.50
10. Have sexual relations.	5.20
11. Participate in moderate recreational activities —golf, bowling, dancing, doubles tennis.	6.00
12. Participate in strenuous sports —swimming, singles tennis, football, basketball, skipping.	7.50

DASI = sum of weights for 'yes' replies

$VO_2max = DASI + 9.6 \times 0.43$

To obtain an objective measurement of a person's aerobic capacity, a graded exercise test should be done with ECG and blood pressure monitoring. The most commonly used treadmill test is the *Bruce Protocol* which involves an increase in both treadmill speed and gradient every 3 minutes. This test is

---

Box 7.5 Physical activity index

I avoid walking if I can and prefer to drive/get a lift/use public transport.	0
I occasionally walk instead of driving/getting a lift/using public transport.	1
I go for short easy walks (< 15 min) at least three to four times a week.	2
I go for short easy walks (< 15 min) at least five to six times a week.	3
I go for 10- to 15-minute brisk walks at least three to four times a week.	3
I use the stairs every day for exercise.	4
I go for 10- to 15-minute brisk walks at least five or more times a week.	4
I go for 15- to 30-minute brisk walks at least three to four times a week.	5
I go for 15- to 30-minute brisk walks at least five or more times a week.	6
I participate in recreational activities of moderate intensity*	
—once or twice a week	6
—three to four times a week	7
—five or more times a week	8
I participate in recreational activities of vigorous intensity[†]	
—once or twice a week	8
—three to four times a week	9
—five or more times a week	10

* Moderate intensity = within individual's exercise capacity—breathing faster than normal but able to sustain comfortably

[†] Vigorous intensity = intense enough to represent a substantial challenge to the person's cardiovascular system

---

often criticized because the first stage is often too hard for unfit patients (starting speed 1.7 m.p.h. and gradient of 10%) and there is a relatively large increase in workload from one stage to the next. For cardiac patients, a modified Bruce Protocol is used. This has two preliminary stages and therefore starts at a much lower intensity. Detailed description of this and various other protocols for exercise testing can be found elsewhere (Dargie 1993, Hayward et al 1995).

Clinically, it is usually not feasible for all patients to undergo such a test; in which case, for uncomplicated low-risk patients (providing there are no contraindications), 'field' tests can be used without the need for ECG monitoring and direct medical supervision.

The 6-minute walking test is the simplest type of maximal exercise test which does not necessitate the use of laboratory equipment. For this test patients are instructed to walk up and down a 10-metre course, aiming to cover as much ground as possible in the time permitted. The examiner then records the distance covered. A criticism of this test is that it is very much dependent on the patient's motivation. This variable limits the reproducibility and validity of the test.

On the other hand, the 12-minute shuttle walking test is a highly reproducible test which is easy to implement. During this test, patients are required to walk a 10-metre course keeping to the speed dictated by audio signals from a cassette player. At first their walking speed is very slow, but after each minute of the test, their walking speed has to increase to keep up with the pace set by the cassette. The test can be maximal (i.e. the test continues until the patient is unable to continue) or submaximal. A submaximal exercise test involves stopping the test at a predetermined heart rate well below the person's age-predicted maximal heart rate, for example setting a heart rate limit of 130 beats per minute. This is only practical if you have the use of a heart rate monitor. An alternative endpoint might be a score of 15 on the perceived exertion scale (i.e. the point at which the person describes the test as becoming 'hard'). Further details of how to implement the test may be found elsewhere (Singh et al 1992). In the future, it is hoped to formally validate this test for use with cardiac patients.

BARRIERS TO THE UPTAKE OF REGULAR EXERCISE

Iliffe et al (1994) remind us that exercise initiatives seem to influence those who would have taken up exercise anyway, the so-called 'worried well'. One of the problems of leading a sedentary lifestyle is that such people rarely place significant demands on their cardiovascular system. Consequently, they have little idea of their true level of fitness and as such have no incentive to improve it. Fitness assessments are one way of motivating individuals to take part in regular aerobic exercise, particularly if they know subsequent retesting is to be carried out. If the person is being expected to carry out an exercise programme unsupervised, regular contact with the health care professional is essential. This can vary from regular telephone contact, to getting the person to complete a weekly exercise diary. Feedback and encouragement are essential for giving patients confidence that they can change. Pollock & Schmidt (1995) remind us that dropout from supervised rehabilitation does not automatically mean that the desired behavioural changes are not being maintained. All too often the reason for non-attendance is unknown (Horgan et al 1992). Finding out the reasons for dropout is crucial.

Membership to health clubs and sports facilities can be outwith the budgets of many patients. Local authorities often have a discount scheme for those who are retired, unemployed, disabled or on a low income. Another reason people give up an exercise programme is that the goals and expectations they were given were unrealistic. Patients who expect sudden, major changes in their health will become discouraged when they fail to see an immediate improvement. In fact, the benefits of secondary prevention may not be evident until 3 or more years after MI (Pollock & Schmidt 1995). Unrealistic goals should be discouraged (for example a previously inactive 50-year-old taking up rock climbing as a hobby).

It is essential to obtain accurate baseline measures of a person's current physical capacity, so that the intensity can be set at the right level. The ideal situation is initially to have the patient undergo a graded exercise test, the results of which can be used to set exercise intensity. Relying on subjective information can be misleading. If open questioning is used, most people tend to overestimate their physical abilities. Exercise scales such as those shown in Boxes 7.4 and 7.5 will give more objective data.

Exercise adherence is highest amongst those who have an individualized exercise programme. This means taking time to find out factors such as the person's likes and dislikes and his or her ease of access to facilities. Information about the existence and location of various organized exercise groups should be prominently displayed. Consideration should be given not only to the mode of exercise, but to the duration and frequency expected. Despite the fact that swimming is known to be a good aerobic exercise, if the swimming pool is not within easy travelling distance, then compliance will be much lower. Campbell et al (1994), on examining the attitudes of postmyocardial infarction patients to cardiac rehabilitation, found that the greatest influence foreseen on attendance was the travelling distance involved. Another reason may be that the exercise is perceived as boring or unexciting.

One example of a highly successful strategy is that employed by general practitioners in Hailsham (Jelley 1993). Here, GPs can prescribe exercise in much the same way as medication. Patients then take their prescription to their local leisure centre and can then attend for a 10-week supervised programme of exercise.

The more complex the behavioural change needed, the harder it is to achieve long-term compliance. Most cardiac patients need to alter several habits. It is essential to introduce change gradually in a positive and realistic manner.

Cardiac patients are often presented with a list of don'ts. It is helpful to reinforce the idea that exercise is a positive step as opposed to being told to refrain from a behaviour perceived as enjoyable. Newton et al (1991) found that exercisers showed much better psychosocial adjustment after MI, confirming the benefits of exercise in restoring self-esteem.

Increasing exercise may not be the first priority. In which case, it is better to try to encourage exercise as part of the normal way of life. Simple changes such as taking the stairs rather than waiting for the lift or elevator, or getting off the bus one or two stops early and walking the rest of the way, soon have a cumulative effect. Equally as important is to enlist the active support of spouses, partners and families. Age should not be a barrier to exercise, since it has the potential not only to enhance a person's well-being, but also to decrease the morbidity and mortality of those over 65 (Pescatello & DiPietro 1993).

The link between inactivity and heart disease needs to be clearly established in the patient's mind. Otherwise their exercise habits are very difficult to change. The health professional's role not only lies in providing education on the health-related benefits of regular exercise and how to realize these safely and effectively, but in being a source of example and motivation.

■ KEY POINTS

• Numerous studies indicate that regular physical activity reduces cardiovascular morbidity and mortality.

• The health-related benefits of regular exercise make it an important strategy in the primary and secondary prevention of CHD.

- Rhythmic, isotonic movement utilizes aerobic pathways for energy.

- Aerobic exercise increases the demands on the oxygen transport system making the heart and respiratory rates rise, ideally to a level which makes the individual slightly breathless.

- Regular aerobic exercise results in desirable changes in the functions of the cardiovascular and musculoskeletal systems.

- The Coronary Prevention Group (1992) state that a minimum of 20 minutes of aerobic exercise at least three times a week is needed to reduce the risks of coronary heart disease.

- 70% of the adult population in the UK do not take enough exercise. If exercise is to maintain its beneficial effects it must be habitual. Fitness cannot be stored. What counts most is current exercise. Athleticism in youth does not confer any additional protection against coronary heart disease in later life.

- Moderate exercise is just as cardioprotective as vigorous exercise.

- The incidence of musculoskeletal and cardiovascular complications is greatest during vigorous activity and competitive exercise.

- Before embarking on an exercise programme, medical clearance should be obtained from the person's GP.

- The exercise prescription should be individualized. Parameters such as type, intensity, duration and frequency should be specified.

- Set realistic exercise objectives.

- The exercise session should be made up of a warm-up, cardiovascular endurance training then a cool-down.

- With all forms of exercise, it is advisable to begin at a relatively easy level and gradually progress as able.

Case study 7.1

Mr A is a 45-year-old who was admitted to hospital with chest pain. Mr A gave no history of ischaemic heart disease and in fact considered himself to be in good health. He had stopped smoking 3 years ago and no other risk factors applied. His ECG showed acute changes in keeping with an inferior MI. Mr A received thrombolytic therapy, made an uncomplicated recovery and was discharged home 6 days later on atenolol and aspirin.

2 weeks later, he had an exercise tolerance test off drug therapy. He exercised for 10 minutes 56 seconds on a Modified Bruce Protocol before stopping with breathlessness. Peak heart rate was 148 beats per minute with a normal BP response and no ECG changes. His functional capacity was calculated to be equal to 6 METs, i.e. VO_2max of 18 ml/kg/min.

As a young man, Mr A had played a lot of football. After a series of minor injuries, his knees prevented him from playing for some time. He slowly got out of the habit of exercising. By this time he had started a new job. His working hours averaged 60 per week with 40% of the time spent at a desk, with another 30% driving. This left him little opportunity to exercise; often the only exercise was a walk to and from the car. Mr A lived in a high rise flat on the 19th floor so he always used the lift. Any time he had to climb the stairs, he became quite breathless, so naturally enough he avoided stairs altogether.

Questions

1. The hospital physiotherapist has given Mr A a walking programme. What guidelines should he be given for controlling his exercise intensity?
2. What advice can you give Mr A to help him incorporate exercise into his day-to-day life?

Answers

1. Mr A is in the early phase of his recovery from his MI, therefore he should be guided towards a daily, light-intensity, moderate-duration exercise plan. Age-predicted target heart rates will not apply because Mr A is taking a beta-blocker.

   The most appropriate advice would be a rating of perceived exertion between 10 and 11—'fairly light'.
2. By setting easily achievable goals. For the first week, he should get off the lift on the floor below and walk up the remaining flight to his flat. Each week the number of flights he walks up should be increased. Perhaps he could walk part of the way into work by getting off the bus one stop earlier. At this stage football is too vigorous a hobby. Competitive exercise is best avoided for 5 months post-event.

PRACTICAL EXERCISE

Make up a directory of local leisure and sports facilities which would be suitable for cardiac patients. The over-50s recreation officer at your local district council may be a good source of information. Identify all the cardiac rehabilitation programmes running in your area. Is there a role for liaison with yourself?

REFERENCES

Allied Dunbar, Health Education Authority, Sports Council 1992 Allied Dunbar National Fitness Survey: a report on activity patterns and fitness levels. Main findings and summary document. Sports Council, Health Education Authority, London

American Association of Cardiovascular and Pulmonary Rehabilitation 1995 Guidelines for cardiac rehabilitation programs, 2nd edn. Human Kinetics, Champaign

American College of Sports Medicine (ACSM) 1991 Guidelines for exercise testing and prescription, 4th edn. Lea & Febinger, Philadelphia

Balady G J 1993 Types of exercise. Arm–leg and static–dynamic. Cardiology Clinics 11: 2 297–308

Bertie J et al 1992 Benefits and weaknesses of a cardiac rehabilitation programme. Journal of the Royal College of Physicians of London 26(2): 147–151

Bhopal R, Unwin N 1995 Cycling, physical exercise and the Millennium Fund. British Medical Journal 311(7001): 344

Birk T J, Birk C 1987 Use of ratings of perceived exertion for exercise prescription. Sports Medicine 4: 1–8

Blair S N et al 1989 Physical fitness and all cause mortality. A prospective study of healthy men and women. Journal of the American Medical Association 262(17): 2395–2401

Blamey A et al 1995 Health Promotion by encouraged use of stairs. British Medical Journal 311(7000): 289–290

British Heart Foundation 1990 Exercise and the heart: report of a British Heart Foundation working party. British Heart Foundation, London

Brill P A 1989 The impact of previous athleticism on exercise habits, physical activity and coronary heart disease risk factors in middle aged men. Research Quarterly for Exercise and Sport 60(3): 209–215

Butler R M et al 1992 Circuit weight training in early cardiac rehabilitation. Journal of the American Osteopathic Association 92(1) 77–89

Campbell R M et al 1994 Cardiac rehabilitation: the agenda set by post myocardial infarction patients. Health Education Journal 53: 409–420

Connelly J B 1992 Strenuous exercise, plasma fibrinogen and factor VII activity. British Heart Journal 67: 351–354

Coronary Prevention Group 1992 Statistics on coronary heart disease. Coronary Prevention Group, London, pp 42–46

Dargie H J 1993 Exercise electrocardiography. Medicine International 21(9): 346–350

DeBusk R F 1990 Training effects of long versus short bouts of exercise in healthy subjects. American Journal of Cardiology 65: 1010–1013

Elwood P C et al 1993 Exercise, fibrinogen and other risk factors for ischaemic heart disease. British Heart Journal 69: 183–187

Fletcher G F 1986 Rehabilitation after coronary angioplasty—is it effective? Archives in Physical Medicine and Rehabilitation 67: 517–519

Fletcher G F et al 1990 Exercise standards: a statement for health professionals from the American Heart Association. Circulation 82: 2286–2322

Froelicher V et al 1985 A randomized trial of the effects of exercise training after coronary artery bypass surgery. Archives in International Medicine 145(4) 689–692

Ghilarducci L E C et al 1989 Effects of high resistance training in coronary artery disease. American Journal of Cardiology 64: 866–870

Greenland P, Chu J S 1988 Efficacy of cardiac rehabilitation services with emphasis on patients after myocardial infarction. Annals of Internal Medicine 109: 650–653

Hall L K 1993 Developing and managing cardiac rehabilitation programs. Human Kinetics, Champaign

Hanson P et al 1985 Exercise capacity and cardiovascular responses to serial exercise testing in men and women after coronary artery bypass graft surgery. Journal of Cardiopulmonary Rehabilitation V(8): 389–397

Haskell W L 1985 Physical activity and health: need to define the required stimulus. American Journal of Cardiology 5: 4D–9D

Hayward M P et al 1995 Physiology and clinical applications of cardiopulmonary exercise testing. British Journal of Hospital Medicine 53(6): 275–282

Hlaty M et al 1989 A brief, self administered questionnaire to determine functional capacity. The Duke Activity Index. American Journal of Cardiology 64: 651–654

Horgan J et al 1992 Working party report on cardiac rehabilitation. British Heart Journal 67: 412–418

Iliffe S et al 1994 Prescribing exercise in general practice. Look before you leap. British Medical Journal 309 (20–27 Aug): 494–495

Jelley S 1993 Prescription for health. Healthline 1 (April): 18–19

Lavie C J 1995 Effects of cardiac rehabilitation and exercise training on exercise capacity, coronary risk factors, behavioural characteristics and quality of life in women. American Journal of Cardiology 75: 340–343

Leon A S et al 1987 Leisure time physical activity levels and risk of coronary heart disease and death. The Multiple Risk Factor Intervention Trial. Journal of the American Medical Association 258(17): 2388–2395

Leon A S et al 1990 Position Paper of the American Association of Cardiovascular and Pulmonary Rehabilitation. Scientific evidence of the value of cardiac rehabilitation services with emphasis on patients following myocardial infarction—Section I: exercise conditioning component. Journal of Cardiopulmonary Rehabilitation 10: 79–87

Lipkin 1991 Is cardiac rehabilitation necessary? British Heart Journal 65: 237–238

Morris C, Froelicher V F 1993 Cardiovascular benefits of improved exercise capacity. Sports Medicine 16(4): 225–236

Morris J N et al 1990 Exercise in leisure time: coronary attack and death rates. British Heart Journal 63: 325–334

Newton M et al 1991 The effects of exercise in a coronary rehabilitation programme. Scottish Medical Journal 36: 38–41

O'Connor G T et al 1989 An overview of randomized trials of rehabilitation with exercise after myocardial infarction. Circulation 80: 234–244

Oldridge N B et al 1988 Cardiac rehabilitation after myocardial infarction. Combined experience of randomized clinical trials. Journal of the American Medical Association 260(7): 945–950

Paffenbarger R S et al 1986 Physical activity, all cause mortality and longevity of college alumni. New England Journal of Medicine 314: 605–613, and 315: 399–401

Pescatello L S, DiPietro L 1993 Physical activity in older adults. An overview of health benefits. Sports Medicine 15(6): 353–364

Pollock M L, Schmidt D H 1995 Heart disease and rehabilitation, 3rd edn. Human Kinetics, Champaign

Powell K E et al 1987 Physical activity and the incidence of coronary heart disease. Annual Review of Public Health 8: 253–287

Raffo J A et al 1980 Effects of physical training on myocardial ischaemia in patients with coronary artery disease. British Heart Journal 43: 262–269

Singh S J et al 1992 Development of a shuttle walking test of disability in patients with chronic airways obstruction. Thorax 47: 1019–1024

Soler-Soler J, Permanyer-Miralder G 1994 How do changes in lifestyle complement medical treatment in heart failure? British Heart Journal Supplement 72: 87–91

Thompson 1994 Cardiac rehabilitation services: the need to develop guidelines. Quality in Health Care 3: 169–172

Todd I C et al 1991 Effects of daily high intensity exercise on myocardial perfusion in angina pectoris. American Journal of Cardiology 68: 1593–1599

Uren N G, Lipkin D P 1992 Exercise training as therapy for chronic heart failure. British Heart Journal 67: 430-433

Audiovisual material

Gaskell J, Mowbray L 1995 Getting it right—the Y's guide to safe and effective exercise. London Central YMCA, London

FURTHER READING

Aliev T A 1993 Role of exercise in rehabilitation of coronary heart disease in cases combined with non insulin dependent diabetes mellitus. Sports Medicine, Training and Rehabilitation 4(1): 53–55

American Association of Cardiovascular and Pulmonary Rehabilitation 1995 Guidelines for cardiac rehabilitation programs, 2nd edn. Human Kinetics, Champaign
Particularly useful chapter for those interested in weight training for cardiac patients.

American College of Sports Medicine 1991 Guidelines for exercise testing and prescription, 4th edn. Lea and Febinger, Philadelphia
A comprehensive manual on exercise testing and prescribing for cardiac patients. Excellent as a quick source of information.

Astrand P-O, Rohdahl K 1986 Textbook of work physiology, 3rd edn. McGraw-Hill, New York
Comprehensive text on exercise physiology.

Douglas P S et al 1992 Exercise and atherosclerositic heart disease in women. Medicine and Science in Sports and Exercise 24(6): 5266–5276
Reviews published research on women and coronary heart disease and gives recommendations for future studies in this area.

National Forum for Coronary Heart Disease Prevention 1995 Physical activity: the agenda for action.
This report draws on the expertise, ideas and suggestions of Forum members to give a response to the Health of the Nation Physical Activity Task Force consultation paper. Points to the need for a coordinating strategy and sets out ideas for action by different sectors at national and local level.

Pollock M L, Schmidt D H 1995 Heart disease and rehabilitation, 3rd edn. Human Kinetics, Champaign
An excellent reference book which reviews all aspects of cardiac rehabilitation. Well referenced.

Wenger N K, Hellersten H K 1992 Rehabilitation of the coronary patient, 3rd edn. Churchill Livingstone, London

Booklets and leaflets
British Heart Foundation:

—Exercise for life! How to enjoy getting fit and staying fit.
This 16-page colour booklet provides information on how the heart works and the various ways you can keep fit.

—Put your heart into walking. How to keep your heart healthy and happy by walking your way to fitness.
This 6-page, A4 size booklet describes how walking can help your heart and provides an 'easy action plan'.

Chest, Heart and Stroke Association:

—Starting a cardiac support group.

A full range of leaflets and posters are available from the Health Promotion Department of your local health board.

USEFUL ADDRESSES

Association of Chartered Physiotherapists in Cardiac Rehabilitation
Chartered Society of Physiotherapy
14 Bedford Row
LONDON WC1R 4ED
Tel: 0171 242 1941

British Association of Cardiac Rehabilitation
Action Heart
Wellesley House
117 Wellington Road
DUDLEY DY1 1UB
Tel: 01384 230222

Cardiac Rehabilitation Interest Group, Scotland
c/o Physiotherapy Department
Stirling Royal Infirmary NHS Trust
Livilands
STIRLING FK8 2AU
Tel: 01786 434000

Scottish Sports Council
Caledonia House
South Gyle
EDINBURGH EH12 9DQ
Tel: 0131 225 8411

Health Education Board for Scotland
Woodburn House
Canaan Lane
EDINBURGH EH10 4SG
Tel: 0131 447 8044

Sports Council (England)
16 Upper Woburn Place
LONDON WC1H 0QP
Tel: 0171 388 1277

Health Education Authority
Hamilton House
Mabledon Place
LONDON WC1H 9TX
Tel: 0171 383 3833

Lifestyle management: behavioural change

Paul Bennett Douglas Carroll

8

Coronary heart disease (CHD) is dependent, to a large extent, on our behaviour and our psychological circumstances. Cigarette smoking, dietary behaviour, exercise levels, and the prevalence and impact of psychological stress are considered key behavioural risks. Major health promotion initiatives have attempted to bring about appropriate behavioural change through programmes targeted at large populations. Increasingly common, however, are programmes targeted at changing the behaviour of individuals identified through screening as being at risk (e.g. Bennett et al 1989).

This chapter will provide a brief overview of some of the processes thought to determine health-related behaviours. It will then examine how these, and a few relatively simple counselling methods, may help promote behavioural change. Space limitations mean that the issues and methods introduced here cannot be considered in great depth. A list of suggested reading, in which they are described in greater detail, is provided at the end of the chapter.

MODELS OF HEALTH BEHAVIOUR

Human behaviour is complex, and difficult to predict. Decisions are frequently a response to chance events and apparently random thought processes. Nevertheless, a number of models of behavioural decision-making have been developed. None pretends to be all encompassing. Rather, they try to provide a parsimonious understanding of at least some of the processes underlying our behaviour. Some of these models are described below. More complex models exist, but this section does not aspire to providing a text on psychology and human decision-making. Rather, it seeks to identify the basic processes to be considered when counselling behavioural change, particularly in relation to behaviours implicated in CHD.

The Health Belief Model

The Health Belief Model (HBM; Becker 1974) suggests that the likelihood of individuals engaging in a particular health-related behaviour is a function of their perceptions of the relationship between that behaviour and illness, their perceived susceptibility to that illness, its seriousness, and the particular costs and benefits involved in engaging in any behaviour. A final influence on the uptake of any behaviour is the presence of cues to action. These may take the form of a reminder to engage in some form of action, including such things as health checks, reminders from doctors on routine visits, and so on.

Although we may ultimately wish to optimize our health, whether or not we engage in behaviours likely to do so is as much, if not more, governed by short-term costs and benefits associated with any behaviour, than by longer-term possible health outcomes. For example, an individual may consider adopting a low-fat diet to reduce his risk of CHD, but be beset by more immediate problems. His family may not wish to change their diet, they may have to learn new cooking methods, eat less-favoured foods, perhaps even increase the cost of their shopping. These short-term costs may override the benefits of potential long-term health gains and prevent appropriate behavioural change. Research conducted with working-class mothers who smoke affords an example (e.g. Jacobson 1981). Many such women chose to smoke cigarettes in the full knowledge of the associated health risks. Those that did frequently reported that smoking helped them cope with adverse life conditions, and that they would be less able to cope with their responsibilities towards their family if they stopped smoking. To promote change in this group of women would clearly involve more than simple advice on the health risks of smoking.

Stages of change

A frequent assumption made in counselling is that the person receiving advice or counselling is willing and able to make use of any information given. This, clearly, is not always the case: people differ over time in their willingness to consider or adopt change. One of the first models to appreciate this was developed by Prochaska & DiClemente (1984). Their model was particularly useful as it identified both the process of change and the counselling strategies most likely to move people toward behavioural change.

Prochaska & DiClemente identified five stages of change. The first stage is known as precontemplation. Here, no or only occasional thought is given to adopting a new behaviour: most smokers, for example, at any one time are not actively considering stopping smoking. The next stage is known as contemplation, in which the individual begins to consider changing his or her behaviour. The movement from precontemplation to contemplation may result from an individual developing a chest infection, hearing of the illness of a fellow smoker, and so on. Reaching this stage does not, however, guarantee behavioural change, and people can still slip back to the pre-contemplation stage (for example, when they recover from illness), and frequently do. However, some may move to a more active consideration of change, even achieving behavioural change. The stages of active consideration and achievement of change are referred to as the 'planning' and 'action' stages. The final stage is one of consolidation and maintenance of any behavioural change. However, a frequent risk at this stage is that the person relapses to the contemplation or even precontemplation stage.

In any counselling process it is important that the counsellor be aware of what stage the client is at. Providing strategies for smoking cessation to a smoker at the precontemplation stage is likely to be ineffective. Rather, strategies should seek to shift the smoker into the contemplation or even planning stage. There is good evidence that such a shift is rarely achieved through direct attempts at persuasion, which often harden attitudes rather than change them (whatever the person may say at the time of interview). However, a technique known as motivational interviewing, described later in the chapter, may be of use here.

Social learning theory

A basic tenet of social learning theory (SLT; Bandura 1977) is that behaviour is guided by its expected consequences. The more positive these are, the more likely one is to engage in any particular behaviour. That said, many behaviours persist when what may seem to be negative health consequences are likely to follow. One reason for this is that in general, short-term outcomes are far more powerful than longer-term ones in determining behaviour. Thus, smokers frequently continue to smoke, although aware of the dangers of smoking, because the short-term rewards of smoking (and fear of immediate negative consequences of quitting, such as withdrawal symptoms) are more salient than long-term probabilistic health gains.

One particularly important aspect of SLT is self-efficacy, which refers to a person's confidence in his or her ability to carry out an action or achieve a particular goal. People are unlikely to attempt change if they do not think they will succeed in doing so. This has powerful implications for counselling. First of all, it suggests that any suggested behavioural change must lie within the perceived capabilities of the individual, by gradual stages if necessary. Secondly, it cautions against decisions concerning behavioural change being determined by epidemiological considerations alone. For example, if a person carries several risk factors for CHD, including smoking, poor diet and lack of exercise, it may be tempting to first try to address the most 'risky' behaviour, in this case probably smoking. However, if the person does not believe he can quit smoking, his consequent lack of success may make him reluctant to try to change other 'risky' behaviours.

The theory of planned behaviour

Throughout much of the 1950s and 1960s psychologists and policy makers operated mainly under the assumption that individuals' attitudes were the primary determinants of their behaviour, and that to change behaviour simply required changing attitudes. Thus, smokers were assumed to smoke because they had a positive attitude towards smoking rather than because of addictive processes or social pressure.

In an attempt to identify key determinants of behaviour which included attitudes as contributing to behavioural decisions but not central to them, Ajzen (1985) developed a model involving three basic processes. In this model, the key determinant of behaviour is one's intention to behave in a certain way. Behavioural intentions are, in turn, derived from three broad influences: the individuals' attitudes to the behaviour, the attitudes they perceive others important to them as having (so-called social norms), and the 'availability' of the behaviour to them. Availability refers to whether or not individuals have access to a given behaviour, recognizing the economic, social, and personal constraints that may exist. This model explains, at least in part, why people do not always behave in accordance with their attitudes. Some ex-smokers, for example, may have a number of negative attitudes towards smoking, but smoke when out with friends who smoke, as the social pressure they encounter may compete with their personal attitudes. What the model does not address are findings that although attitudes, social norms and availability strongly predict intentions to behave in certain ways, intentions frequently do not predict behaviour: 'the road to hell is paved with good intentions'.

Comment

These models provide some understanding of the decision-making process related to health behaviours. None provides a complete account. Between them, however, they offer some insight into the processes which govern health-related decisions. The most important message is that while potential health gain informs behaviour and behaviour change, it is only part of the explanation.

CHANGING BEHAVIOUR

The process of helping people change their behaviour can vary in complexity from simple provision of information to dealing with complex issues and adverse emotional responses to hearing health risk information. The approach that needs to be followed will be determined by, amongst other things, the length of time available for counselling, the characteristics of the individual being screened, and the 'depth' to which the counsellor is prepared to explore issues relevant to the patient. The following section will examine three issues: motivating behavioural change; facilitating behavioural change through information giving; and helping people cope with the adverse emotional effects of receiving risk information.

Some basic skills

Whatever approach is adopted, some basic skills are necessary to involve people in the counselling process. A key predictor of adherence to recommended therapeutic regimens is an individual's level of satisfaction with his or her care. This in turn is strongly influenced by the quality of communication with professional staff. Friendliness and warmth are obvious prerequisites. Ideally, the participants should sit at approximately right angles with no obstacles such as a desk in the way. This arrangement allows each person to see the other person fully, and to make and break eye contact as necessary. Direct face-to-face contact makes it difficult to look away and can be seen as confrontational. An open posture, sitting very slightly forward, emphasizes interest and listening.

Motivating behavioural change

There is a clear goal to screening: to identify and, where possible, change risk factors for CHD. However, it should not be assumed that those attending screening are motivated and willing to change. For this reason, identification of a person's willingness to make behavioural change is an important part of assessment. Following assessment of CHD risk, it is useful to identify at what stage of change the person is in relation to each risk behaviour, and to attempt to move him or her towards appropriate behavioural change. As previously noted, this is usually not best achieved through direct attempts at persuasion; rather, people may best be moved towards change or consideration of change through their own analysis of the advantages and disadvantages of their present behaviour and any possible behavioural change. For individuals in the precontemplative stage, a goal of this approach may simply be to shift them to the contemplation stage; for others, it may serve to increase their motivation to make a change in behaviour that they had already intended.

A key strategy is to focus people's attention on both the 'good' and 'less good' aspects of the behaviour they may benefit from changing. By inviting the people to consider both 'good' and 'less good' aspects of their behaviour, they may experience dissonance and begin to consider change, without the pressure resulting from more direct attempts at persuasion. Focusing first on the 'good things' about their behaviour reduces threat or confrontation. Individuals can then be asked to identify the 'less good'. Open questioning techniques may facilitate exploration of these issues. Finally, the counsellor can summarize both good and less good aspects of the behaviour, so they are starkly identified:

- What are the good things about your (lack of exercise)?
- What are the less good things about your (lack of exercise)?
  —How does it affect you?
  —What don't you like about it?
- Summary of the information given, in 'you' language: e.g. 'So, not exercising gives you time to . . . . On the other hand . . .'.

Following this phase, it may be useful to ask whether the individual would like information about the issues raised in this discussion. The decision whether to offer information or not must depend on the individual's response to this inquiry. Some will make it clear that they are not interested, whereas others may be neutral or willing to consider change.

Information exchange

To maximize the effectiveness of any information given, it is important that it is presented in a manner which makes it easy to understand and remember. Unfortunately, this is not always the case. When dealing with a variety of behaviours, advice is often presented piecemeal. Issues related to smoking are dealt with after taking a smoking history, dietary advice is given following discussion of eating habits, and so on. Such an approach necessarily interrupts the acquisition of information with discussion of new issues, interfering with memory and consideration of any information given. Accordingly, advice on behavioural change should generally be presented at the end of any screening interview. Some simple guidelines can ensure maximal impact of any information given. These are described by Nichols (1987), who identified three stages in the process of giving information:

- initial check on the person's present level of knowledge
- information provision
- accuracy check: ensuring any information has been remembered and understood.

Information check

Before giving information it is important to find out what the person knows and, indeed what he or she wants to know. Unnecessary reiteration can thus be avoided and information pitched at a level consistent with the individual's present knowledge. It will also allow the counsellor to identify any misconceptions the person has about his or her risk or risk behaviours.

Information provision

The language used should be appropriate to the person to whom the information is being given. Jargon should be avoided. This sounds simple, yet words and phrases that are routine to health care workers may be totally alien to others. Equally, vague phrases, such as, 'Your blood pressure is a little high' are best avoided. These frequently confuse and can lead to a misunderstanding of the nature of the problem.

Where a number of risk factors are identified, it may be best to focus on only one of them, and to suggest that the person returns to discuss the others. In addition, it is important to identify which of any risk or preventive behaviours the person would like to know about. Basing the choice of information solely on epidemiological risk ('Your smoking is probably causing you the most risk for heart disease. Perhaps I could give you some advice on how to cut down . . .') is likely to be of little benefit. Asking people what they wish to know about is more likely to identify behaviours amenable to change. Once the areas of information have been chosen, a few rules of thumb may help effective information exchange:

- do not overload people with information; if necessary, they can come back for more
- information should be given clearly in short and simple sentences
- the language used should mirror that of the person

- information should be given issue by issue, not as a jumble of related and unrelated information
- repetition increases memory—in the words of a famous researcher in doctor–patient recall: 'Tell what you're going to tell 'em, tell 'em, tell 'em what you've told 'em'.

Some of these points are exemplified in the following dialogue between a practice nurse and a smoker with a high serum cholesterol level:

Nurse: As you know, we've found some things which increase your risk of having a heart attack. It's no news to you that you smoke, and you know this raises your risk. But you didn't know that your cholesterol levels were high. If you would like to reduce your risk of heart attack, it would be helpful to cut out your smoking and reduce your cholesterol levels. I wonder how you feel about doing either of these . . .

Mr J: Well, I've tried to stop smoking so many times. I know its bad for me, but it's really difficult to stop. My cholesterol reading was a bit of a shock, though—perhaps I could have a go at changing that.

Nurse: OK; let's talk about how to reduce your cholesterol now. If you would like to look at some ways of cutting down smoking, perhaps we could do that another time. What do you think that you are eating or doing that is making your cholesterol levels high?

Later:

Nurse: From what you've told me, I think there are a number of things you could do to reduce your cholesterol levels. Firstly, you could cut down the amount of fatty meat you eat and eat more vegetables. Secondly, you could change how you cook some of your food. Finally, you could reduce the amount of crisps and chocolate you eat, perhaps by replacing them with a lower-fat snack. Let's look at each of those in turn . . . .

In this condensed and brief dialogue the nurse has gone through some of the key stages in appropriate advice giving. First of all, he identified what Mr J wanted advice on at present, while making it clear that advice on other issues could be given another time should Mr J wish it. He then explored Mr J's understanding of the causes of his high cholesterol levels. Finally, at the end of this process, the nurse broke down the type of information to be given into three clear categories: cutting down fatty meat; changing cooking methods; changing snacks. This explicit categorization, followed by more detailed information on each issue, increases the likelihood that the information will be remembered.

Accuracy check

People may nod their heads in the right places, but nevertheless, not have understood all that they have been told. It is important to check explicitly that they have understood any information given. If nothing else, such a check will serve to strengthen memory. It will also reduce the risk of inappropriate action arising from misunderstanding. Care must be taken not to patronize, but an accuracy check can be achieved with some subtlety by, for example, asking patients whether they have any questions, whether explanations were clear, or which of any suggestions made they may find useful to try out.

The impact of adverse health information

Although for the professionals involved, the identification of risk factors for CHD and facilitating appropriate change are routine procedures, some individuals will inevitably respond to information with alarm and anxiety. Indeed, one study found that over one-third of people who had their cholesterol measured and were found to have 'safe' levels still reported significantly increased health anxieties many months after the screening procedure. Not surprisingly, then, the impact of receiving adverse health information can, in a substantial number of persons, result in significant anxiety. This may have a number of outcomes. As well as the obvious distress, anxiety may interfere in a number of ways with how people use any information given following such knowledge.

The most immediate effect is that people may take little notice of what they are told following this information. Anxiety interferes with concentration and memory, so people may simply not take in or retain any information given in a counselling session. In the longer term, anxiety may result in the individual feeling overwhelmed and not able to use any advice given. Conversely, it may result in excessive and inappropriate behavioural change (see Case Study 8.1).

Coming to terms with bad news

The first part of helping people deal constructively with adverse risk information is to help them come to some sort of understanding of the risk they have to deal with and give them some time to process the information.

Case Study 8.1

Mr F was screened for CHD risk as part a local screening programme. He was advised to cut down his saturated fat intake and to take more exercise in order to reduce his risk. 3 months later he was seen by the dietitian to monitor progress. Despite not being overweight at the time of initial counselling, in the 3 months following screening he had lost over 2 stones in weight. He looked haggard and his clothes were, almost literally, hanging off him. He told the dietitian that he had cut his fat intake drastically, through eating vegetables, salad and very little else. He was frightened to eat anything which he thought contained fat. His family were experiencing problems as they could not cope with the diet he had imposed on himself, and his wife was preparing his food separately from that for the rest of the family. He was exercising constantly, and spent up to 2 hours a day exercising by riding his bicycle. He was also very anxious about his cholesterol and fretted about it on a daily basis. The changes he had made, while apparently complying with the advice given, were excessive and had resulted in his and his family's misery. Appropriate care at the time of initial counselling may have prevented this rather worrying response.

Having informed an individual of his or her risk, some pause in the counselling process may be advisable. To find out how the person feels, a simple question may suffice. If any factual concerns are expressed, these may be allayed by provision of information. If the person expresses more serious upset, time may be required to permit expression of any fears or anxieties. It is important at this stage that the person is made to feel that it is acceptable to express upset or concern.

Tempting as it may be, the goal of the counsellor is not to try to reassure inappropriately, but to allow the individual to talk about his or her feelings and emotions. Listening quietly may be the counsellor's only response at this stage. If concerns are felt, but not expressed, individuals may be too distracted by their own thoughts to process any information given. Only after a period in which anxieties are expressed, may some people be receptive to information concerning how they may reduce their risk for CHD.

A PROBLEM-SOLVING APPROACH

While many individuals will require relatively simple advice, and act upon it appropriately, the advice necessary and how this may be implemented may not always be obvious. Consider the case of Mrs T (Case Study 8.2).

The case history, while being perhaps somewhat unusual in its specifics, highlights a common problem resulting from inappropriate or casual advice

---

Case Study 8.2

Mrs T, a 43-year-old obese woman, attended a screening programme for CHD risks conducted in her local GP's surgery. She was found not only to be significantly overweight, but also to have raised serum cholesterol levels. As a consequence she attended a clinic where she was seen by a dietitian. She was given advice on 'healthy eating' and a diet sheet, and asked to come back in 1 month. When her weight and cholesterol levels were measured 1 month later, they were found to be unchanged; if anything, they had increased.

At this point the dietitian explored in depth some of the issues preventing change. Mrs T actually had a good idea of what comprised a 'healthy' and 'unhealthy ' diet and had been placed on similar diets to the one prescribed a number of times previously, but all to no avail. Further discussion revealed that the main reason for her eating excessively and consuming high-fat food was lack of support within her family. Her two sons, who had flats of their own, but who used the family home much as a hotel would frequently arrive home from the pub late at night and demand a 'fry up'. She, reluctantly, accepted the role of provider and cooked their food, but found it difficult not to nibble while she did so. As a result, although she may have eaten carefully during the day, she frequently finished the day eating high-fat foods. Not only did this increase her calorific intake, it also reduced her motivation to diet the following day, as she saw herself as having 'ruined' her diet. This recurring process significantly eroded her motivation to diet over the longer term. Thus, the problem now needing solving was not what to eat, but how to manage within this particular context.

giving. The person may (or may not) wish to comply with the advice given, but other things get in the way. A more thorough process of engendering change may be to facilitate identification of both what changes are desired and how they may be achieved.

One way that this may be achieved is through a process of counselling developed by Gerald Egan. Central to Egan's approach is that the job of the counsellor (or helper as he phrases it) is not to act as an expert solving the person's problems. Instead, the counsellor's role is to mobilize the individual's own resources both to identify problems accurately and to arrive at strategies of solution. Counselling is problem oriented. It is focused specifically on the issues at hand and in the 'here and now'. Egan's model of counselling involves three phases:

- problem exploration and clarification
- goal setting
- facilitating action.

Some people may not need to work through each stage of the counselling process. Others may be able to work through all the phases in one session. Yet others may require more than one session.

Problem exploration and clarification

The goal of the first stage of counselling is to help the person identify the problems he or she is facing (or may face) in achieving change. The problem can be merely lack of information, in which case provision of information may be all that is required. However, individuals can face other problems. Some of these may surface immediately on receiving initial health information ('I'm not sure how I'm going to sort these dietary changes with my family') or later ('I don't know—I tried to carry out your advice on cutting down fat, but my weight still seems to be going up'). Responses of this sort should prompt further probing. The goal is to clarify *exactly* what the problems faced are.

It is important to deal with each stage sequentially and thoroughly. Flitting from stage to stage will serve only to confuse both the counsellor and the individual, while thoroughness will reduce the risk of identifying incorrect problems or solutions, as in the case of Mrs T. Some skills or strategies that are particularly pertinent to this stage of counselling are listed below:

- direct questioning and prompts
- silence and minimal prompts
- empathic feedback.

The most obvious way of eliciting information is to ask direct questions. These should be open-ended, in order to discourage one-word answers. Questions such as 'What do your family eat on a typical weekend?' are likely to elicit much more information than 'How often do your family eat green vegetables?' A second approach similar to direct questioning is known as prompting. Here, requests for information take the form of prompts and probes requesting information: 'Tell me about . . .', 'Describe . . .'.

It is important to mix direct questioning with other techniques of encouraging the person to explore relevant issues. One such method involves the use of silence or minimal prompts ('uh-huh'). By its very nature, problem exploration leads individuals to consider matters they have not previously addressed. The process cannot be rushed, and filling silences with new questions may interrupt their thoughts and impede the proper exploration of problems.

A further method of encouraging problem exploration is through the use of empathic feedback. Reflecting back to people an understanding of their situation or feelings through a simple phrase can be highly effective. Such feedback also serves to verify the counsellor's understanding.

Take the example of Mrs T:

Mrs T: Well it's disappointing that my cholesterol levels haven't changed, but I really have no willpower. As soon as I just look at food I seem to put on weight.

Counsellor: That seems nothing short of miraculous! It may help us to find out what you are eating that's causing the problem. What do *you* think is keeping your weight on?

Mrs T: I don't know (*pause*). Well I know what to eat, and when to eat. It seems so difficult to stick to a diet sometimes, though. Sometimes I stick to the diet, but often the whole things seems to collapse. I don't know—nothing seems to work with me.

Counsellor: You seem quite despondent. But, you can eat appropriately at times. Tell me about the things that get in the way of dieting.

Mrs T: Oh, there's lots of things. But I suppose one thing that really gets me down is the way my boys treat the house like a hotel and expect me to cook for them all the time. And they always want fry ups!

Here, the counsellor has managed through direct questioning to move from a situation where everything and nothing seems to be contributing to Mrs T's failure to lose weight to identification of a key factor. She also highlighted the success Mrs T did report, in an attempt to focus on her success and to increase her confidence that change is achievable.

Goal setting

Once particular problems have been identified, some people may feel they have the resources to deal with them and may need no further help in making appropriate changes. Others, however, may need further support in arriving at some ideas about how to cope with such obstacles. The first stage in change is for the individual to decide the goals he or she wishes to achieve, and to help the individual frame his or her goals in specific rather than general terms (e.g. 'I will go to the gym on Tuesday and Thursday evenings' versus 'I must do more exercise').

If the final goal seems too difficult to achieve in one step, the elaboration of sub-goals working towards the final goal should be encouraged. Short-term success in achieving modest, short-term goals is more likely to motivate further change than pursuing difficult-to-attain, long-term goals. It is easier to lose 2 pounds of weight per week than to strive for a 3-stone weight loss over an ill-defined time period.

Goals must pay heed to people's resources, and their social and environmental circumstances. Even a short walk lasting 10 minutes two or three times a week may be a sufficient initial goal for a 'couch potato'. Goals which are too adventurous may prove impossible to achieve, and the resultant failure foster a general unwillingness to attempt future change: 'I knew it would happen; I tried and I failed'. In the case of Mrs T, the aim at this stage of counselling would be to identify goals both in terms of weight loss and not cooking 'fry ups' for her sons. How she sets about achieving these can then be explored in detail in the third stage of counselling.

Some goals may be apparent following the problem exploration phase. However, should this not be the case, Egan identified a series of strategies designed to help the client identify and set goals:

- summarizing
- providing relevant information
- challenging to provide new perspectives.

A good summary provides a concise and structured means for focusing on the changes required.

Counsellor: Let's look at what we've got now. You've identified a number of things which are contributing to your weight problem. You find it difficult to keep long-term targets, such as losing 2 stones of weight before Christmas, you don't exercise as much as you used to, and you've developed a liking for ice cream . . .

Mrs F: Yes, that about sums it up. I guess I do need to do something about these things. I suppose I could set about doing more exercise . . .

Challenge involves inviting the person to explore new perspectives. It is particularly useful when the person appears locked into old ways of thinking or feels little can be done. Several types of challenge have been identified, including invitations to explore new solutions and 'identification of possibilities'.

As noted in the section on motivational interviewing, direct challenges, however well phrased (Well, why don't you try to lose 2 pounds of weight a week?), are likely to result in resistance to change or feelings of defeat. Therefore, the person should be invited to explore new solutions, deploying phrases like:

- Perhaps it would be useful to look at some different ways of looking at solutions to this problem.
- I wonder if there are any other things you could do to deal with this problem.

Facilitating action
Once goals have been established in the second phase of counselling, some individuals may feel they need no further support in achieving them. Others,

who by this stage may have a good idea of what they want to achieve, can remain unsure of how to achieve them. Discussion between the counsellor and the person may still be necessary. One useful strategy at this stage is to brainstorm. This involves thinking through as many possibilities as possible, forsaking quality for quantity. Once a list has been generated, these possibilities can then be sifted and focused strategies developed:

Counsellor: Be as adventurous as you like—just think of as many solutions as you can. We can weed out the good ideas in a few minutes. You never know, some of the 'crazy' solutions may turn out to be the answer to the problem.

Consider the possibilities simply for establishing a new 'fitness plan':

- join a local gymnasium
- attend aerobic classes at a leisure centre
- walk or cycle to work
- join up with friends to form an exercise group
- set up a crèche with friends to take it in turns to look after children while you exercise
- go for a brisk walk during the lunch hour
- buy a bicycle
- attend a course of lessons in a new sport
- buy an aerobics videotape
- walk to the local shops instead of taking the car.

Exercises

To practise listening skills
Sit with a friend for a period of 10 minutes, and use the various strategies to explore an interest they have or an issue they wish to explore. Try not to interrupt or interject your own ideas or things you wish to say, and to keep them focused on the issue at hand. The goal is simply to listen and allow the other person to talk about *one* issue. Sounds simple, but this exercise can be extremely difficult.

More advanced practise
To practise more skills, it may be helpful to role play with a colleague a problem presented by a client you have seen recently. Explicitly stage the process through the three phases of counselling and stop after each phase to discuss how the experience of being counselled felt from the client's perspective. The goal is not to provide expert feedback, but that of the client. This, after all, is the most important aspect of counselling, and can provide important insights into your own skills and methods.

STRESS AND STRESS MANAGEMENT TRAINING

As noted previously, helping people cope with the stress of receiving 'bad news' can involve listening to them express their anxieties and concerns, so these can be dealt with constructively. However, many people report having to cope with long-term stress resulting from their life situation. Although there are a number of stress management techniques that may help people cope with stress, these should not be seen as distinct from the approach developed by Egan. To achieve some goals, it may be necessary to learn new skills and coping strategies. Stress management skills may be seen as falling into this category.

Most stress management strategies are based on the model of stress developed by Lazarus & Folkman (1984). This model suggests that stress is a process, and can be described as a series of stages. The first stage of the stress process is usually (but not exclusively) an environmental event. But we do not all respond to such events in the same way. Some may respond to a high stress work situation with enthusiasm and enjoyment; others may feel overwhelmed and distressed. The trigger event, therefore, forms the beginning of a complex chain of internal events, and cannot be seen simply as the 'stress' in itself. The next stage in the process involves an appraisal of the environmental stimulus. If regarded as something the person feels confident he or she can cope with, an event is likely to have minimal impact. A stress response will occur when the event is viewed as demanding or having potential harm to the individual, *and* the individual feels he or she will have difficulty in coping. The response may involve increased autonomic arousal, increased muscular tension, feeling 'stressed' or anxious, and some degree of 'stressed' behaviour.

Stress management involves dealing with each of the stages in the stress process. Stress may be obviated by changing environmental circumstances. It may be reduced by modifying the individual's various responses to these circumstances. Relaxation is the stress management skill most frequently taught. It can be useful for a number of reasons. First of all, it can reduce unpleasant physical sensations and chronic tiredness. Secondly, it provides individuals with a means of gaining some control over their response to stress. Finally, relaxation is relatively easy to teach and use. This section will concentrate on teaching these skills. Other techniques involved in stress management are discussed in Meichenbaum (1985) and, in the context of CHD, by Bennett (1993).

Relaxation training

The aim of relaxation training is to help people be as relaxed as possible throughout the day and, in particular, at times of stress. Although learning relaxation involves lying or sitting quietly for some minutes away from the hustle and bustle of everyday life, its ultimate value is in its application at times of stress. There is little to be gained by becoming increasingly tense during the day and only unwinding at night in a comfy chair. However expert someone may become in this sort of relaxation, it will do little to ameliorate the effects of daily stress. Learning to use relaxation skills appropriately involves developing awareness of stress evidenced through physical tension throughout the day and learning to minimize this tension. It is best achieved using three, interacting, approaches:

- learning relaxation skills
- learning to monitor tension in daily life
- learning to use relaxation skills at times of stress.

Learning relaxation skills

The acquisition of relaxation skills is best achieved in stages. The first involves learning to relax under optimal conditions. Ideally, the person should be talked through a series of relaxation instructions by the counsellor before practising at home. Time, and other considerations, often preclude this, and home practice with a tape has to suffice. The most effective tapes promote gradual relaxation throughout the body, by means of tensing and relaxing specific muscle groups systematically. The order in which the muscles are relaxed varies, but a typical exercise may involve the following stages (the tensing procedure is described in brackets):

- hands and forearms (making a fist)
- upper arms (touching fingers to shoulder)
- shoulders and lower neck (hunching shoulders)
- back of neck (pushing back against support)
- lips (pushing them together)
- forehead (frowning)
- abdomen/chest (holding deep breath)
- abdomen (tensing stomach muscles)
- lower legs and feet (pointing foot up and toward head, not lifting leg).

Each muscle group should be tensed just sufficiently to feel the effects, affording practice at recognizing and relaxing away 'normal' levels of tension.

Relaxation is best practised in a situation where the person can relax fully and easily. However, in order to apply relaxation at times of actual stress, regular daily practice is essential. Individuals need to overlearn the skill, so that it becomes a habitual response and can be performed 'to order'. As they become more practised, they can cut down the tensing component, focusing instead on the immediate relaxation of the muscle groups. The regularity of practice can be reduced with developing expertise.

Monitoring physical tension

While learning relaxation skills, individuals can begin to monitor their levels of physical tension. As they learn to relax, most people become increasingly aware of periods during the day when they are particularly tense, or incidents in the day which may trigger tension. Formal stress management programmes often ask people to record their tension at regular intervals during the day or when they are feeling particularly tense, as this helps to identify likely triggers and any pattern of stress that may occur (see Table 8.1). This may feel too formal for many counsellors, but can be a useful exercise. Note in the example that the stressors identified are those of everyday life, the stressors most people have to deal with using stress management techniques.

Using relaxation skills

To be useful, relaxation needs to be integrated into daily life. After 1 or

Table 8.1 A typical 'tension diary'

Time	Level of tension (0–10)	Trigger
08.00	9	Rushing to get kids to child minder
09.00	6	Driving and arriving at work—still feel rushed
10.00	4	General tension at work
11.00	2	Coffee break—bliss!
12.00	3	General work
13.00	7	Annoyed—had to work over lunch

2 weeks of monitoring tension and learning relaxation, patients can begin to gradually incorporate relaxation into their daily lives. This can be done by using tension as a cue to attempt to relax. Use can be made of coffee and other breaks during the day to relax fully. However, the goal of relaxation training is to help people relax as fully as is appropriate while maintaining their daily routine or when dealing with particular stressors. This level of relaxation takes practice and time to achieve. Accordingly, relaxation is best used to reduce even relatively low levels of excess tension. Accumulated minor stresses during the day can be more wearing than occasional larger stresses. In addition, the consistent use of relaxation techniques can prepare the person to cope with times of greater stress: without practice, use of relaxation skills at such times may be difficult if not impossible.

CONCLUSIONS

Facilitating behavioural change in those at risk for CHD should reduce risk of disease. However, while optimizing health is a goal of screening, individuals' motivation and ability to change are frequently more rooted in the 'here and now'. Some people may not place a high value on possible future health gain some years hence and be unwilling or unready to change. Others may be motivated and able to act on information provided during the screening process. Yet others may wish to change, but lack the confidence or problem-solving skills to enable this.

The goal of the counsellor is to identify where in this continuum of change people lie and to tailor any intervention accordingly. Those who are un-motivated may benefit from the opportunity simply to consider the pros and cons of change, with the goal of counselling being no more than to facilitate this process. Those in the second group will benefit from clear and structured information provision. The final group will benefit most from a problem-solving approach such as that developed by Egan.

Use of the strategies for facilitating behavioural change suggested here may mean that the screening process takes longer than many of the original (e.g. Fullard et al 1983) models of screening and counselling. It is difficult, if not impossible, to conduct the form of information-giving or counselling described here within the 20 minutes per person time constraints initially considered to be about the optimum. However, the probability of achieving lasting behavioural change in any but the most motivated and self-confident individual is significantly greater than that likely to be achieved by the simple educational techniques advocated by these models. Accordingly, while they may appear time-consuming, their 'cost-effectiveness' is likely to be high.

■ KEY POINTS

• Decisions concerning health-related behaviours are not simply based on their health consequences. Other factors involved include the immediate costs and benefits of engaging in any behaviour and the availability of the behaviour to the individual.

• At any one time an individual may be more or less motivated to change his or her behaviour. A key aspect of counselling is to identify what 'stage of change' the individual is at, and to tailor any intervention accordingly.

• The quality of communication in the counselling process is central to facilitating appropriate behavioural change.

• Even where any behavioural change required is relatively simple, time should be given to exploring motivational factors and enhancing motivation to change.

• Facilitating some behavioural change may simply require the provision of appropriate information. This process involves: an initial check on present knowledge; the provision of information; and an accuracy check.

• Information given should be structured and relevant to the individual's level of knowledge and the individual's own desired behavioural change.

• Care should be taken to detect and pre-empt inappropriate levels of anxiety following the provision of adverse health information.

• Facilitating behavioural change may require more complex counselling. This may involve three stages: problem exploration and clarification; goal setting; facilitating action.

• Skills and strategies primarily involved in the problem exploration stage are: direct questioning and prompts; silence and minimal prompts; and empathic feedback.

• Goals must be concrete and within the resources of the individual. Some strategies which may help individuals define their goals are: summarizing; providing relevant information; challenge.

• One useful way of facilitating plans for achieving goals is the use of 'brainstorm' techniques.

• Stress is a process, with identifiable, interacting, 'stages': a 'trigger event'; cognitive appraisal; and a stress response including stressed behaviour and physical tension.

• Relaxation focuses on one part of this process, reducing physical tension. Learning relaxation involves three stages: learning relaxation skills; learning to monitor tension in daily life; and learning to use relaxation skills at times of stress.

REFERENCES

Ajzen I 1985 From intentions to action: a theory of planned behavior. In: Kuhl J, Beckman J (eds) Action control: from cognitions to behaviors. Springer, New York

Bandura A 1977 Social learning theory. Prentice Hall, Engelwood Cliffs, NJ

Becker M H 1974 The health belief model and personal health behaviour. Health Education Monographs 2: 324–508

Bennett P, Blackall M, Clapham M, Little S, Williams K 1989 South Birmingham Coronary Prevention Project: a district approach to the prevention of heart disease. Community Medicine 11: 90–96

Egan G 1990 The skilled helper: models, skills, and methods for effective helping. Brooks/Cole Publishing, Monterey

Fullard E, Fowler A, Gray J A M 1983 Facilitating prevention in primary care. British Medical Journal 289: 1585–1587

Jacobson B 1981 The ladykillers: why smoking is a feminist issue. Pluto, London

Lazarus R S, Folkman S 1984 Stress, appraisal and coping. Springer, New York

Prochaska J O, DiClemente C C 1984 The transtheoretical approach: crossing traditional foundations of change. Don Jones, Irwin, Homewood, IL

FURTHER READING

Bennett P 1993 Counselling for heart disease. British Psychological Society, Leicester

Covers the issues discussed in the present chapter in more detail, as well as examining others, such as Type A behaviour and smoking cessation methods.

Egan G 1990 The skilled helper: models, skills, and methods for effective helping. Brooks/Cole Publishing, Monterey

Arguably, the *text on counselling behavioural change. Perhaps more detailed than some would wish for, but nevertheless an excellent text.*

Meichenbaum D 1985 Stress inoculation training. Pergamon Press, Oxford

A simple, easy to follow, text with lots of examples of the use of stress management principles and techniques.

Nichols K A 1987 Psychological care in physical illness. Croom Helm, London

Rollnick S, Heather N, Bell A 1992 Negotiating behaviour change in medical settings: the development of brief motivational interviewing. Journal of Mental Health 1: 25–37

A simple introduction to the techniques of motivational interviewing.

Medical management of coronary heart disease

Keith G. Oldroyd

■ CONTENTS

At the time that a patient is shown to have coronary heart disease (CHD), primary prevention, if any ever took place, has by definition failed. Two related issues then confront the patient and his/her clinician. Firstly, how best to address the current manifestations (symptoms) of the disease and secondly, what to do to prevent further clinical events or deterioration in symptoms in the future, i.e. secondary prevention. This chapter will concentrate on the use of drug therapy and various forms of mechanical revascularization to procure these twin goals.

ANGINA

Angina has three cardinal features. These are retrosternal chest discomfort, provocation by exertion or stress and prompt relief by rest or the administration of nitrates. Patients with two out of three of these characteristics are considered to have atypical chest pain and patients with only one out of three should be described as having non-cardiac chest pain. Thus angina is a clinical diagnosis and the typical history is easy to recognize. The majority of patients with genuine angina have CHD but it is important to remember that a significant minority have other forms of cardiovascular disease such as valvular heart disease, particularly aortic stenosis and cardiomyopathy. A small number of patients with angina have no currently identifiable cardiac disease.

Drug treatment of angina

Nitrates

Nitrates in their various forms are an essential component of the drug therapy of angina. Their main mode of action is venous dilatation with consequent reductions in preload and myocardial oxygen demand. At higher doses direct arterial dilatation can be produced. The vascular effects of nitrates are not dependent on the presence of an intact endothelium. Sublingual glyceryl trinitrate is used for rapid relief of acute anginal attacks. Tablets are much less expensive than sprays in frequent users. The cost difference narrows in less-frequent users, since opened tablets should be replaced after 8 weeks. Isosorbide dinitrate or mononitrate can be used for prophylaxis of angina. An asymmetric regimen (8 a.m., 2 p.m. and 6 p.m. for dinitrate and 8 a.m. and 2 p.m. for mononitrate) is recommended to avoid tolerance. Transdermal nitrate patches are available as are once-daily modified-release oral nitrate preparations. The latter are designed to prevent the development of tolerance but they are very expensive and some authorities recommend their use only for individual patients unable to comply with asymmetric regimes. Buccal administration of nitrates avoids problems of variable absorption and may be a viable alternative to intravenous therapy in patients with unstable angina or heart failure. The main adverse effects of nitrates are headache, flushing and postural hypotension which can be particularly troublesome in the elderly (Table 9.1).

Beta-adrenoceptor blockers

Beta-blockers (Table 9.2) reduce myocardial oxygen consumption by slowing the heart rate both at rest and on exercise and by reducing the force of contraction of the myocardium. So-called cardioselective beta-blockers have

Table 9.1 Side effect profiles of antianginal drugs

	Bradycardia AV block	Worsening of LV dysfunction	Headache flushing	Gastro-intestinal symptoms	Broncho-constriction
Beta-blockers	+++	++	0	+	+++
Nifedipine	0	0	+++	+	0
Diltiazem	+	+	+	+	0
Verapamil	++	++	+	++	0
Nitrates	0	0	+++	+	0

Table 9.2 Selected properties and maintenance doses of a variety of beta-blockers

	Cardioselective	Vasodilatation	Usual daily dose in angina (mg)
Atenolol	+	–	50–100
Metoprolol	+	–	100–200
Bisoprolol	+	–	5–10
Timolol	–	–	20–40
Propranolol	–	–	120–240
Sotalol	–	–	160–240
Labetolol	Beta$_2$ agonist	+	400–800
Carvedilol	–	+	25–50

less activity at beta$_2$-receptors but they are not cardiospecific and will still provoke bronchoconstriction in patients with reversible airways obstruction. Beta-blockers are often the agents of first choice for the treatment of angina. They are very effective and have additional cardioprotective effects although this has only been demonstrated in patients with a prior history of myocardial infarction (MI). The main adverse effects are excessive bradycardia, worsening of ventricular dysfunction and bronchoconstriction (Table 9.1). Some beta-blockers have additional vasodilatory effects. Sotalol has additional Class III antiarrhythmic activity. Although there is no correlation between lipid solubility and central nervous system side effects, if these are a problem switching to a drug with low lipophilicity such as atenolol may help. Beta-blockers with partial agonist activity (intrinsic sympathetic activity, ISA) are generally avoided as they have not been shown to possess the cardioprotective effects of beta-blockers without this property. One drawback of beta-blockers without ISA is their potential to adversely affect lipid profiles with a tendency to increase triglyceride and lower HDL-cholesterol levels.

Calcium channel blockers

There are three distinct types of calcium antagonist in common use; the dihydropyridines of which nifedipine was the first of the several currently available, diltiazem and verapamil. The dihydropyridines act mainly on vascular smooth muscle producing coronary and systemic arterial vasodilatation. Verapamil has its main effects on the myocardium including the atrioventricular node and is in effect like a beta-blocker without any propensity to cause bronchoconstriction. Although diltiazem is often thought of as a half-way house between the two, it shares more of the properties of verapamil than nifedipine (Table 9.3). All of these drugs are available in a range of different delivery systems. The pharmacokinetic profiles of the available sustained-release preparations differ slightly and it is recommended that they should be prescribed by brand name. The main adverse effects vary among the three sub-types and are summarized in Table 9.3.

Table 9.3 Cardiovascular effects of the three different classes of calcium channel blocker

	Vasodilatation	Heart rate	Contractility
Nifedipine	++	↑↓	−
Diltiazem	+	↓	↓
Verapamil	−	↓↓	↓↓

Potassium channel openers

These new agents are a chemically diverse group which share the ability to relax vascular smooth muscle. Nicorandil is the first example of this new type of drug to become available for use clinically. The predominant effect is systemic and coronary vasodilatation without any change in contractility. Interestingly, even in diseased segments of coronary artery, nicorandil appears able to produce some dilatation.

Appropriate selection of drug therapy in angina

Initial therapy. The choice of drug(s) should be based on the pattern of angina experienced by the patient and on any concomitant medical conditions.

1. Effort angina with consistent ischaemic threshold usually reflects increased oxygen demand—beta-blocker.
2. Variable ischaemic threshold may reflect variable coronary vasomotor tone/oxygen supply—diltiazem/verapamil.
3. Variant angina—pain at rest particularly with ST segment elevation during ischaemic episodes—diltiazem/verapamil/nitrates.
4. Coexistent ventricular dysfunction/CHF—nitrates, amlodipine.
5. Asthma/COAD—diltiazem/verapamil/nitrates.
6. Silent ischaemia—beta-blocker > calcium channel blockers.
7. Coexistent aortic stenosis—nitrates; avoid dihydropiridine calcium channel blockers.

Combinations. If a single drug fails to control symptoms adequately, a second and if necessary a third drug from different anti-anginal groups may be added (triple therapy). Some general guidelines are outlined below.

1. Maximize the dose of the initially selected drug before adding a second agent.
2. The addition of a beta-blocker to either diltiazem or verapamil does not usually improve anti-anginal efficacy.
3. Dihydropiridines are unattractive as monotherapy but work well in conjunction with beta-blockers.
4. Caution should be exercised when using diltiazem and beta-blockers together. Verapamil and beta-blockers together are contraindicated.

Common questions patients ask about anti-anginal therapy

Question. Which GTN preparation is better—spray or tablets?

Answer. If GTN is used infrequently, a spray is better. If GTN is used frequently, tablets are preferable. If the patient experiences dizziness with the spray, switch to tablets and advise that as soon as he/she feels either dizziness or the angina easing he/she should spit the tablet out.

Question. How should I use my GTN tablets/spray?
Answer. When a diagnosis of angina has been established it is preferable to use GTN before any activities which regularly provoke angina. Tell the patients not to worry about the GTN losing its effect—this is rarely a problem.

Question. I am on regular (mono-) nitrate tablets—when should I take them?
Answer. In mainly effort-related angina, take the tablets on waking and after lunch with no evening dose. If there are frequent symptoms at night, take the tablets before bed and on waking with no dose in between.

Question. The tablets have helped my angina but I have swollen legs by night-time (nifedipine, amlodipine, etc.). Should I continue with them? Should I be on a water tablet?
Answer. Unless the swollen legs are a sign of heart failure there is no need to prescribe diuretics. Usually elevating the legs above waist level when resting or if necessary a reduction in drug dose controls this problem. If the swelling persists and is very troublesome, the offending drug may have to be substituted with another. Only if this is not felt to be an option should the use of a very small dose of a weak diuretic be considered.

Question. The tablets have helped my angina but I feel very tired (beta-blockers). Will this get better?
Answer. It may do. Some beta-blockers cause sleep disturbance and if this is the case, withdrawal of therapy is usually required. Some patients with CHD have sleep disturbance as part of a depressive mood disorder and this may require separate specific therapy. Other causes of fatigue should be considered, e.g. occult heart failure, anaemia or hypothyroidism. If all of these have been excluded and the fatigue continues to be very troublesome, then dose-reduction or withdrawal should be considered.

Appropriate investigation of patients with CHD

Most patients with angina have CHD. Other causes of angina such as aortic stenosis and anaemia should be easily excluded by clinical examination and simple blood tests. Patients with CHD should proceed to diagnostic coronary angiography with a view to some form of mechanical revascularization under the following circumstances:

- patients with medically refractory angina (usually on maximum tolerated doses of nitrate, calcium channel blocker and beta-blocker plus aspirin, plus heparin if unstable)
- patients with angina (and/or a previous MI) and a strongly positive exercise test suggestive of prognostically significant CHD
- patients with a previous MI and a strongly positive exercise test suggestive of prognostically significant CHD

- most patients with a non-Q-wave MI particularly if there is evidence of inducible ischaemia.

Non-surgical revascularization

Percutaneous transluminal coronary angioplasty (PTCA) using an inflatable balloon was the original technique of non-surgical revascularization. PTCA success and complication rates vary according to the type of lesion being dilated but many centres now report overall success rates in excess of 90% for all lesions treated. The success rate for chronic total occlusions has always been lower, averaging around 70%. However, even here, current balloon technology is improving the performance of PTCA (Fig. 9.1). A number of new non-balloon devices are finding a role in particular situations. These include:

- directional atherectomy—combined balloon and rotating blade device which removes plaque and allows it to be retrieved for analysis; good in certain anatomical locations
- rotational atherectomy—very high speed rotating burr which ablates plaque into microparticles; good for calcified lesions
- extraction atherectomy—spinning propeller with suction which 'hoovers' out material from the vessel lumen; good for thrombus
- laser angioplasty—vaporizes tissue using laser energy; becoming easier to use with good potential in totally occluded vessels.

None of these techniques has been convincingly demonstrated to be any better than conventional balloon PTCA in any given situation. However, this is not the case for intra-coronary stents which have undoubtedly been a major advance in the treatment of CHD.

Intra-coronary stents

Stents are devices which are implanted percutaneously in coronary and other arteries to create a scaffold and maintain the patency of the vessel lumen. Dotter implanted the first vascular stents in canine popliteal arteries in 1969.

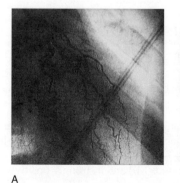 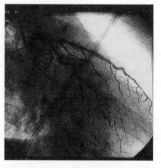

A   B

Figure 9.1 PTCA of a chronic total occlusion of the left anterior descending artery: (A) before PTCA; (B) after PTCA.

Currently there are several commercially available metallic vascular stents suitable for implantation in the coronary arteries, and many more in the pipeline (Fig. 9.2). Stenting has been successful because it addresses the two main problems of conventional PTCA—abrupt vessel closure (AVC) and restenosis.

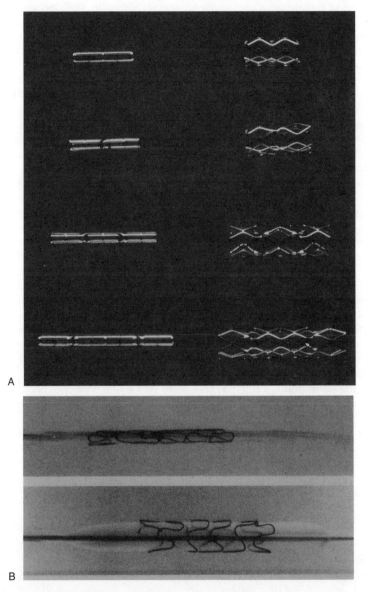

Figure 9.2 (A) Four different sizes of the Palmaz–Schatz intra-coronary stent. (B) A Wiktor intra-coronary stent before and after balloon inflation.

AVC is the phenomenon whereby a vessel subjected to PTCA occludes during or in the first few hours after the procedure. It is to a certain extent an unpredictable adverse event, occurs in up to 5% of patients and often leads to a myocardial infarction or a need for urgent coronary bypass surgery. Placement of a stent into a vessel which has acutely occluded or has the features of threatened acute closure usually stabilizes the situation and often no other therapy is required.

Restenosis is due to a combination of inadequate initial dilatation, elastic recoil of the artery, neointimal proliferation and (probably) chronic vascular remodelling. The individual contribution of each of these phenomena varies from lesion to lesion and patient to patient. Two large randomized multi-centre trials have shown conclusively that elective implantation of the Palmaz–Schatz stent reduces restenosis compared to conventional balloon angioplasty (Table 9.4) (Fischman et al 1994, Serruys et al 1994). Of even greater importance was the demonstration that there were parallel highly significant reductions in adverse clinical end-points and the rate of reintervention.

Widespread adoption of intra-coronary stenting has been hampered by two considerations—cost and the complications associated with the anti-coagulation required to prevent stent thrombosis during the first few weeks after implantation. Currently, using any of the commercially available stents in the UK adds around £1000 to the cost of the angioplasty. Depending on the anticoagulant strategy the patient's stay in hospital may be prolonged by up to 6–7 days compared to routine PTCA. However, using a decision-analytic model Cohen et al (1994) have suggested that despite a higher initial cost, elective stenting for single-vessel disease may be a cost-effective option. It must be remembered that the model used incorporated the published costs and procedural and complication rates of stent implantation as of the early 1990s. There is no doubt that the actual practice of stent implantation has changed dramatically since then and an up-to-date analysis may well place elective stenting in an even more favourable light.

In the stent group of BENESTENT there was a 10% incidence of bleeding compared to 1.6% in the PTCA group (Serruys et al 1994). A particularly intensive antithrombotic regimen was employed in an attempt to prevent stent thrombosis but we now know that this was probably unnecessary. Some centres have implanted large numbers of stents without the use of oral

Table 9.4 Effect of elective implantation of the Palmaz–Schatz stent on restenosis (defined as a diameter stenosis of > 50% at 6 months) in two randomized clinical trials of stenting versus conventional PTCA

| | | Restenosis | | | |
	n	PTCA	Stent	% reduction	p
STRESS	410	43	29	33	0.01
BENESTENT	520	33	22	33	< 0.03

anticoagulants with excellent outcomes (Colombo et al 1995). This strategy was based on the observation, made using intravascular ultrasound, that in around 70% of cases, the apposition between the stent and the vessel wall is suboptimal when the stent is deployed using conventional balloon pressures. High pressure (~ 17–18 atmospheres) dilatations following stent implantation optimize deployment and allow patients to go home the following day on antiplatelet therapy alone (aspirin and/or ticlopidine). Special balloons are required for the high pressure inflations which may add to the cost of the procedure but this has to be set against much earlier discharge and lower bleeding complications.

Surgical revascularization

Current techniques of coronary artery bypass surgery (CABG) usually involve the placement of one or more arterial conduits. This is based on data showing that the long-term patency of arterial grafts is superior to that of saphenous veins. The left internal mammary artery (LIMA) is used in most cases to bypass the left anterior descending (LAD) coronary artery. The LIMA is almost always left attached to the subclavian artery (pedicled graft) so that only a single surgical anastomosis is required. Some surgeons may also use the right internal mammary artery to bypass either the circumflex or right coronary arteries. In this case, the graft may be pedicled or it may be detached and used as a free graft. There is some evidence that the latter technique produces better results. Other arterial conduits which can be used include the radial, gastro-epiploic and inferior gastric arteries. Complete arterial revascularization, even for three-vessel coronary disease is becoming more common. Nonetheless, most patients receive one or more venous conduits and a common approach is to use the LIMA for the LAD and two vein grafts for the circumflex and right coronary arteries.

Indications for mechanical revascularization

Patients are offered mechanical revascularization either to relieve symptoms refractory to maximum medical therapy or in the belief that revascularization will improve prognosis (secondary prevention); often both indications apply in the same patient.

Selection of patients for PTCA

The ideal patient for PTCA has single-vessel, single-lesion disease and these were the only patients offered PTCA in the early days of the technique. Now, because of improvements in operator experience, catheter technology and imaging quality many patients with multivessel disease are treated by PTCA. If it is considered that complete revascularization of every stenosed artery is not necessary, some of these patients may be treated by single-vessel PTCA to the most severe or 'culprit' lesion and this will usually substantially relieve angina. In others, multivessel PTCA may be performed in one or more stages. Comparisons between the effects of different treatment strategies on the prognosis of CHD have been undertaken but as this is such a rapidly evolving field the results are often of historical interest only.

Medical therapy versus surgery

The 10-year results of the randomized trials comparing CABG and medical (drug) therapy in the management of CHD have been the subject of a recent meta-analysis (Yusuf et al 1994). These trials recruited patients with stable disease, i.e. patients with stable angina not severe enough to warrant surgery or patients with a previous MI. In reality, they compared a strategy of immediate surgery versus one of medical therapy with surgery later if symptoms worsened. After 10 years, 41% of patients randomized to initial medical therapy had actually undergone CABG compared to 93% of those randomized to CABG. The CABG group had significantly lower total mortality than the medical-treatment group at all time points though the absolute benefit decreased as time progressed (Table 9.5 and Fig. 9.3). This waning of the initial effects of surgery mirrors the natural history of graft occlusion. Sub-group analysis suggested that the benefits of surgery were greatest in those

Table 9.5 Summary of results of a meta-analysis of randomized trials comparing coronary artery bypass grafting (CABG) and medical therapy in stable coronary heart disease (adapted from Yusuf et al 1994)

Follow-up	Reduction in mortality with CABG	95% confidence intervals
5 years	39%	23–52
7 years	32%	17–44
10 years	17%	2–30

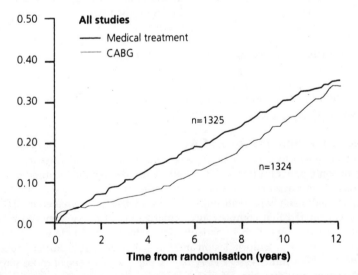

Figure 9.3 Long-term survival in all of the randomized studies of medical therapy versus CABG for patients with coronary heart disease and angina not in itself severe enough to warrant surgery (adapted from Yusuf et al 1994).

with left main stem stenosis or proximal three-vessel disease. In two-vessel disease with involvement of the LAD artery the odds ratio for reduction in mortality with surgery was of borderline significance (0.34–1.01); without LAD involvement there was no significant mortality benefit with surgery. In univariate analysis, the relative benefits of surgery over medical therapy were not significantly affected by other risk factors such as left ventricular dysfunction, previous MI, abnormal exercise test and age. However, when these factors are considered together the absolute survival benefit did increase with increasing risk. In other words, if a patient with left main stem stenosis or proximal three-vessel disease also has one or more of the above risk factors, this increases the likelihood that that patient's survival will be improved by surgery rather than medical therapy. Nonetheless, the mean extension of survival with CABG over 10 years was only 4.3 months. Even in the highest risk groups as assessed by standard risk scoring the mean extension of survival was only 8–10 months. Advocates of surgery will contend that current results of CABG would be better, due to a number of factors:

- much higher frequency of arterial revascularization
- greater use of aspirin with consequently lower early graft occlusion
- improvements in the techniques of cardiopulmonary bypass and myocardial preservation
- improved control of risk factors following CABG.

However, it is also worth noting that there have been substantial improvements in medical therapy since the time of these trials and at least three interventions not widely used then have been shown to reduce mortality in CHD—aspirin, angiotensin-converting enzyme inhibitors and effective lipid lowering. In addition, the CABG trials were almost exclusively men only and none recruited patients aged more than 65. Further trials are required to compare modern medical and surgical therapy in women, the elderly and in the subgroups in whom no clear advantage of surgery was demonstrated.

Medical therapy versus PTCA

The ACME trial suggested that over a 6-month follow-up period PTCA resulted in better relief of angina and a greater improvement in exercise capacity compared to medical therapy in patients with initially mild symptoms and single-vessel disease (Parisi et al 1992). In clinical practice, however, PTCA is not usually used as an alternative to medical therapy. It is reserved for suitable patients who have medically refractory angina incompatible with their desired lifestyle. There is as yet no randomized clinical trial comparing the long-term outcome and mortality of PTCA and medical therapy in any category of CHD patient. In a non-randomized cohort study, the 3- to 5-year clinical outcome of 627 patients undergoing PTCA at a single high-volume centre and 865 patients from the CASS registry treated medically has been presented by Ellis et al (1989). These patients all had one- or two-vessel coronary disease with involvement of the LAD coronary artery. Overall no differences were seen in relative risk of death or MI. The relative risk of death increased with medical therapy with either ejection fraction

< 50% or two-vessel disease. There was a trend towards a reduction in relative risk of MI with PTCA if the LAD stenosis was 90–99%. Angina, activity and employment status were all better with PTCA; however, the likelihood of later CABG increased with PTCA.

PTCA versus CABG

The early follow-up data from several trials comparing PTCA and CABG have been reported. Most have excluded single-vessel disease as there is general agreement that if possible this should be dealt with non-surgically with the option of CABG being reserved for the future (almost inevitable) development of more diffuse disease. However, patients with single-vessel disease were included in the Randomized Intervention Treatment of Angina (RITA) trial and in the Lausanne trial of patients with isolated disease of the proximal LAD artery (RITA Trial Participants 1993, Goy et al 1994). Some of the trials demanded that the operators attempt complete revascularization of all target vessels, whilst others were less stringent. Despite these differences and consequently less complete revascularization in multivessel disease with PTCA, total mortality and rates of myocardial infarction have not been significantly different over the first 1–3 years following randomization (Hamm et al 1994, King et al 1994). Patients randomized to PTCA have consistently lower event-free survival, primarily because of repeat procedures required for restenosis. In the RITA trial, the initial average cost of treating a patient randomized to PTCA was about 52% of that for CABG. Despite reinterventions, total costs in the PTCA group were still 20% less than with CABG at 2 years (Schulpher et al 1994). In addition, very few of the patients randomized to PTCA in RITA and the other trials of PTCA versus CABG received intra-coronary stents which would have undoubtedly improved the outcome in the non-surgical group. As follow-up progresses, late graft closure will start to impact on the surgical results and will certainly necessitate reintervention (often PTCA) in a proportion of patients. Future studies will be required to compare current state-of-the-art techniques of non-surgical revascularization including elective stenting with CABG.

MYOCARDIAL INFARCTION

In a sense, secondary prevention begins as soon as a patient presents with acute MI. The most effective means of preventing the late consequences of MI is to attempt to limit the initial extent of damage by restoring normal myocardial perfusion as rapidly as possible. The vast majority of MI is due to thrombus formation in a coronary artery, usually at the site of a pre-existing atheromatous plaque. There are two main methods of dealing quickly with this occlusive coronary thrombus—intravenous administration of one or more thrombolytic agents or PTCA.

Thrombolytic therapy in MI

A series of large randomized clinical trials have been performed in an attempt to establish the best thrombolytic regimens. The early placebo-controlled studies clearly showed the benefits of thrombolytic therapy with significant reductions in mortality in the ISIS-2 trial using streptokinase (SK) (ISIS-2 Collaborative Group 1988), in the APSAC trial using anistreplase (AIMS Trial Study Group 1988) and in the ASSET trial using recombinant tissue plasminogen activator (rt-PA) (Wilcox et al 1988). The ISIS-3 and GISSI-2 trials which directly compared SK, anistreplase and rt-PA showed no differences between these three agents in 30-day mortality and provided support for the existing practice in the UK of using SK as the drug of first choice (ISIS-3 Collaborative Group 1993, Gruppo Italiano per lo Studio della Sopravivenza nell'Infarto Miocardico 1990). rt-PA has usually been reserved for patients with prior exposure to SK who have circulating antibodies to SK which reduces its efficacy and may also provoke serious allergic reactions. This result surprised many investigators as previous small studies employing angiography to determine infarct-related artery patency had shown that more arteries were open earlier with rt-PA than with SK. These studies had also indicated the need to follow up the administration of rt-PA with intravenous heparin rather than subcutaneous heparin as was employed in ISIS-3. Primarily because of this criticism the GUSTO trial was conducted. The rt-PA arm of this study employed an accelerated or 'front-loaded' regimen in which a bolus dose was given and the remaining dose was administered in 90 minutes as opposed to the previously used 3-hour infusion without a bolus. It was then followed up with intravenous heparin for at least 24 hours. The other treatment groups were SK with subcutaneous heparin as in ISIS-3, SK with intravenous heparin and a hybrid regimen involving reduced doses of both SK and rt-PA. GUSTO showed an overall reduction in absolute mortality of 1% with accelerated rt-PA and intravenous heparin compared to the two SK regimens combined (GUSTO Investigators 1993). Following the demonstration of this modest but statistically significant effect, the use of rt-PA has increased, particularly in patients presenting early (< 4 hours) with extensive antero-lateral infarctions in whom subgroup analysis suggested the greatest differential benefit.

PTCA in acute MI

Some patients have relative or absolute contraindications to thrombolytic therapy and in certain patient subgroups such as those presenting with cardiogenic shock thrombolytic therapy is ineffective. In such patients consideration should be given to employing PTCA as a means of achieving reperfusion. Direct comparisons of intravenous thrombolytic therapy with primary PTCA in randomized trials have shown higher rates of reperfusion with PTCA and a recent meta-analysis has confirmed a significantly higher event-free survival at short-term follow-up (Michels & Yusuf 1995). This emphasizes the secondary preventive effect of rapid and full restoration of coronary flow at the time of the initial MI.

SECONDARY PREVENTION IN CORONARY HEART DISEASE

Strategies for secondary prevention in patients with CHD have almost exclusively involved studies of various drug interventions in patients with a prior MI. There are virtually no data on the effects of most current therapies on the outcome of patients with stable angina pectoris but without any history of prior MI. Extrapolation of the data from postinfarct studies to this latter group of patients is problematical as the two groups have undoubtedly different natural histories and event rates. From a public health point of view, one of the difficulties of applying even accepted secondary prevention strategies to patients with prior myocardial infarction is that epidemiological studies suggest that up to one-third of such patients in the community are unrecognized, i.e. they have had silent infarctions (Sugurdsson et al 1995). In a patient known to have had a previous MI, a wide range of options for secondary prevention exist.

Aspirin

Aspirin is a critical component of the acute therapy of MI and produces the same magnitude of mortality reduction as streptokinase given alone (ISIS-2 Collaborative group 1988). In patients with no history of vascular events (primary prevention), who are by definition at low risk, it has been difficult to show conclusively that aspirin reduces cardiovascular mortality. However, in secondary prevention the data from the Antiplatelet Trialists' Collaboration confirm that antiplatelet therapy, mainly aspirin, significantly reduces vascular events (vascular death, non-fatal stroke and myocardial infarction) in patients at high risk, i.e. those with a prior history of vascular disease or other conditions associated with an increased risk of occlusive vascular disease such as atrial fibrillation and valvular heart disease (Table 9.6) (Antiplatelet Trialists' Collaboration 1994a). These reductions were significant in middle and old age, in men and women, in hypertensive and normotensive patients and in diabetic and non-diabetic patients. There was no evidence that any other antiplatelet agent or higher doses of aspirin were more effective than aspirin at 75–325 mg daily. The optimal duration of treatment in each patient category remains undetermined but is at least 2–3 years. Similar meta-

Table 9.6 Summary of secondary preventive effects of antiplatelet therapy (mainly aspirin) from the Antiplatelet Trialists' Collaboration

	n	Vascular events prevented per 1000 patients treated	2p value
Acute MI	~ 20 000	40 at 1 month	< 0.0001
Previous MI	~ 20 000	40 at 2 years	< 0.0001
Previous stroke/TIA	~ 10 000	40 at 3 years	< 0.0001
Unstable angina	~ 4000	50 at 6 months	< 0.0001
Other cardiovascular disease*	~ 14 000	20 at 1 year	< 0.0001

* Stable angina, vascular surgery, angioplasty, atrial fibrillation, valvular heart disease, peripheral vascular disease
Key: MI: myocardial infarction; TIA: transient ischaemic attack

analysis has confirmed the beneficial effects of aspirin on graft or arterial patency following vascular surgery/angioplasty and the ability of aspirin to reduce the incidence of venous thrombosis and pulmonary embolism in both medical and surgical patients (Antiplatelet Trialists' Collaboration 1994b, 1994c).

Heparin

In the acute therapy of MI intravenous heparin is routinely administered for 24–48 hours after the use of rt-PA. There is no clear evidence of any additional benefit of either intravenous or high-dose (12 500 units twice daily) subcutaneous heparin after the use of streptokinase. In unstable angina associated with electrocardiographic evidence of ischaemia, intravenous heparin therapy significantly reduces the frequency of ischaemic episodes compared to aspirin with bolus heparin or thrombolytic therapy (Serneri et al 1990).

In the early 1970s it was shown that low-dose (5000 units three times daily) subcutaneous heparin substantially reduced the incidence of deep venous thrombosis in patients with MI (Wray et al 1973). However, it is not known whether this benefit would still be apparent in the 1990s in patients who have received thrombolytic therapy and have been mobilized much more rapidly than used to be the case. In patients with MI at high risk of venous or systemic thrombo-embolism, e.g. past history of thrombo-embolism, atrial fibrillation, persistent heart failure, cardiogenic shock or ventricular aneurysm formation, full intravenous and subsequently oral anticoagulation should be considered. The usual contraindications should be observed with particular caution being required in patients with any evidence of postinfarction pericarditis.

Warfarin

A number of trials have addressed the question of whether oral anticoagulant therapy can reduce the late mortality following MI. In the most recent of these, 1214 patients were randomized at a mean of 27 days following the index event. After a mean follow-up period of around 3 years both total mortality and reinfarction were significantly reduced (Smith et al 1990). Again the difficulty of applying these data to current clinical practice relates to the low use of thrombolytic therapy and aspirin in these trial patients. There is no doubt that thrombolysis in itself reduces the incidence of mural thrombus and subsequent thrombo-embolic complications of MI and this may negate any of the benefits of oral anticoagulants shown in non-thrombolysed populations. Warfarin and aspirin have never been directly compared in a secondary prevention trial after MI. In practice, all patients receive aspirin unless contraindicated and warfarin may be added for specific indications such as atrial fibrillation associated with atrial dilatation and/or left ventricular dysfunction or the demonstration of mural thrombus on echocardiography.

Angiotensin-converting enzyme inhibitors (ACEI)

Rationale for the use of ACEI in MI

The original hypothesis that ACEI would favourably influence the outcome after MI was based on animal studies which showed that ACEI could modify ventricular remodelling. This is the term used to describe the complex changes in ventricular size and shape involving expansion of both the infarcted and non-infarcted regions of the myocardium which follow MI. Around one-third of patients demonstrate significant remodelling after MI, the best predictors of this being the presence of a large transmural antero-apical infarction (Pirolo et al 1986) and also the presence of heart failure. Although the initial few weeks of ventricular remodelling may help to maintain cardiac function, mortality at 8 weeks is higher in patients experiencing infarct expansion (Eaton et al 1979). The magnitude of the increase in left ventricular volume may be the single best predictor of an adverse prognosis following MI (Hammermeister et al 1979, White et al 1987).

In the first animal studies of the effects of ACEI on ventricular remodelling, rats subjected to coronary artery ligation were treated with captopril. This resulted in a smaller left ventricle at follow-up compared to placebo (Pfeffer et al 1985). Mortality was also reduced in the treated groups versus placebo with the maximal improvement in survival being seen in animals with the greatest attenuation of ventricular enlargement. The mechanism of action, at least in this species, is not solely related to afterload reduction as hydrallazine is ineffective despite an equal lowering of blood pressure (Raya et al 1989). In the first reported human study, Pfeffer et al (1988) started treatment with captopril an average of 20 days after a first anterior myocardial infarction and continued therapy for 1 year. In the study group as a whole, no beneficial effects were seen. In a subgroup with large infarcts or a persistently occluded infarct-related artery, captopril attenuated the increase in left ventricular volume seen in the placebo group. In a similar study with treatment commencing an average of 9 days after the index event, Sharpe et al (1988) showed that captopril attenuated left ventricular dilatation. Angiotensin levels are elevated within 2–3 days of myocardial infarction and so it was postulated that starting treatment earlier might enhance the therapeutic effect of ACEI (McAlpine et al 1988). In 100 patients with MI randomized to captopril or placebo within 24 hours of admission, favourable effects on ventricular remodelling were seen within 2 months, which was somewhat earlier than in the two previous studies cited above (Oldroyd et al 1991).

Mortality trials with ACEI in MI

These preliminary animal and clinical studies provided the impetus for the design and execution of several large trials aimed at determining whether ACEI could reduce the mortality of patients with MI (Table 9.7). All of these randomized placebo-controlled trials showed a significant reduction in mortality at a variety of follow-up times except the CONSENSUS II trial which was halted prematurely because of a non-significant excess mortality in the enalapril group. The study authors themselves believed that this was due to the early administration of intravenous enalaprilat which may have provoked an excess incidence of harmful hypotension (Swedberg et al 1992). The pattern of results in all of the trials is similar to that seen in the beta-blocker trials, i.e. the relative risk reduction is greatest in the AIRE trial which selected the highest-risk group of patients (Fig. 9.4) (Acute Infarction

Table 9.7 Postinfarction trials of angiotensin-converting enzyme inhibitors (ACEI)

	n	Entry criteria	ACEI target dose	Mortality effect (95% CI)
SAVE	2231	Ejection fraction < 40%. No heart failure or ongoing ischaemia. Mean time to start of therapy: 11 days	Captopril 50 mg t.i.d.	↓ by 19% (3–32%) at 42 months
CONSENSUS II	6090	Within 24 hours. No clear contraindication to ACEI	i.v. enalaprilat 1 mg, enalapril 20 mg o.d.	↑ by 10% (− 7 to 29%) at 6 months
AIRE	2006	Stable patients with clinical and/or X-ray evidence of CHF. Days 3–10, mean day 5	Ramipril 5 mg b.i.d.	↓ by 27% (11–40%) at 15 months
GISSI 3	19 394	Within 24 hours. No clear contraindication to ACEI	Lisinopril 10 mg o.d.	↓ by 12% (1–21%) at 6 weeks
ISIS 4	58 050	Within 24 hours. No clear contraindication to ACEI	Captopril 50 mg b.i.d.	↓ by 7% (1–73%) at 35 days

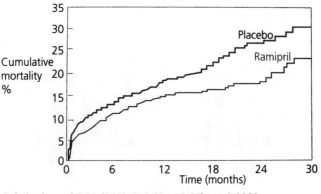

Relative hazard 0.73 (95% CI 0.60 to 0.89) p = 0.0002

Figure 9.4 Reduction in the risk of death from all causes in the AIRE study (Acute Infarction Ramipril Efficacy (AIRE) Study Investigators 1993).

Ramipril Efficacy (AIRE) Study Investigators 1993). These patients were also identified without the need for any sophisticated measurements of ejection fraction. In the GISSI-3 (1994) and ISIS-4 (1995) trials which recruited essentially all patients with MI and so avoided the issue of patient selection, smaller risk reductions were seen. This may in fact represent a similar magnitude of effect in patients similar to those recruited in AIRE and little or no effect in patients at low risk. The SAVE trial which recruited patients at intermediate risk produced an intermediate risk reduction (Pfeffer et al 1992).

Mechanisms of post-MI mortality reduction with ACEI
The SAVE echo sub-study indicated that there is a relationship between adverse events and progressive ventricular dilatation. There were 91 adverse events in the 419 patients with analysable echo studies. Of these, 57 occurred in 216 patients on placebo and 34 in 203 patients on captopril, a 36% increase with placebo. Within the captopril group, adverse events occurred in those patients who despite drug therapy had demonstrated progressive ventricular enlargement (St John Sutton et al 1994). In both SAVE and AIRE there were significant reductions in the incidence of severe heart failure which would be expected to translate into reductions in mortality. The question of whether ACEI reduce mortality by reducing reinfarction is unresolved. A reduction in reinfarction was shown with long-term therapy in SAVE (Fig. 9.5) and SOLVD but not in AIRE nor with short-term therapy in GISSI-3 and ISIS-4. Thus although reinfarction may be reduced in some patient subgroups, current data do not allow us to identify those most likely to benefit or the ACEI regimen required to produce the effect.

Beta-adrenoceptor blockade
Several studies have confirmed the ability of beta-blockers to improve the prognosis of patients with MI. However, they have all been performed in

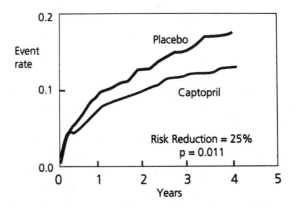

Figure 9.5 Reduction in the incidence of recurrent myocardial infarction in the SAVE study (Pfeffer et al 1992).

the pre-thrombolytic era. Both cardioselective and non-cardioselective drugs appear to work, though agents with partial agonist activity such as oxprenolol are much less effective (Yusuf et al 1985). There have been three different strategies tested in the beta-blocker trials: intravenous therapy on admission followed by oral therapy for 1–2 years; intravenous therapy followed by oral therapy for 1 week; and oral therapy started pre-discharge and continued for 1–2 years. All have been shown to be effective and, unlike the results seen with calcium channel blockade, the greatest effect of beta-blockade is seen in patients at highest risk of subsequent mortality, i.e. those with extensive infarctions or heart failure at presentation. There are no randomized placebo-controlled studies of the additional benefits of beta-blockade in a thrombolysed population. In the TIMI II trial, patients were randomized to early intravenous or late oral beta-blockade following treatment with rt-PA. Early therapy reduced the incidence of recurrent ischaemia and reinfarction but did not alter 1-year survival (TIMI Study Group 1989).

Calcium channel blockade

Nifedipine
Several trials have confirmed that nifedipine has no beneficial effects on survival when used routinely in patients with prior myocardial infarction (Held et al 1989). In fact, the trend is for mortality to be increased. Accordingly, whilst routine use following MI is clearly contraindicated, monotherapy with nifedipine in postinfarction angina should also be avoided.

Diltiazem
In the Multicenter Diltiazem Postinfarction Trial (MDPIT) no benefits of treatment with diltiazem were seen. On the contrary, there was evidence of a harmful effect in patients with significant left ventricular dysfunction (MDPIT Research Group 1988). The late follow-up of this trial confirmed that in the subgroup of patients with either pulmonary congestion at the time

of randomization, left ventricular ejection fraction < 40% or Q-wave antero-lateral infarction who received diltiazem, the frequency of heart failure was significantly greater than with placebo. In addition, 2-year mortality in the diltiazem group was 35% versus 22% with placebo: $p = 0.055$ (Goldstein et al 1991). In a randomized trial restricted to patients with non-Q-wave infarction, diltiazem in a high dosage of 360 mg daily produced a significant reduction in reinfarction (Gibson et al 1986).

Verapamil

In the first Danish Verapamil Infarction Trial (DAVIT I), verapamil 0.1 mg/kg intravenously was administered at the time of admission and followed by 120 mg three times daily for up to 6 months in over 1400 patients with acute myocardial infarction. No significant effect on mortality was seen. A retro-spective analysis suggested a lower mortality in the verapamil group between day 22 and 180. Accordingly, a second trial (DAVIT II) was conducted in which patients were only randomized in the second week after the index infarction and treatment was continued for up to 18 months. Again, no significant effect on mortality was seen though there was a significant reduc-tion in the combined end-point of death and reinfarction. A retrospective analysis of this trial suggested that the benefit was limited to patients without any evidence of heart failure during their admission (see Table 9.8) (Danish Study Group on Verapamil in Myocardial Infarction 1990). An important feature of the protocol in these two trials was that patients requiring beta-blocker therapy because of angina, arrhythmias or hypertension were excluded and elective use of beta-blockade for secondary prevention was not allowed.

Table 9.8 Outcome data from the DAVIT II study

	Verapamil	Placebo	Hazard ratio (95% CI)*
n	878	897	
Death (%)	11.1	13.8	0.80 (0.61–1.05)
Death/reinfarction (%)	18.0	21.6	0.80 (0.64–0.99)
No heart failure			
n	587	574	
Death (%)	7.7	11.8	0.64 (0.44–0.94)
Death/reinfarction (%)	14.6	19.7	0.70 (0.52–0.93)
Heart failure			
n	291	323	
Death (%)	17.9	17.5	1.05 (0.72–1.54)
Death/reinfarction (%)	24.9	24.9	0.98 (0.72–1.39)

* If the 95% confidence intervals of the hazard ratio do not include 1 this denotes a statistically significant effect.

Nitrates

Despite the theoretical attractions of nitrate therapy two mega-trials have failed to show any mortality reductions in patients treated with intravenous followed by transdermal nitrates (GISSI-3 1994) or oral nitrates (ISIS-4 1995) for 4–6 weeks after MI. This is one of the therapies in which the large randomized clinical trials failed to produce the result predicted by meta-analysis of the pooled data from previous smaller studies. A confounding factor in the analysis of GISSI-3 was that 44% of the control group received intravenous nitrates on day 1 and some authorities believe that the question of a possible benefit of early intravenous nitrate therapy in acute MI is still unresolved. In any case, nitrates are still widely used in acute MI for specific indications such as persistent myocardial ischaemia, heart failure and control of hypertension both before and after thrombolytic therapy.

Lipid-lowering drugs

The role of lipid-lowering drug therapy in the primary and secondary prevention of CHD has been clarified recently in the West of Scotland Coronary Prevention Study (Shepherd et al 1994) and in the Scandinavian Simvastatin Survival Study (Scandinavian Simvastatin Study Group 1994). Epidemiological studies have always shown a direct relationship between total (T-C) and low density lipoprotein cholesterol concentrations in the population and the prevalence of CHD. Early clinical studies with relatively weak lipid-lowering drugs had been unable to demonstrate reductions in total mortality, partly due to an unexplained (random) statistically non-significant excess of non-cardiac mortality. However meta-analysis of these older trials indicated that the average T-C reduction achieved of around 10% (0.6 mmol/l) sustained for 2–5 years resulted in an 18% reduction in the combined end-point of death and non-fatal MI (Law et al 1994). Moreover, the data suggested that the lower the cholesterol the greater the effect, the implication being that if more substantial cholesterol reductions could be obtained, beneficial effects on total mortality would be seen. In this decade the availability of a series of HMG CoA reductase inhibitors (statins) which typically reduce T-C by around 25% has allowed this hypothesis to be tested.

Lipid-lowering trials

The West of Scotland Study is described in detail on pages 47–49. Meta-analysis of a number of small secondary prevention trials using mono-therapy with a statin suggested a risk reduction of mortality of around 40%. However, the Scandinavian Simvastatin Survival Study has provided the definitive confirmation that these drugs can reduce total mortality when given to patients with a prior history of angina and/or myocardial infarction. In this trial, 4444 patients with total cholesterol levels between 5.5 and 8.0 mmol/l received either simvastatin 20–40 mg daily or a matching placebo. After an average follow-up period of 5.4 years T-C had, as expected, been reduced by around 25%. Again, as predicted from the meta-analysis of the original lipid-lowering trials, this was associated with a reduction in major

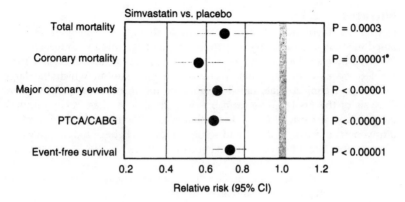

Figure 9.6 Odds ratios (95% confidence intervals) and their respective *p* values for the major end-points in the 4S study (Scandinavian Simvastatin Survival Study Group 1994).

adverse cardiac events of 44% and a reduction in total mortality of 30% (Fig. 9.6) (Scandinavian Simvastatin Survival Study Group 1994). The benefits of simvastatin in this study were similar in both sexes, in patients above and below the age of 65, in patients with or without a previous MI and in patients treated concomitantly with aspirin versus those not taking aspirin. As an additional bonus, the simvastatin group also demonstrated 30% reductions in the incidence of unstable angina, the need for revascularization (by surgery or PTCA) and the incidence of transient cerebral ischaemia or stroke. By so doing this secondary preventive measure becomes very cost-effective. Simvastatin was very well tolerated with the withdrawal rate from the study being similar in the treatment and placebo groups and there was no excess incidence of non-cardiac death as had been reported in earlier trials.

Mechanism of mortality reduction with lipid lowering

The exact mechanism by which lipid lowering can reduce the incidence of acute vascular events in as little as 2 years from the onset of therapy remains speculative. In the Pravastatin Limitation of Atherosclerosis in the Coronary arteries (PLAC-I) and the Pravastatin, Lipids and Atherosclerosis in the Carotid arteries (PLAC-II) trials, quantitative coronary angiography (PLAC-I) and B-mode ultrasound (PLAC-II) were used to measure the effects of the drug on plaque burden (Pitt et al 1994, Crouse et al 1995). Despite effective lipid lowering the changes seen in arterial wall thickness or lumen diameter were usually no more than 0.1–0.2 mm per diseased segment. It should be borne in mind that quantitative angiography, even using automated computer-enhanced edge detection, is by no means the gold standard for assessing plaque/atheroma regression. Atheroma is a disease of the arterial wall and angiography looks at the lumen. Whilst many plaques do impinge on the lumen of the vessel, many do not. Diseased arteries remodel and may maintain their lumen dimensions despite the presence of significant atheroma

(Glagov et al 1987). In the future, studies employing intravascular ultrasound or perhaps magnetic resonance imaging may provide a better measure of atheroma regression. Nonetheless, in the pooled data from these two trials, the small changes shown were associated with a significant reduction in clinical events (Pitt et al 1994). A clue to the mechanism comes from the observation that the major effects were seen on the progression of minimal lesions and the development of new lesions. It is known that many acute coronary artery occlusions occur in arteries in which the pre-existing stenoses were only mild to moderate. These 'young' plaques are lipid-rich and prone to plaque rupture with subsequent thrombosis formation. Cholesterol-lowering may regress or stabilize these culprit plaques and thereby reduce acute ischaemic events. An additional, recently described effect of lipid-lowering therapy is the restoration of normal coronary endothelial function in patients with coronary artery disease (Treasure et al 1995, Anderson et al 1995). Normally functioning endothelium secretes a number of substances which exert antithrombotic effects, are important in the maintenance of normal perfusion and may protect against plaque rupture. The restoration of coronary endothelial function may also explain the results of recent studies which have shown that even short-term lipid lowering reduces both the symptoms of angina in patients with CHD and also the objective extent of myocardial ischaemia as assessed by ambulatory electrocardio-graphic recording or positron emission tomography (Gould et al 1994, Andrew et al 1994). As such, effective lipid lowering as well as having a role in secondary prevention in CHD may also become an important part of anti-anginal medication.

CONGESTIVE HEART FAILURE

Coronary heart disease and particularly MI is now the major cause of congestive heart failure (CHF) in the developed world. As such, the primary prevention of coronary heart disease by risk factor modification should ulti-mately feed through into a reduction in the incidence of CHF. In similar fashion, more rapid and complete restoration of adequate myocardial per-fusion in patients who have sustained an acute MI, with newer thrombolytic regimes and/or primary angioplasty, should also reduce the subsequent development of CHF. Meanwhile, the incidence of CHF is rising and by the time it has developed the coronary artery disease process is usually so advanced that there is very little scope left for secondary prevention. The medical management of CHF centres around the use of three groups of drugs—digoxin, diuretics and vasodilators (usually ACEI).

Digoxin

Digoxin has been around for over 200 years but its exact role in the treat-ment of CHF has still not been defined. In the large number of patients with CHF who are in atrial fibrillation, digoxin is the drug of first choice to slow atrioventricular conduction and control the ventricular rate. In patients with sinus rhythm there has always been controversy as to whether digoxin could add anything to patients adequately treated with diuretics and some form of vasodilator. Recently, two trials have been conducted in which patients with mild to moderate CHF who were stable on their current therapy of digoxin and diuretics (PROVED) or digoxin, diuretics and an ACEI (RADIANCE) were randomly assigned in a double blind manner to either continue with their digoxin or to switch to a placebo (Uretsky et al 1993, Packer et al 1993). Both studies clearly demonstrated using both subjective and objective assessments that the patients switched to placebo did significantly less well. Neither of these trials was large enough to address the question of whether digoxin improves survival in patients with CHF but such a trial (DIG-TRIAL) is ongoing and it will also quantify the benefit of adding digoxin to patients who are stable on diuretics and ACEI. It has long been thought that the beneficial effects of digoxin in CHF are related to its ability to increase the force of contraction of cardiac muscle, i.e. a positive inotropic action. However, digoxin is a relatively weak inotrope and recently it has been suggested that it may be acting by modulating the neuroendocrine response and restoring normal cardiovascular reflex function in CHF. The reduction in circulating concentrations of catecholamines seen in patients with CHF treated with digoxin is similar to that seen with ACEI. As this is one of the mechanisms postulated to explain the beneficial effects of ACEI on survival in patients with CHF it may be that digoxin will also ultimately be shown to have a favourable effect on outcome.

Diuretics

No clinical trials have addressed the question of whether diuretics have any effect on disease progression or survival in patients with CHF. There is no doubt that diuretic therapy improves symptoms and thereby quality of life in patients with CHF, and even in mild CHF, trials attempting to use ACEI alone have not been successful. As such, they are an essential part of the treatment and will probably never be the subject of survival studies. There are, however, a number of adverse features associated with diuretic therapy which may unfavourably influence disease progression and survival. These include electrolyte disturbances and activation of the renin–angiotensin system. Some of these may be offset in part by the concomitant use of ACEI. Generally, it is good practice to maximize ACEI dosages in the hope that this will allow the use of the minimum dosage of diuretics commensurate with keeping the patient's clinical condition stable.

Angiotensin-converting enzyme inhibitors

There is no doubt that ACEI improve symptoms and effort capacity in patients with congestive heart failure and as such they are an essential part of therapy. In terms of CHD prevention there is also ample evidence to support their use.

Cooperative North Scandinavian Enalapril Survival Study (CONSENSUS I)

This trial of the use of enalapril in severe Class IV heart failure showed, for the first time, that a therapy for heart failure could improve the prognosis.

Indeed the effect was so marked that the trial was stopped prematurely (CONSENSUS Trial Group 1987).

Studies of Left Ventricular Dysfunction (SOLVD)

This was two trials in one. In the treatment arm, patients with mild to moderate Class II–III CHF and an ejection fraction < 35% were randomized to enalapril or placebo in addition to their previous therapy, usually digoxin and diuretics. Patients with an ejection fraction < 35% but no symptoms of CHF, i.e. asymptomatic left ventricular dysfunction or functional Class I were recruited into the prevention arm. This study differs from the postinfarction trials described above in that patients with recent (< 1 month) myocardial infarction were excluded. However, around 70% of the patients did have ischaemic heart disease. In the treatment arm, over an average follow-up period of 41 months there was a 16% (95% CI: 5–26%) reduction in mortality with the bulk of this effect being due to a reduction in death from progressive heart failure as opposed to any reduction in sudden death (SOLVD Investigators 1991). In the prevention arm with a lower-risk group of patients, enalapril produced no significant reduction in either total or cardiovascular mortality. The combined end-point of death and the development of CHF was significantly reduced (SOLVD Investigators 1992).

Veterans Administration Cooperative Vasodilator-Heart Failure Trials (V-HeFT)

In V-HeFT I the combination of hydrallazine and nitrates had been shown to reduce mortality when compared to both prazosin and placebo in patients with Class II–III CHF (Cohn et al 1986). In V-HeFT II this combination was compared to enalapril in patients with Class II–IV CHF. Total mortality was significantly lower with enalapril but unlike the SOLVD data, this appeared to be due to a reduction in sudden death (Cohn et al 1992). This may be a real difference between studies but it may also relate to the difficulty of defining and confirming sudden cardiac death.

Newer therapies

A number of combined inotropic/vasodilator drugs have been used in a variety of heart failure trials. Improvements in symptoms and exercise capacity have been consistently shown but some trials have shown an excess mortality in the treated group. This has led to the withdrawal of certain drugs, most notably flosequinan. Such therapies which improve the quality of life but may in some cases shorten life expectancy pose a dilemma for patients with heart failure and for those directing their treatment. Given the choice, individual patients may elect to take a particular drug if it markedly improves symptoms even if it adversely affects the long-term outcome.

ARRHYTHMIAS

Many patients with CHD have arrhythmias, some of which are clinically silent. It is crucially important to establish the correct electrocardiographic diagnosis. Frequent ambulatory recordings may be required and if doubt remains it may be necessary to proceed to electrophysiological study. Drug therapy of arrhythmias in patients with CHD is often complicated by co-existent ventricular dysfunction or heart failure which can be worsened by the negative inotropic effect of many antiarrhythmic drugs. It is beyond the scope of this chapter to discuss details of the management of specific arrhythmias but some generally applicable comments relevant to patients with CHD are made below.

Symptomatic arrhythmias requiring therapy

Atrial fibrillation

This may not require specific antiarrhythmic therapy. If it is chronic and the ventricular rate is rapid, it can be slowed by any drug which slows conduction through the atrioventricular (AV) node, i.e. digoxin, beta-blocker or verapamil. The choice is often determined by any coexisting disease. Consideration should be given to attempting to restore sinus rhythm in all patients. If this is not possible or fails, lifelong therapy with either aspirin or warfarin is required to reduce the risk of cardiac thrombo-embolism. In patients with significant ventricular function or a prior history of cardiac thrombo-embolism, warfarin is usually preferred. Paroxysmal atrial fibrillation is often treated with sotalol or amiodarone.

Other supraventricular arrhythmias

Most narrow complex regular tachycardias are due to re-entry circuits involving the AV node. As such they are not caused by CHD but they may coexist. Drugs which modify AV node conduction are effective but it is sometimes necessary to use other agents such as flecainide, propafenone or amiodarone. A permanent cure can often be provided by radio-frequency ablation. Atrial flutter can be more difficult to deal with and is often associated with CHD. Again the main role of drug therapy is to slow the ventricular rate. Pharmacological or more often electrical cardioversion to sinus rhythm is usually successful.

Ventricular tachycardia

Patients with a history of prior MI and ventricular tachycardia occurring beyond the first 48 hours after MI are a high-risk group for sudden death. Late ventricular tachycardia is usually due to electrical instability in and around the scar tissue of the original infarct. If acute ischaemia or other potential provoking factors are excluded then therapy will be required. The ESVEM study suggested that serial ambulatory ECG recordings predicted long-term therapeutic efficacy in such patients better than serial electrophysiological testing and sotalol was probably the drug of first choice (Mason 1993a, 1993b). Amiodarone was not tested in this trial which has been the subject of fierce debate. Many centres continue to prefer electrophysiological testing when they are trying to identify effective antiarrhythmic therapy for ventricular tachycardia. Failure of drug therapy indicates a need to consider implantation of an automatic cardioverter defibrillator.

Out-of-hospital cardiac arrest

The diffusion of cardiopulmonary resuscitation skills into the community and the provision of defibrillators in ambulances has dramatically increased the chances of patients with CHD surviving out-of-hospital cardiac arrest. Most of these arrests are due to ventricular fibrillation and, in the absence of any evidence of acute myocardial ischaemia/infarction, antiarrhythmic therapy is indicated. If a sustained ventricular tachycardia can be induced by programmed stimulation, this can be used to guide pharmacological therapy. If there is no inducible arrhythmia or if drug therapy fails, current practice is to consider implantation of an automatic cardioverter defibrillator. These devices have also allowed trials of different drug therapy to be safely performed in survivors of cardiac arrest and ongoing studies are comparing the use of empirical amiodarone and beta-blockade.

Asymptomatic arrhythmias

Observational studies have previously shown a relationship between adverse outcome and the presence of complex ventricular ectopy following MI and in patients with CHF.

Postmyocardial infarction

The CAST study showed that the use of Class I antiarrhythmic therapy in patients with prior MI and asymptomatic complex ventricular ectopy caused rather than prevented sudden death (Cardiac Arrhythmia Suppression Trial (CAST) Investigators 1989). This finding is probably related to the ability of all antiarrhythmic drugs to also exert proarrhythmic effects. There is some preliminary evidence that empirical use of amiodarone following MI may be of some benefit (Cairns et al 1991, Nademanee et al 1993).

Congestive heart failure

In severe heart failure many deaths are sudden and are assumed to be due to ventricular arrhythmias. The GESICA study demonstrated that over 2 years of follow-up, amiodarone 300 mg/day reduced total mortality by 28% (95% CI: 4–45%) in patients with severe CHF and no symptomatic ventricular arrhythmias (Doval et al 1994). The patients in this trial were already on best optimal therapy for CHF including ACEI. The VA trial showed no reduction in sudden death or overall mortality with amiodarone in 674 patients with CHF and 10 or more ventricular ectopic beats per hour on Holter monitoring (Singh et al 1995). The different outcomes of these two trials may be related to the different patient groups studied. In GESICA, only 30% of the patients had CHD, whereas in the VA trial, only 30% of the patients did not have CHD. A subgroup analysis in the VA trial suggested a favourable trend towards improved survival with amiodarone in the non-ischaemic patients which would be consistent with the GESICA result.

■ KEY POINTS

• Beta-blockers, calcium channel blockers and nitrates all relieve angina but there is no evidence that any of these therapies can improve the survival of patients with angina and no history of myocardial infarction.

• Patients with medically refractory angina should be considered for either PTCA or CABG.

• Randomized studies performed in the late 1970s showed that compared to medical therapy CABG improves the survival of patients with significant stenosis of the left main coronary artery or significant proximal stenosis of all three epicardial coronary arteries.

• Randomized studies performed in the 1990s have shown that for many categories of CHD there is no difference in survival or subsequent rates of myocardial infarction between patients treated by PTCA and those treated by CABG.

• Restenosis following PTCA results in a much higher incidence of repeat procedures compared to CABG but restenosis can be reduced by elective implantation of intracoronary stents.

• In acute MI, aspirin and prompt reperfusion of the occluded coronary artery by either thrombolytic drugs or PTCA improve survival.

• Following MI, all patients should continue on aspirin. Beta-blockers, ACEI and simvastatin have all been shown to improve survival in certain groups of patients. Amiodarone and warfarin may be of benefit in specific subgroups.

• Digoxin, diuretics and ACEI all improve the symptoms of CHF.

• ACEI reduce mortality in all categories of CHF. If ACEI cannot be tolerated (rare), patients with mild to moderate CHF may benefit from a combination of hydrallazine and nitrates.

• In some patients with CHF, amiodarone may reduce the incidence of sudden death. Unfortunately, this therapy appears to be less effective in patients with CHF secondary to CHD.

• Survival from sudden out-of-hospital cardiac arrest has been improved by the teaching of cardiopulmonary resuscitation to members of the public.

Case Study 9.1

A 55-year-old male is admitted with an acute myocardial infarction. On admission, he receives aspirin and streptokinase. Examination reveals some signs of congestive heart failure but these clear by day 2 following treatment with diuretics. His subsequent recovery is uneventful and a pre-discharge exercise test is negative. Further investigations show a left ventricular ejection fraction of 38% and total cholesterol 6.7 mmol/l.

Questions
1. Would you start this patient on a beta-blocker or an angiotensin-converting enzyme inhibitor?
2. What would you do about this patient's hyperlipidaemia?

Answers
1. Probably both. The presence of signs of heart failure on admission indicates that this patient would benefit from treatment with an angiotensin-converting enzyme inhibitor as demonstrated in the AIRE trial. Ramipril would be the appropriate drug. However, transient heart failure is not a contraindication to beta-blockade and, with cautious dose titration, it is likely that he will tolerate a beta-blocker. As yet, there are no randomized data comparing beta-blockers and angiotensin-converting enzyme inhibitors or the combination against either alone in post-MI patients.
2. A 2-month trial of dietary therapy. If still > 5.5 mmol/l and normal triglycerides, start therapy with simvastatin 20 mg/day (see Scandinavian Simvastatin Survival Study Group 1994).

REFERENCES

Acute Infarction Ramipril Efficacy (AIRE) Study Investigators 1993 Effect of ramipril on mortality and morbidity of survivors of acute myocardial infarction with clinical evidence of heart failure. Lancet 342: 821–828

AIMS Trial Study Group 1988 Effect of intravenous APSAC on mortality after acute myocardial infarction: Preliminary report of a placebo-controlled clinical trial. Lancet I: 547

Anderson T J, Meredith I T, Yeung A C, Frei B, Selwyn A P, Ganz P 1995 The effect of cholesterol-lowering and antioxidant therapy on endothelium-dependent coronary vasomotion. New England Journal of Medicine 332: 488–493

Andrew T C, Selwyn A P, Ganz P et al 1994 The effect of cholesterol lowering on myocardial ischaemia. Circulation 90: 11–27 (Abstract)

Antiplatelet Trialists' Collaboration 1994a Collaborative overview of randomised trials of antiplatelet therapy—I: prevention of death, myocardial infarction, and stroke by prolonged antiplatelet therapy in various categories of patients. British Medical Journal 308: 81–106

Antiplatelet Trialists' Collaboration 1994b Collaborative overview of randomised trials of antiplatelet therapy—II: maintenance of vascular graft or arterial patency by antiplatelet therapy. British Medical Journal 308: 159–168

Antiplatelet Trialists' Collaboration 1994c Collaborative overview of randomised trials of antiplatelet therapy—III: reduction in venous thrombosis and pulmonary embolism by antiplatelet prophylaxis among surgical and medical patients. British Medical Journal 308: 235–246

Cairns J A, Connolly S J, Gent M, Roberts R 1991 Post-myocardial infarction mortality in patients with ventricular premature depolarizations. Canadian Amiodarone Myocardial Infarction Arrhythmia Trial pilot study. Circulation 84: 550–557

Cardiac Arrhythmia Suppression Trial (CAST) Investigators 1989 Preliminary report: effect of encainide and flecainide on mortality in a randomized trial of arrhythmia suppression after myocardial infarction. New England Journal of Medicine 321: 406–412

Cohen D J, Breall J A, Kalon K L H et al 1994 Evaluating the potential cost-effectiveness of stenting as a treatment for symptomatic single-vessel coronary disease. Use of a decision-analytic model. Circulation 89: 1859–1874

Cohn J N, Archbald D G, Ziesche S et al 1986 Effect of vasodilator therapy on mortality in chronic congestive heart failure: results of a Veterans Administration Cooperative Study. New England Journal of Medicine 314: 1547–1552

Cohn J N, Johnson G, Ziesche S et al 1992 A comparison of enalapril with hydralazine-isosorbide dinitrate in the treatment of congestive heart failure. New England Journal of Medicine 327: 669–677

Colombo A, Hall P, Nakamura S et al 1995 Intracoronary stenting without anticoagulation accomplished with intravascular ultrasound guidance. Circulation 91: 1676–1688

CONSENSUS Trial Group 1987 Effects of enalapril on mortality in severe congestive heart failure. Results of the Cooperative North Scandinavian Enalapril Survival Study. New England Journal of Medicine 316: 1429–1435

Crouse J R, Byington R P, Bond M G, Espeland M A, Craven T E, Sprinkle J W, McGovern M E, Furberg C D 1995 Pravastatin, lipids, and atherosclerosis in the carotid arteries. (PLAC-II). American Journal of Cardiology 75: 455–459

Danish Study Group on Verapamil in Myocardial Infarction 1990 Effect of verapamil on mortality and major events after acute myocardial infarction (The Danish Verapamil Infarction Trial II—DAVIT II). American Journal of Cardiology 66: 779–785

Dotter C T 1969 Transluminally-placed coilspring end arterial tube grafts: long term patency in canine popliteal artery. Investigative Radiology 4: 329–332

Doval H C, Grancelli H O, Perrone S V et al 1994 Randomised trial of low-dose amiodarone in severe congestive heart failure. Lancet 344: 493–498

Eaton L W, Weiss J L, Bulkley B H, Garrison J B, Weisfeldt M L 1979 Regional cardiac dilatation after acute myocardial infarction. New England Journal of Medicine 300: 57–62

Ellis S G, Fisher L, Dushman-Ellis S et al 1989 Comparison of coronary angioplasty with medical treatment for single- and double-vessel coronary disease with left anterior descending coronary involvement: long-term outcome based on an Emory-CASS registry study. American Heart Journal 118: 208–220

Fischman D L, Leon M B, Baim D S et al 1994 A randomized comparison of coronary-stent placement and balloon angioplasty in the treatment of coronary artery disease. New England Journal of Medicine 331: 496–501

Gibson R S, Boden W E, Theroux P et al 1986 Diltiazem and reinfarction in patients with non-Q-wave infarction. New England Journal of Medicine 315: 423–429

Glagov S, Weisenberg E, Zarins C, Stankunavicius R, Kolerris G J 1987 Compensatory enlargement of human atherosclerotic coronary arteries. New England Journal of Medicine 316: 1371–1375

Goldstein R E, Bocuzzi S J, Cruess D et al 1991 Diltiazem increases late-onset congestive heart failure in postinfarction patients with early reduction in ejection fraction. Circulation 83: 52–60

Gould K L, Martucci J P, Goldberg D I et al 1994 Short-term cholesterol lowering decreases size and severity of perfusion abnormalities by positron emission tomography after dipyridamole in patients with coronary artery disease. A potential non-invasive marker of healing coronary endothelium. Circulation 89: 1530–1538

Goy J-J, Eeckhout E, Burnard B et al 1994 Coronary angioplasty versus left internal mammary artery grafting for isolated proximal left anterior descending artery stenosis. Lancet 343: 1449–1453

Gruppo Italiano per lo Studio della Sopravivenza nell'Infarto Miocardico 1990 GISSI-2: A factorial randomised trial of alteplase versus streptokinase and heparin versus no heparin among 12 490 patients with acute myocardial infarction. Lancet 336: 65–71

Gruppo Italiano per lo Studio della Sopravivenza nell'Infarto Miocardico 1994 GISSI-3: Effects of lisinopril and transdermal glyceryl trinitrate singly and together on 6 week mortality and ventricular function after acute myocardial infarction. Lancet 343: 1115–1122

GUSTO Investigators 1993 An international randomized trial comparing four thrombolytic strategies for acute myocardial infarction. New England Journal of Medicine 329: 673–682

Hamm C W, Reimers J, Ischinger T et al 1994 A randomized study of coronary angioplasty compared with bypass surgery in patients with symptomatic multivessel disease. New England Journal of Medicine 331: 1037–1043

Hammermeister K E, DeRouen T A, Dodge H T 1979 Variables predictive of survival in patients with coronary disease: Selection by univariate and multivariate analyses from the clinical, electrocardiographic, exercise, arteriographic and quantitative angiographic evaluations. Circulation 59: 421–430

Held P H, Yusuf S, Furberg C D 1989 Calcium channel blockers in acute myocardial infarction and unstable angina: an overview. British Medical Journal 229: 1187–1192

ISIS-2 (Second International Study of Infarct Survival) Collaborative Group 1988 Randomized trial of intravenous streptokinase, oral aspirin, both, or neither among 17,187 cases of suspected acute myocardial infarction: ISIS-2. Lancet 2: 349–360

ISIS-3 (Third International Study of Infarct Survival) Collaborative Group 1993 ISIS-3: a randomized comparison of streptokinase vs tissue plasminogen activator vs anistreplase and of aspirin plus heparin vs aspirin alone among 41 229 cases of suspected acute myocardial infarction. Lancet 339: 753–770

ISIS-4 (Fourth International Study of Infarct Survival) Collaborative Group 1995 ISIS-4: A randomised factorial trial assessing early oral captopril, oral mononitrate, and intravenous magnesium sulphate in 58,050 patients with suspected acute myocardial infarction. Lancet 345: 669–681

King S B III, Lembo N, Weintraub W et al 1994 A randomized trial comparing coronary angioplasty with coronary bypass surgery. New England Journal of Medicine 331: 1044–1050

Law M R, Wald N J, Thompson S G 1994 Serum cholesterol reduction and health: by how much and how quickly is the risk of ischaemic heart disease lowered? British Medical Journal 308: 367–372

McAlpine H M, Morton J J, Leckie B, Rumley A, Gillen G, Dargie H J 1988 Neuroendocrine activation after acute myocardial infarction. British Heart Journal 60: 117–124

Mason J W for the Electrophysiologic Study Versus Electrocardiographic Monitoring (ESVEM) Investigators 1993a A comparison of electrophysiologic testing with Holter monitoring to predict antiarrhythmic-drug efficacy for ventricular tachyarrhythmias. New England Journal of Medicine 329: 445–451

Mason J W for the ESVEM Investigators 1993b A comparison of seven antiarrhythmic drugs in patients with ventricular tachyarrhythmias. New England Journal of Medicine 329: 452–58

Michels K B, Yusuf S 1995 Does PTCA in acute myocardial infarction affect mortality and reinfarction rates? Circulation 91: 476–485

Multicenter Diltiazem Postinfarction Trial Research Group 1988 The effect of diltiazem on mortality and reinfarction after myocardial infarction. New England Journal of Medicine 319: 385–392

Nademanee K, Singh B N, Stevenson W G, Weiss J N 1993 Amiodarone and post-myocardial infarction patients. Circulation 88: 764–773

Oldroyd K G, Pye M, Ray S G, Christie J, Ford I, Cobbe S M, Dargie H J 1991 Effects of early captopril administration on infarct expansion, ventricular remodelling and exercise capacity after acute myocardial infarction. American Journal of Cardiology 68: 713–718

Packer M, Georghiade M, Young J et al 1993 Withdrawal of digoxin from patients with chronic heart failure treated with angiotensin converting enzyme inhibitors. New England Journal of Medicine 329: 1–7

Parisi A F, Folland E D, Hartigan P 1992 A comparison of angioplasty with medical therapy in the treatment of single-vessel coronary artery disease. New England Journal of Medicine 326: 10–16

Pfeffer J M, Pfeffer M A, Braunwald E 1985 Influence of chronic captopril therapy on the infarcted left ventricle of the rat. Circulation Research 57: 84–95

Pfeffer M A, Braunwald E, Moye L A et al 1992 Effect of captopril on mortality and morbidity in patients with left ventricular dysfunction after myocardial infarction. New England Journal of Medicine 327: 669–677

Pfeffer M A, Lamas G A, Vaughan D E, Parisi A F, Braunwald E 1988 Effect of captopril on progressive ventricular dilatation after anterior myocardial infarction. New England Journal of Medicine 319: 80–86

Pirolo J S, Hutchins G M, Moore G W 1986 Infarct expansion: pathologic analysis of 204 patients with a single myocardial infarct. Journal of American College of Cardiology 7: 349–354

Pitt B, Furberg C D, McGovern M on behalf of the PLAC-I and II Investigators 1994 Reduction in cardiovascular events during treatment with pravastatin: pooled analysis from coronary and carotid atherosclerosis intervention trials. European Heart Journal 15 (Abstract Suppl.): 487

Pitt B, Mancini G B J, Ellis S G, Rosman H S, McGovern M E for the PLAC-I Investigators 1994 Pravastatin limitation of atherosclerosis in the coronary arteries (PLAC-I). Journal of American College of Cardiology 131A: 1A–484A

Raya T E, Gay R G, Aguirre M, Goldman S 1989 Importance of venodilatation in prevention of left ventricular dilatation after chronic large myocardial infarction in rats: a comparison of captopril and hydralazine. Circulation Research 64: 330–337

RITA Trial Participants 1993 Coronary angioplasty versus coronary artery bypass surgery: the Randomised Intervention Treatment of Angina trial. Lancet 341: 573–580

Scandinavian Simvastatin Survival Study Group 1994 Randomised trial of cholesterol lowering in 4,444 patients with coronary heart disease: the Scandinavian Simvastatin Survival Study. Lancet 344: 1383–1389

Schulpher M J, Seed P, Henderson R A et al 1994 Health service costs of coronary angioplasty and coronary artery bypass surgery: the Randomised Intervention Treatment of Angina (RITA) Trial. Lancet 344: 927–930

Serneri G G N, Gensini G F, Poggesi L et al 1990 Effect of heparin, aspirin or alteplase in reduction of myocardial ischaemia in refractory unstable angina. Lancet 335: 615–618

Serruys P W, de Jaegere P, Kiemeneij F et al 1994 A comparison of balloon-expandable-stent implantation with balloon angioplasty in patients with coronary artery disease. New England Journal of Medicine 331: 489–495

Sharpe N, Murphy J, Smith H, Hannan S 1988 Treatment of patients with symptomless left ventricular dysfunction after myocardial infarction. Lancet i: 255–259

Shepherd J, Cobbe S M, Ford I, Isles C G, Lorimer A R, Macfarlane P W, McKillop J H, Packhard C J 1995 Prevention of coronary heart disease with pravastatin in men with hypercholesterolaemia. New England Journal of Medicine 333: 1301–1307

Singh S N, Fletcher R D, Gross Fisher S et al 1995 Amiodarone in patients with congestive heart failure and asymptomatic ventricular arrhythmias. New England Journal of Medicine 333: 77–82

Smith P, Arnesen H, Holme I 1990 The effect of warfarin on mortality and reinfarction after myocardial infarction. New England Journal of Medicine 323: 147–152

SOLVD Investigators 1991 Effect of enalapril on survival in patients with reduced ejection fractions and congestive heart failure. New England Journal of Medicine 316: 293–302

SOLVD Investigators 1992 Effect of enalapril on mortality and the development of heart failure in asymptomatic patients with reduced left ventricular ejection fractions. New England Journal of Medicine 327: 685–691

St John Sutton M, Pfeffer M A, Plappert T et al 1994 Quantitative two-dimensional echocardiographic measurements are major predictors of adverse cardiovascular events after acute myocardial infarction. The protective effects of captopril. Circulation 89: 68–75

Sugurdsson E, Thorgeirsson G, Sigvaldason H, Sigfusson N 1995 Unrecognized myocardial infarction: epidemiology, clinical characteristics, and the prognostic role of angina pectoris. The Reykjavik Study. Annals of Internal Medicine 122: 96–102

Swedberg K, Held P, Kjekshus J et al on behalf of the CONSENSUS II Study Group 1992 Effects of early administration of enalapril on mortality in patients with acute myocardial infarction. Results of the Cooperative North Scandinavian Enalapril Survival Study II (CONSENSUS II). New England Journal of Medicine 327: 678–684

TIMI Study Group 1989 Comparison of invasive and conservative strategies after treatment with intravenous tissue plasminogen activator in acute myocardial infarction. Results of the Thrombolysis in Myocardial Infarction (TIMI) Phase II Trial. New England Journal of Medicine 320: 618–622

Treasure C B, Klein J L, Weintraub W S et al 1995 Beneficial effects of cholesterol-lowering therapy on the coronary endothelium in patients with coronary artery disease. New England Journal of Medicine 332: 481–487

Uretsky B F, Young J B, Shahidi F E et al 1993 Randomized study assessing the effect of digoxin withdrawal in patients with mild to moderate chronic congestive heart failure: results of the PROVED trial. Journal of American College of Cardiology 22: 955–962

White H D, Norris R M, Brown M A, Brandt P W T, Whitlock R M L, Wild C J 1987 Left ventricular end-systolic volume as the major determinant of survival after recovery from myocardial infarction. Circulation 76: 44–51

Wilcox R G, Olsson C G, Skene A M et al 1988 Trial of tissue plasminogen activator for mortality reduction in acute myocardial infarction. Anglo-Scandinavian Study of Early Thrombolysis (ASSET). Lancet ii: 525

Wray R, Maurer B, Shillingford J 1973 Prophylactic anticoagulant therapy in the prevention of calf-vein thrombosis after myocardial infarction. New England Journal of Medicine 288: 815–820

Yusuf S, Peto R, Lewis J et al 1985 Beta blockade during and after myocardial infarction: an overview of the randomized trials. Progress in Cardiovascular Disease 27: 335

Yusuf S, Zucker D, Peduzzi P et al 1994 Effect of coronary artery bypass graft surgery on survival: overview of 10 year results from randomised trials by the Coronary Artery Bypass Graft Surgery Trialists Collaboration. Lancet 344: 563–570

FURTHER READING

The management of coronary heart disease and its many complications is a rapidly changing field. The delay between completion of clinical trials and their publication sometimes means that even journal items can be somewhat behind the times. Nevertheless, the most up-to-date information can be obtained by perusing one or more of the following journals:

- *General cardiology:* New England Journal of Medicine; Lancet; British Medical Journal
- *Specialist cardiology:* Circulation; American Journal of Cardiology; Journal of American College of Cardiology; American Heart Journal; Heart.

Braunwald E 1988 Heart disease. A textbook of cardiovascular disease. Saunders, Philadelphia

A large and comprehensive textbook with predominantly North American contributors. Very well illustrated and referenced.

Julian D G, Camm A J, Fox K, Hall R J C, Poole-Wilson P A 1996 Diseases of the heart. Baillière Tindall, London

British version of Braunwald and as such offers some differing opinions on various issues. Not quite so comprehensive but very readable.

Swanton R H 1994 Cardiology. Blackwell Scientific Publications, Oxford

In the Pocket Consultant series. A condensed and concise version of the larger textbooks. Lots of practical information on the management of CHD.

Lipid-lowering drug therapy

Allan Gaw

10

INTRODUCTION

The important link between elevated plasma lipid concentrations and coronary heart disease (CHD) has been bolstered in recent years by repeated demonstration of the benefits of lipid-lowering therapy in preventing atherosclerotic disease. The findings of some of the major trials of lipid-lowering drug therapy are discussed in Chapter 3. This chapter will deal with the lipid-lowering drugs themselves and will outline their mechanism of action, their effects and their potential side effects.

The lipid-lowering drugs can be divided conveniently into four classes—resins, statins, fibrates and others—each with its distinctive therapeutic profile. Resins and statins are used mainly to lower plasma cholesterol in individuals with primary hypercholesterolaemia. Fibrates, on the other hand, are most often employed in patients with raised plasma triglyceride levels or mixed hyperlipidaemia. The final category represents a miscellaneous group of drugs most of which only have a single representative on the pharmacy shelf. Included in this group are drugs such as nicotinic acid and maxepa (fish oil), which are usually prescribed in situations where other compounds have failed to work, in particular, in the treatment of severe hypertriglyceridaemia. Table 10.1 summarizes the major effects of the lipid-lowering drugs on the plasma lipoprotein profile.

Table 10.1 Lipid-lowering drugs

Class	Marketed agents	UK trade names	Indication	Range of response to therapy
Bile acid sequestrant resins	Cholestyramine Colestipol	Questran (Questran-Light) Colestid	Raised LDL	10–25% decrease in LDL
Statins	Fluvastatin Pravastatin Simvastatin	Lescol Lipostat Zocor	Raised LDL	15–35% decrease in LDL
Fibrates	Bezafibrate Clofibrate Ciprofibrate Fenofibrate Gemfibrozil	Bezalip Mono Atromid-S Modalim Lipantil Micro Lopid	Raised LDL Raised TG	LDL change + 40% to – 35% TG decrease 15–70%
Nicotinic acid & derivatives*	Acipimox Nicofuranose	Nicotinic acid (generic) Olbetam Bradilan	Raised LDL Raised TG	LDL decrease 10–20% TG decrease 15–70%
Fish oil		Maxepa	Raised TG	TG decrease 10–50%
Probucol		Lurselle	Raised LDL	LDL decrease 0–20%

In the discussion that follows on the different lipid-lowering therapies it is imperative for the reader to note that drug doses, regimens and indications are subject to change. The reader must always consult the current data sheet for each drug appropriate to his or her own country before prescribing these drugs or making management decisions.

BILE ACID SEQUESTRANT RESINS

Mechanism of action

The bile acid sequestrant resins are able to lower LDL-cholesterol by 20–25% when given at the highest recommended dose. They are considered very safe drugs since they are not absorbed systemically and have been in clinical use for several decades. Furthermore, they are one of the few lipid-lowering compounds recommended for use in children with severe hypercholesterol-aemia. The principal drawback to their more widespread prescription is the fact that they are difficult to take and patient compliance is often very poor. Approximately half of the subjects who begin resin therapy stop because of their inability to tolerate the side effects.

Each day 10–20 g of bile acids (cholic acid, chenodeoxycholic acid and their salts) pass through the liver and intestine in an enterohepatic circulation

(Danielson & Sjoval 1975). These compounds are essential for the efficient absorption of dietary fat in the duodenum and upper jejunum and, having facilitated this process, are reabsorbed in the terminal third of the ileum, returning to the liver in the portal circulation. Their production from cholesterol by a pathway which is initiated by the enzyme cholesterol-7-alpha-hydroxylase is under feedback inhibition particularly by chenodeoxycholic acid (Danielson & Sjoval 1975). Two strategies have been used to interrupt this enterohepatic circulation and cause increased faecal loss of bile acids. The first is surgical removal of the terminal 200 cm of ileum, the site of active resorption (Moore et al 1969); the second is administration of sequestrant resins which bind bile acids strongly. The effects of these manoeuvres on plasma lipid levels are secondary to the liver's compensatory response of generating more bile acids to maintain efficient lipid absorption from the intestine. Loss of bile acids from the portal return to the liver leads to activation of cholesterol-7-alpha hydroxylase. Synthesis of bile acids goes up several-fold and the result is a decrease in intracellular cholesterol levels. The resulting shortfall in cholesterol is corrected by the hepatocyte in two ways: first, synthesis from acetate is promoted by stimulation of the rate-limiting enzyme, 3-hydroxyl-3-methyl glutaryl coenzyme A (HMG CoA) reductase; and second, the cell makes membrane receptors which are able to bind low density lipoprotein (LDL) and facilitate its endocytosis (see Ch. 3). LDL receptors which possess specific binding sites for apolipoprotein B, the major protein on the surface of LDL, play an essential role in maintaining cellular cholesterol balance. Following interaction of the receptor with the lipoprotein, the complex is drawn into the cell and delivered to the lysosomal compartment where digestive enzymes release the particles' cholesterol to meet cellular requirements. It was in the 1980s that evidence was obtained for the key role of the receptor in the hypocholesterolaemic action of bile acid sequestrant resins. The drugs were shown by Shepherd and his colleagues (1980) to promote receptor-mediated catabolism of LDL in subjects with heterozygous familial hypercholesterolaemia (FH) who have a genetic deficiency of functional LDL receptors. Moreover, using hepatic biopsies, it was demonstrated directly that LDL-receptor activity was increased in individuals given cholestyramine (Reihnér et al 1990). Thus resins promote the hepatocytes' own ability to take up LDL from extracellular fluid and the result is a shift of cholesterol from the plasma to the liver, thus causing a sharp fall in plasma LDL-cholesterol levels. The central role of the receptor in the action of sequestrant resins is further exemplified by the inability of the drugs to lower plasma cholesterol in homozygous familial hypercholesterolaemics who are completely deficient in functioning LDL receptors (Goldstein & Brown 1983).

Sequestrant resins have additional actions on plasma triglyceride and HDL levels. Bile acids returning to the liver in the enterohepatic circulation suppress not only cholesterol synthesis but also triglyceride production (Angelin et al 1978). The release of this inhibition by resin therapy causes an immediate rise in triglyceride synthesis and a promotion of VLDL secretion so that within days of initiating therapy, VLDL triglyceride levels can increase twofold. Subsequently, the plasma triglyceride concentration falls back towards baseline values through an adaptation brought about by increased lipolysis. Resins are, therefore, not indicated in individuals who have moderately or severely elevated plasma triglyceride levels.

Prescribing information

These drugs are contraindicated in biliary obstruction and their side effects are very common, including nausea, vomiting, constipation, diarrhoea, dyspepsia, flatulence, and abdominal pain. Because they bind bile acids and at least partially prevent the absorption of the fat-soluble vitamins, A, D and K, prolonged use of the resins may lead to an increased bleeding tendency due to hypoprothrombinaemia related to vitamin K deficiency. Because of this, fat-soluble vitamin and folate supplements may need to be given especially if patients are on prolonged high-dose therapy, or if the resins are being used in children or continued through pregnancy.

Most commonly, the resins are supplied as granular 'sand-like' preparations in sachets. Each sachet of Questran or Questran Light contains 4 g of anhydrous cholestyramine while each sachet of Colestid contains 5 g of colestipol hydrochloride. For lipid-lowering therapy, up to six sachets per day in divided doses may be required. Because of the common frequency of unpleasant gastrointestinal side effects, the dose should be titrated up slowly over a period of weeks and possibly months. The patient should be aware that the cholestyramine or colestipol granules do not dissolve in liquids but are made more palatable when mixed with fruit juices or sprinkled on some foods. Long-term compliance is very difficult with these drugs and a variety of aids in the form of recipe books and mixing glasses are available from the manufacturers to encourage patients to vary the way they take the resin.

An important note must be made to counsel patients when starting bile acid sequestrant therapy that these agents will bind to other therapeutic drugs with potentially very serious results. Thyroxine used in the management of hypothyroidism and the oral contraceptive pill are just two examples of drugs which will be prevented from complete absorption when taken with a resin. In order to avoid this interaction all other medications should be taken at least 1 hour before or 4-6 hours after cholestyramine or colestipol is taken.

Despite being one of the oldest forms of lipid-lowering drug therapy, the resins remain the most expensive. These drugs should therefore not simply be used as a default prescription for first-line treatment of hypercholesterolaemia but should be reserved for those patients who are either intolerant of other lipid-lowering therapies or those whose form of hyperlipidaemia requires combination therapy.

HMG COENZYME A REDUCTASE INHIBITORS OR STATINS

Mechanism of action

Approximately half of the body's cholesterol is obtained from the diet while the remainder is synthesized from the simple molecule acetate, principally in the liver and intestine. Suppression of the pathway of endogenous cholesterol production offers significant potential for regulating whole body cholesterol balance. Thus, the discovery of a class of drugs which inhibit the pacemaker enzyme in cholesterol synthesis, HMG CoA reductase, was a landmark in the lipid-lowering therapeutic area. Reductase inhibitors, or 'statins' as they are more simply called, can be given in milligram doses to produce reductions in LDL-cholesterol of up to 35% (Table 10.1). They are remarkably effective, easy to take and their introduction into clinical practice has revolutionized the treatment of hypercholesterolaemia (Feussner 1994).

Investigation of the influence of statins on LDL metabolism has revealed that in subjects with heterozygous FH, the major effect of the drug is to promote LDL receptor activity in a manner similar to that observed with bile acid sequestrant resins (Bilheimer et al 1983). This finding indicates that statins and resins work through a common pathway (Fig. 10.1), namely increased receptor synthesis in liver cells in response to a depleted intra-cellular cholesterol level. This proposed mechanism of action implies that resins and statins may have additive effects when given in combination and this has been shown to be the case. LDL reductions of up to 60% are observed (Mabuchi et al 1983) as the liver attempts to compensate for both increased faecal bile acid loss and inhibited cholesterol synthesis. This combined therapy is the most effective lipid-lowering regimen available at the present time.

Metabolic investigations in hyperlipidaemic subjects who do not suffer from FH have shown that statins can also affect the production rate of LDL. As described in Chapter 3, LDL is derived from VLDL by a process of delipidation and remodelling. Originally it was thought that all VLDL was converted to LDL; however, it is now clear that both VLDL and the transient intermediate in LDL production, intermediate density lipoprotein (IDL), have the capacity to interact with LDL receptors and so these precursors have two possible metabolic fates, receptor-mediated catabolism and lipolysis to LDL (Fig. 10.1). Recently, it was demonstrated that simvastatin therapy, while not altering the production rate of VLDL, diverted VLDL and IDL particles towards clearance by the LDL receptor and this led to a significant reduction in LDL production (Gaw et al 1993). This further action of the statins helps explain their almost universal efficacy. In FH heterozygotes where the LDL receptor is defective (Bilheimer et al 1993), statins activate the remaining normal receptor gene and promote LDL clearance, whereas in moderately hypercholesterolaemic subjects where the elevation in LDL is due to over-production of the lipoprotein (Gaw et al 1995), the drugs can also diminish this pathway.

At first statins were thought to have little effect on plasma triglyceride and HDL levels; a not unreasonable assumption given their mechanism of action. However, it is now established from abundant trial data (Feussner 1994) that plasma triglyceride levels fall on therapy by approximately 10–20%. The decrease appears to be independent of the dose given and seems to be common to all statins. Furthermore, there is a small but significant rise in HDL-cholesterol of the order of 5–10%. This may be secondary to the decrease

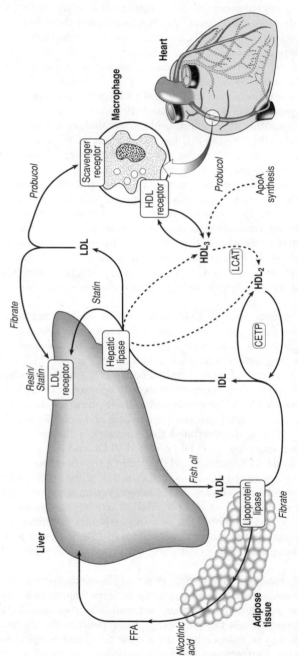

Figure 10.1 Principal mechanisms of action of lipid-lowering drugs. Free fatty acids (FFA) released from adipose tissue promote the secretion of VLDL by the liver. This lipoprotein, via the action of lipoprotein and hepatic lipases, is converted to IDL and finally to LDL. LDL is catabolized by specific receptors, principally in the liver. If this pathway is overwhelmed, then excess LDL is cleared by scavenger receptors on macrophages. Oxidation of LDL is required before the lipoprotein is taken up by macrophages, which may be resident in the coronary artery wall as well as other tissues. HDL can assimilate excess unesterified cholesterol from cells. The cholesterol is then trapped in the lipoprotein by the action of lecithin : cholesterol acyl transferase (LCAT). Cholesteryl ester in HDL is carried back to the liver either directly or following transfer of the lipid to apoB-containing lipoproteins via the activity of cholesteryl ester transfer protein (CETP). The main sites of action of the lipid-lowering drug classes are illustrated.

in plasma triglyceride levels since the two are linked metabolically, but a separate effect of statins on HDL metabolism cannot be ruled out. The mechanism by which statins lower plasma triglyceride is as yet unknown.

Recently a new member, atorvastatin, has been added to this drug class (Nawrocki et al 1995), but at the time of writing this drug is not yet available for routine clinical use. This compound has increased potency in that it lowers LDL-cholesterol by 60–70% when given at 40 mg/d, an effect that cannot be matched by other statins even when given in high doses. This observation suggests that atorvastatin may be affecting LDL through mechanisms additional to those seen with other statins, a hypothesis supported by the finding that atorvastatin reduces plasma triglyceride by 20–30%.

Prescribing information

The statins are all available as tablets of varying strength. The main contra-indication is active liver disease. The statins should also be avoided in pregnancy and breast-feeding and in patients with porphyria. There are some reports of statin use in children with severe hyperlipidaemia but in general these drugs should not be used in children. Most of the side effects of the statins are relatively mild, including gastrointestinal upsets—constipation, flatulence, dyspepsia, abdominal pain and diarrhoea—as well as headaches, insomnia, fatigue and skin rashes. Much more serious but very rare are rhabdomyolysis and hepatitis. A frequent finding is an increase in the serum level of creatine kinase (CK). This is a marker of muscle damage and if markedly raised (more than three times the upper limit of normal), the statin should be discontinued. Similarly, if a clinical diagnosis of myopathy is made, the drug should be stopped. However, in major trials this potentially serious side effect of rhabdomyolysis has not turned out to be a significant problem (Feussner 1994, Scandinavian Simvastatin Survival Study Group 1994). From a practical point of view, remember that in patients of African descent serum CK levels are normally higher than Caucasian values and this in itself is not an indicator of muscle damage, drug-induced or otherwise.

Because of the potential muscle and hepatic toxicity with these drugs it is considered prudent to check the liver function tests and CK prior to treatment and at intervals during therapy. Female patients should be advised to avoid pregnancy during treatment and for at least 1 month after stopping the drug. Again, because of the potential hepatotoxicity of the statins, they should be avoided in patients who abuse alcohol.

The dose of a statin is dependent on which member of the class is prescribed. Simvastatin is available in 10 and 20 mg tablets and the usual dose is 10–40 mg per day usually given at night. The rationale for night-time dosing is that the statins exert their effect by inhibiting cholesterol synthesis in the body. Normally cholesterol synthesis rates exhibit a diurnal rhythm with maximal rates at night. Therefore by giving the enzyme inhibitor at the time of peak enzyme activity it is hoped that the most effective lipid-lowering is achieved. Pravastatin is available in 10 and 20 mg tablets and the usual dose is again 10–40 mg per day at night. Fluvastatin is available in 20 and 40 mg tablets and the usual dose is 20–40 mg per day, again given at night.

FIBRATES

Mechanism of action

The parent compound of the fibric acid derivatives or fibrates as they are commonly known is para-chloro-phenoxyisobutyric acid, which was synthesized in the 1950s. As the first therapeutically useful and clinically acceptable hypolipidaemic agent, its production was a milestone. Clofibrate, as its ester is known, is an effective lipid-lowering agent in humans and was employed in many trials world-wide over a period of 20 years, but the poor results of the WHO trial (described in Ch. 3) have led to a decline in its use. A new generation of more powerful analogues have been developed including bezafibrate, ciprofibrate, fenofibrate and gemfibrozil and these have largely superseded clofibrate. These agents share a similar lipid-lowering profile, reducing plasma triglyceride levels usually by 20–50% and plasma cholesterol by 10–25%. HDL-cholesterol is normally increased 10–30% by fibrates depending on the pretreatment level (patients with lower basal HDL respond with greater increases). The dyslipidaemic syndrome characterized by raised plasma triglyceride and low HDL-cholesterol is associated with high risk of CHD. Individuals with this lipid profile, i.e. plasma triglyceride > 2.3 mmol/l and an LDL to HDL ratio of > 5, have been shown to benefit most from fibrate therapy (Manninen et al 1992).

The mechanism of action of fibrates has been studied for many years. Since they perturb all lipoprotein classes it is predictable that they have a number of effects. The plasma concentration of VLDL is reduced up to 50% on therapy and the decrease is primarily in the largest triglyceride-rich VLDL species. Two main mechanisms have been proposed to explain the influence of fibrates on VLDL metabolism. The first is a fall in the return of free fatty acids to the liver secondary to suppression of their release from adipose tissue (Kissebah et al 1974). It is known from recent in vitro studies that the supply of fatty acids to hepatocytes is a principal determinant of the rate of VLDL assembly and secretion (Dixon & Ginsberg 1993). When cells are deprived of this lipid source, apoB, which is made continuously, is degraded intracellularly; an abundant supply of fatty acids, on the other hand, stabilizes apoB and promotes the formation of large, triglyceride-rich particles. The second perturbation proposed to explain the drug-induced reduction in VLDL is stimulation of lipoprotein lipase activity (Simpson et al 1990), the enzyme which governs triglyceride hydrolysis in plasma. Kinetic studies indicate that both mechanisms operate in vivo. It has been shown that bezafibrate therapy in Type III subjects inhibits the formation of large VLDL (Packard et al 1986), while in Type IV subjects evidence was obtained that the drug promotes the conversion of larger VLDL to smaller VLDL consistent with an effect on lipoprotein lipase activity (Shepherd et al 1984). Other studies have reported enhanced chylomicron clearance during fibrate therapy which can again be explained by an action of the drug on lipase (Simpson et al 1990).

Fibrates have a complex effect on the concentration, composition and metabolism of LDL. It has been known for a number of years that in subjects with elevated LDL, fibrates can induce a fall in the level of this lipoprotein, while in those where the initial concentration is low (usually hypertriglyceridaemic subjects), therapy causes LDL to rise. The basis for the paradoxical influence of the drugs on plasma LDL concentration has been defined with the help of metabolic studies. First, it was shown in hypercholesterolaemic patients that a fibrate promotes removal of LDL by receptor-mediated catabolism, possibly due to an effect of the drug on the activity of receptors (Stewart et al 1982). Second, it was found in hypertriglyceridaemic subjects that a fibrate-induced increase in LDL circulating mass was due to suppression of hypercatabolism by receptor-independent pathways; accelerated clearance by this route is a characteristic of patients with high plasma triglyceride levels (Shepherd et al 1985). In reconciling these drug actions it was concluded that fibrate treatment 'normalizes' LDL metabolism in both types of patients.

Recently, the action of fibrates on LDL has been re-examined in the light of evidence that the lipoprotein class is heterogeneous. Traditionally, LDL was thought to exist as a population of particles that differed little from each other. However, with the development of high-resolution separation techniques, it has become clear that LDL is composed of a number of distinct subfractions, namely:

- LDL I—the least dense, most lipid-rich
- LDL II—the most abundant
- LDL III—the smallest and densest subfraction.

A preponderance of LDL III in the LDL profile is associated with a three- to sevenfold increase in the risk of coronary heart disease (Griffin et al 1994). It has been shown that fibrates perturb the LDL subfraction pattern, shifting the distribution from smaller to larger particles (Franceschini et al 1995) probably as a result of the alteration in plasma triglyceride, since the concentration of this lipid has a profound influence on the LDL subfraction profile. Small, dense LDL bind poorly to receptors whereas the larger LDL species have a higher affinity; thus when fibrates shift the spectrum away from small, dense LDL the nature of the binding lipoprotein changes and, conceivably, it is this action that promotes clearance of the lipoprotein through the LDL receptor pathway.

Less work has been done on the effects of fibrates on HDL and the precise mechanism by which the fibrates exert their powerful HDL-cholesterol-raising effect is not yet fully understood.

Prescribing information

The principle contraindication to the fibrate group is severe renal impairment. All fibrates will cause a myositis-like syndrome in these patients. In addition, because some of the fibrates have been associated with increased incidence of gallstone, these drugs should be avoided in patients with a history of gallstones. As with most lipid-lowering drugs the fibrates should also be avoided in pregnancy and lactation and should not be given to patients with severe hepatic impairment. The only fibrate currently licensed for use in children is fenofibrate.

The fibrates are generally well-tolerated drugs and rarely is withdrawal of treatment necessary. Before commencing therapy it is prudent to record a number of baseline laboratory safety parameters including a full blood count and liver and kidney function tests. Pretreatment assessment of renal function is useful to alert the clinician to the possibility of overdosage due to drug accumulation in renal impairment. The most common side effects that are seen in clinical practice are gastrointestinal disturbances such as nausea and diarrhoea. More uncommon side effects include impotence and loss of libido, skin rashes, increased appetite and weight gain. Clofibrate has also been noted to cause increases in serum CK and the aminotransferases associated with malaise, myalgia and myaesthenia.

The fibrates bind extensively to plasma albumin and this in turn displaces other acidic drugs from these plasma protein binding sites. The clinical consequence of this is that the coadministration of a fibrate with other drugs such as the oral anticoagulant warfarin may potentiate the effect of the latter. This potentially hazardous drug interaction is common to all fibrates and may prompt the use of other lipid-lowering drugs in situations where the fibrates would have been drugs of first choice. Alternatively, the dose of the anti-coagulant should be reduced by about one-third at the commencement of fibrate therapy and then gradually adjusted as required. Possible similar interactions with oral hypoglycaemic agents should also be kept in mind.

The usual daily doses of the fibrates are dependent on which member of the class is prescribed. Bezafibrate, fenofibrate and ciprofibrate are available as once-daily preparations while clofibrate and gemfibrozil have to be taken in divided doses. It is usually recommended that the fibrates are taken either with or after food to minimize their gastrointestinal side effects.

OTHER LIPID-LOWERING DRUGS

A number of other pharmacological agents have been used, with varying success, in reducing plasma lipid levels. These include nicotinic acid, pro-bucol and fish oils. Their mechanisms of action are known to some extent and it is clear that their effects are distinct from those of the major classes noted above.

NICOTINIC ACID AND ITS DERIVATIVES

Mechanism of action

Nicotinic acid operates primarily to block free fatty acid release from the adipocyte (Fig. 10.1) by indirectly inhibiting the activity of hormone-sensitive lipase in fat tissue. This reduces free fatty acid flux to the liver and, as a consequence, depresses VLDL synthesis and secretion (Kissebah et al 1974). The drug is also postulated to inhibit hepatic lipase and this is the likely cause of the rather remarkable change in total HDL and the increase in the particularly anti-atherogenic subfraction, HDL_2, seen on medication (Shepherd et al 1979). Thus, the drug has a favourable effect on all lipoprotein species but its use is limited by the unpleasant side effects described below.

Prescribing information

Nicotinic acid is contraindicated in pregnancy and lactation and care must be taken when it is used in patients who have diabetes mellitus, hepatic impairment, gout or peptic ulceration. This drug is associated with a number of prostaglandin-mediated symptoms such as flushing of the head and neck, dizziness, headache, palpitation and pruritus. These symptoms can be partially controlled by starting with low doses taken with food and increasing slowly over a period of weeks to the desired final dose. Alternatively, the administration of aspirin (300 mg) half an hour before the nicotinic acid may be used in patients who find the symptoms particularly troubling. Other side effects include nausea and vomiting and more rarely hepatic failure.

Nicotinic acid is available in 50 mg tablets. The dose of nicotinic acid prescribed has to be titrated up over a period of time to avoid unpleasant side effects and to ensure patient compliance. Starting at 100–200 mg three times daily the dose is increased gradually to 1–2 g three times daily if necessary.

The nicotinic acid derivative acipimox has a similar but attenuated side effect profile and is given in smaller doses. The 250 mg capsules are given at a dose of 500–750 mg per day. Similarly, nicofuranose is used as an alternative to nicotinic acid because its prostaglandin-mediated side effects are less severe. This compound is available in 250 mg tablets and is prescribed at an initial dose of 500 mg three times daily rising gradually to 1 g three times daily.

PROBUCOL

Mechanism of action

Probucol is a powerful antioxidant that was found to have cholesterol-reducing properties. It has been used to a varying degree but recently has fallen out of favour because the HDL concentration is profoundly and adversely affected by the drug; up to 50% of the reduction in total plasma cholesterol is in the high density fraction (Atmeh et al 1983). The amount of LDL lowering with probucol is highly variable and no consistent perturbation in LDL metabolism has been detected on therapy. In contrast, the drug substantially inhibits the synthesis of the apolipoproteins associated with HDL (Atmeh et al 1983) which accounts in part for the fall in HDL. There is, in addition a relative depletion of cholesterol in HDL particles on therapy. The significance of these findings is not yet clear and it may even be argued that during probucol therapy the reduction in HDL-cholesterol is simply a reflection of the fact that there is less of the sterol in peripheral tissues for HDL to extract in the process of reverse cholesterol transport (Fig. 10.1). One other important effect of probucol is its ability to protect LDL from oxidation. The lipoprotein isolated from subjects given the drug is highly resistant to oxidation in vitro (Parthasarathy et al 1986) and in animal models probucol was able to slow significantly the progression of atherosclerosis (Kita et al 1987).

Probucol is contraindicated in patients who are breast-feeding and it is recommended that pregnancy should be avoided during treatment and for

6 months after stopping therapy. Before commencing therapy an ECG should be recorded in patients who have had recent myocardial damage or who have experienced cardiac arrhythmias.

The side effects most commonly noted are gastrointestinal, with diarrhoea, nausea and vomiting, but these are often mild and transient. More importantly there may be ventricular arrhythmias and there are rare reports of angioedema.

Probucol is available as 250 mg tablets and the usual dose is 500 mg twice daily, with food.

FISH OIL

Mechanism of action

Fish oil, principally its docosahexaenoic and eicosapentaenoic acid constituents, has a triglyceride-lowering effect in man with VLDL levels falling 30–50% on therapy. This has been shown to be due to suppression of VLDL triglyceride production in the liver (Harris et al 1990). There is a concomitant, beneficial increase in HDL but also in many subjects, a significant and adverse increase in LDL. The latter phenomenon has been ascribed to the fact that fish oils promote the release of smaller VLDL particles from the liver (Sullivan et al 1986) which have been shown to be better precursors for LDL than their larger counterparts (Packard et al 1984). Thus, the benefits of fish oils in terms of triglyceride and VLDL lowering are, at least partially, offset by the rise in plasma LDL levels.

Prescribing information

The commercial fish oil preparation Maxepa is available as capsules, as a liquid, or as an emulsion. This oil in capsule or liquid form contains as a percentage of total fatty acids 18% eicosapentaenoic acid and 12% docosahexaenoic acid, while the emulsion contains 9% and 6% respectively. The usual dose is five capsules, 5 ml of liquid, or 10 ml of emulsion per day, taken with food.

There are no strong contraindications but caution is advised in the use of fish oils in subjects with bleeding disorders or who are taking anticoagulants. The main side effects are nausea and belching which may be troublesome enough to limit patient compliance.

COMBINATION THERAPY

Lipid-lowering drugs have been used in combined regimens with the expectation that two or more drugs may act synergistically to correct aberrant lipoprotein metabolism or that they may serve to offset each other's unwanted effects on the lipid profile.

Almost every combination of lipid-lowering drugs has been tried, often empirically over the last 30 years. Some regimens have been highly successful in achieving their therapeutic goals, while others may be potentially dangerous. In the latter category is the combination of a statin and a fibrate. In designing new combined regimens, an exciting combination was thought initially to be that of a fibrate plus a statin. Enthusiasm for such a regimen was, however, curbed when reports of myopathy associated with lovastatin plus gemfibrozil therapy were published (Pierce et al 1990). Despite this, and because the combination had shown such early promise other studies have demonstrated the efficacy and safety of this regimen in different types of hyperlipoproteinemia (e.g. Illingworth & O'Malley 1990). However, caution is still urged by many investigators who suggest careful follow-up of these patients on combined fibrate and statin protocols with serial CK measurements and liver function tests.

LIPID-LOWERING DRUGS IN PRACTICE

Lipid-lowering, or more correctly lipid-regulating, drugs have an important place in the management of the lipid related risk of CHD. However, they occupy this place only after dietary management of dyslipidaemia has been tried and found inadequate. All patients who have a firm diagnosis of dyslipidaemia should receive detailed and tailored dietary advice as outlined in Chapter 6. There are varying opinions on how long dietary management alone should be tried in an individual before drug therapy is considered. Most practitioners would suggest a trial of not less than 3 months before resorting to drug therapy. It is important to note that drug therapy is then prescribed as an adjunct to dietary therapy and not as an alternative. The patients' lifestyle changes in terms of diet should be continued and patients must be made to realize that the initiation of drug therapy does not mean that their efforts, which are sometimes considerable, have been in vain.

Another important point to be considered by both patient and prescriber is that lipid-lowering drug therapy is lifelong and requires understanding and cooperation from the patient if it is to be effective and worthwhile. Like the management of hypertension, the drug treatment of dyslipidaemia does not carry any immediate and obvious benefit or 'feel-good factor'. The concept of CHD risk should be explained to the patient along with the rationale for prevention. In the secondary prevention situation, where the patient has already suffered a coronary event, this is much easier and the patient is invariably well focused on the issue. However, in primary prevention more time may need to be spent in explaining the reasons for commencing drug therapy and the long-term benefits that are expected.

The choice of lipid-regulating drug is dictated by the patient's form of dyslipidaemia and past medical history, the cost, and to some extent the practitioner's experience. It is not the remit of this chapter to suggest specific drug regimens; nor is this the place for a discussion of the relative costs of lipid-regulating drugs, but some useful statements can be made.

Although there can be many underlying causes of dyslipidaemia, patients usually present with one of three broad categories: hypercholesterolaemia, hypertriglyceridaemia, or a mixed hyperlipidaemia. In hypercholesterolaemia the first-line drugs were until recently the resins, but these are being superseded by the statins whose good safety and efficacy record is now widely acknowledged. In moderate hypertriglyceridaemia the first-line agents are usually members of the fibrate or nicotinic acid families, with the fish oils as second line. In those with mixed hyperlipidaemia, the fibrates are usually first line with the nicotinic acid derivatives as reserves. There is of course considerable overlap in this scheme, e.g. the modern fibrates are potent LDL-cholesterol-lowering agents and therefore have a place as first-line agents in hypercholesterolaemia while the statins have triglyceride-lowering effects and may well be considered in a mixed hyperlipidaemia.

CONCLUSIONS

The correction of raised plasma lipid levels is a problem that faces the health care team on a daily basis. There is now abundant evidence that individuals with high CHD risk factor scores require intervention to lower their plasma lipid levels. Diet is always the cornerstone of therapy and drugs should only be considered when this has been demonstrated to be inadequate. A range of hypolipidaemic pharmacologic agents is now available and the mechanisms of action of most of these are now well understood.

■ KEY POINTS

• The first-line management of dyslipidaemia is dietary management.

• Lipid-lowering drugs should be considered in patients who have dyslipidaemia resistant to dietary management and whose overall risk factor profile for CHD is poor.

• The lipid-lowering drugs may be divided conveniently into four classes: resins, statins, fibrates and others.

• The resins bind and remove bile acids from the body, thus forcing the liver to resort to plasma LDL-cholesterol for its needs. This in turn lowers plasma LDL-cholesterol.

• The statins inhibit the rate-limiting enzyme in the body's cholesterol production, thus again forcing the liver to resort to plasma LDL-cholesterol for its needs.

• The fibrates have a variety of actions including increasing the activity of lipoprotein lipase, decreasing the return of free fatty acids from adipose tissue to the liver, and shifting the size and density of LDL particles towards a form more readily removed from the plasma by the LDL receptor.

• Like all drugs, the lipid-lowering drugs have a range of side effects and contraindications which must be considered before their use.

• Most lipid-lowering drugs should be avoided in children, in pregnancy, and in hepatic or renal failure. There are, however, important exceptions to these rules.

• Lipid-lowering drug therapy is lifelong and will only be successful with the full cooperation and understanding of the patient.

Case study 10.1

Mr A B is a 48-year-old man who presents at his GP complaining of tiredness and lethargy. He has a long history of thyroid disease and has been on thyroxine replacement therapy for over 10 years. Recently he was also diagnosed as having hypercholesterolaemia, for which he was given dietary advice and subsequently started on cholestyramine four sachets (4 g each) per day.

Questions
1. What investigations should be performed?
2. What do you think may have happened?

Answers
1. Because of the patient's history of hypothyroidism it is likely that his present symptoms may be due to under-replacement with thyroxine. To check this, his thyroid function tests should be performed, which in this man showed a low serum T_4 and a high TSH consistent with hypothyroidism.
2. The most common cause of recurring hypothyroidism in patients on replacement therapy is poor compliance with medication. Mr A B, however, was adamant that he had taken his thyroxine tablets faithfully along with his newly prescribed cholestyramine. Therein lies the problem. Cholestyramine is a bile acid sequestrant resin which binds to bile acids in the gut. It will also bind to other compounds including some therapeutic drugs, thus preventing their absorption. The two most important of these are thyroxine and the oral contraceptive pill. It is important to elicit a full drug history from anyone who is to be prescribed a bile acid sequestrant resin as this important drug interaction must be highlighted. Patients who must take both drugs should space them apart as much as possible but preferably alternative lipid-lowering drugs should be used.

PRACTICAL EXERCISE

Some patients remain on specific therapies for years without review because of the repeat prescription system. This is unfortunate, especially if a patient remains unnoticed on what has become an obsolete drug. In the field of lipid-lowering many patients remain on clofibrate with relatively little clinical benefit or are continued on bile acid sequestrant resins even though their compliance is poor or even non-existent.

Review the lipid-lowering therapy of the patients in your care and find out more about those on clofibrate or the bile acid sequestrant resins. Some patients will be happy on these drugs, but others may benefit from a therapy update.

REFERENCES

Angelin B, Einarsson K, Hellström K, Leijd B 1978 Effects of cholestyramine and chenodeoxycholic acid on the metabolism of endogenous triglyceride in hyperlipoproteinemia. Journal of Lipid Research 19: 1017–1024

Atmeh R F, Stewart J M, Boag D E, Packard C J, Lorimer A R, Shepherd J 1983 The hypolipidemic action of probucol: a study of its effects on high and low density lipoproteins. Journal of Lipid Research 24: 588–595

Bilheimer D W, Grundy S M, Brown M S, Goldstein J L 1983 Mevinolin and colestipol stimulate receptor-mediated clearance of low density lipoprotein from plasma in familial hypercholesterolemia heterozygotes. Proceedings of the National Academy of Science of the USA 80: 4124–4128

Danielson H, Sjoval J 1975 Bile acid metabolism. Annual Review of Biochemistry 44: 233–253

Dixon J L, Ginsberg H N 1993 Regulation of hepatic secretion of apolipoprotein B-containing lipoproteins: information from cultured liver cells. Journal of Lipid Research 34: 167–169

Feussner G 1994 HMG CoA reductase inhibitors. Current Opinion in Lipidology 5: 59–68

Franceschini G, Lovate M R, Manzoni C et al 1995 Effect of gemfibrozil treatment in hypercholesterolemia on low density lipoprotein (LDL) subclass distribution and LDL-cell interaction. Atherosclerosis 114: 61–71

Gaw A, Packard C J, Murray E F, Lindsay G M, Griffin B A, Caslake M J, Vallance B D, Lorimer A R, Shepherd J 1993 Effects of simvastatin on apoB metabolism and LDL subfraction distribution. Arteriosclerosis and Thrombosis 13: 170–189

Gaw A, Packard C J, Lindsay G M, Griffin B A, Caslake M J, Lorimer A R, Shepherd J 1995 Overproduction of small very low density lipoproteins (Sf 10–60) in moderate hypercholesterolemia: relationships between apolipoprotein B kinetics and plasma lipoproteins. Journal of Lipid Research 36: 158–171

Goldstein J L, Brown M S 1983 Familial hypercholesterolemia. In: Stanbury J B, Wyngaarden J B, Fredrickson D S, Goldstein J L, Brown M S (eds) The metabolic basis of inherited disease, 5th edn. McGraw Hill, New York, pp 672–712

Griffin B A, Freeman D J, Tait G W, Thomson J, Caslake M J, Packard C J, Shepherd J 1994 Role of plasma triglyceride in the regulation of plasma low density lipoprotein (LDL) subfractions: relative contribution of small, dense LDL to coronary heart disease risk. Atherosclerosis 106: 241–253

Harris W S, Connor W E, Illingworth D R, Rothrock D W, Foster D M 1990 Effects of fish oil on VLDL triglyceride kinetics in humans. Journal of Lipid Research 31: 1549–1558

Illingworth D R, O'Malley J P 1990 The hypolipidemic effects of lovastatin and clofibrate alone and in combination in patients with type III hyperlipidemia. Metabolism 39: 403–409

Kissebah A H, Adams P W, Harrigan W V 1974 The mechanism of action of clofibrate and tetranicotinylfructose on the kinetics of plasma free fatty acid and triglyceride transport in Type IV and Type V hypertriglyceridemia. European Journal of Clinical Investigation 4: 163–174

Kita T, Nayano Y, Yokode M, Ishie K, Kume N, Ooshima A, Yoshida H, Kawai C 1987 Probucol prevents progression of atherosclerosis in Watanabe heritable hyperlipidemic rabbits: an animal model for familial hypercholesterolemia. Proceedings of the National Academy of Science of the USA 84: 5928–5931

Mabuchi H, Sakai T, Sakai Y, Yoshimura A, Watanabe A, Wakasugi T, Koizumi J, Takeda R 1983 Reduction of serum cholesterol in heterozygous patients with familial hypercholesterolemia. Additive effects of compactin and cholestyramine. New England Journal of Medicine 308: 609–613

Manninen V, Tenkanen L, Koskinen P et al 1992 Joint effects of serum triglyceride and LDL cholesterol and HDL cholesterol concentrations on coronary heart disease risk in the Helsinki Heart Study: implications for treatment. Circulation 85: 37–45

Moore R B, Frantz I D, Buchwald H 1969 Changes in cholesterol pool size, turnover rate and fecal bile acid and sterol excretion after partial ileal bypass in hypercholesterolemic patients. Surgery 65: 98–108

Nawrocki J W, Weiss S R, Davidson M H, Sprecher D L, Schwartz S L, Lupien P-J, Jones P H, Haber H E, Black D M 1995 Reduction of LDL cholesterol by 25% to 60%

in patients with primary hypercholesterolemia by atorvastatin a new HMG-CoA reductase inhibitor. Arteriosclerosis, Thrombosis and Vascular Biology 15: 678–682

Packard C J, Munro A, Lorimer A R, Gotto A M, Shepherd J 1984 Metabolism of apolipoprotein B in large triglyceride-rich very low density lipoproteins of normal and hypertriglyceridemic subjects. Journal of Clinical Investigation 74: 2178–2192

Packard C J, Clegg R J, Dominiczak M H, Lorimer A R, Shepherd J 1986 Effects of bezafibrate on apolipoprotein B metabolism in Type III hyperlipoproteinemic subjects. Journal of Lipid Research 27: 930–938

Parthasarathy S, Young S G, Witztum J L, Pittman R C, Steinberg D 1986 Probucol inhibits oxidative modification of low density lipoprotein. Journal of Clinical Investigation 77: 641–644

Pierce L R, Wysowski D K, Gross T P 1990 Myopathy and rhabdomyolysis associated with lovastatin-gemfibrozil combination therapy. Journal of the American Medical Association 264: 71–75

Reihnér E, Angelin B, Rudling M, Ewerth S, Björkhem I, Einarsson K 1990 Regulation of hepatic cholesterol metabolism in humans: stimulatory effects of cholestyramine on HMG-CoA reductase activity and low density lipoprotein receptor expression in gallstone patients. Journal of Lipid Research 31: 2219–2226

Scandinavian Simvastatin Survival Study Group 1994 Randomised trial of cholesterol lowering in 4444 patients with coronary heart disease: The Scandinavian Simvastatin Survival Study (4S). Lancet 344: 1383–1389

Shepherd J, Packard C J, Patsch J R, Gotto A M, Taunton O D 1979 Effect of nicotinic acid on plasma high density lipoprotein subfraction distribution and composition and on apolipoprotein A metabolism. Journal of Clinical Investigation 63: 858–867

Shepherd J, Packard C J, Bicker S, Lawrie T D V, Morgan H G 1980 Cholestyramine promotes receptor mediated low density lipoprotein catabolism. New England Journal of Medicine 302: 1219–1222

Shepherd J, Packard C J, Stewart J M, Atmeh R F, Clark R S, Boag D E, Carr K, Lorimer A R, Ballantyne D, Morgan H G, Lawrie T D V 1984 Apolipoprotein A and B (Sf 100–400) metabolism during bezafibrate therapy in hypertriglyceridemic subjects. Journal of Clinical Investigation 74: 2164–2177

Shepherd J, Caslake M J, Lorimer A R, Vallance B D, Packard C J 1985 Fenofibrate reduces low density lipoprotein catabolism in hypertriglyceridemic subjects. Arteriosclerosis 5: 162–165

Simpson H S, Williamson C M, Olivecrona T, Pringle S, Maclean J, Lorimer A R, Bonnefous F, Bogaievsky Y, Packard C J, Shepherd J 1990 Postprandial lipemia, fenofibrate and coronary artery disease. Atherosclerosis 85: 193–202

Stewart J M, Packard C J, Lorimer A R, Boag D E, Shepherd J 1982 Effects of bezafibrate on receptor mediated and receptor independent low density lipoprotein catabolism on type II hyperlipoproteinemic subjects. Atherosclerosis 44: 355–364

Sullivan D R, Sanders T A B, Trayner I M, Thompson G R 1986 Paradoxical elevation of LDL apoprotein B levels in hypertriglyceridemic patients and normal subjects ingesting fish oil. Atherosclerosis 61: 129–134

FURTHER READING

British National Formulary 1995 British Medical Association & the Royal Pharmaceutical Society of Great Britain, London
The standard work giving details of all lipid-lowering drugs with prescribing notes and details of side effects and contraindications.

Durrington P N 1989 Hyperlipidaemia: diagnosis and management. Wright, London
This is an excellent book covering all aspects of clinical lipidology and has good sections on the lipid-lowering drugs.

Gaw A, Cowan R A, O'Reilly D St J, Stewart M J, Shepherd J 1995 Clinical biochemistry: an illustrated colour text. Churchill Livingstone, Edinburgh

This textbook includes useful fully illustrated sections on lipids and coronary heart disease.

Havel R J, Rapaport E 1995 Drug therapy. Management of primary hyperlipidemia. New England Journal of Medicine 332: 1491–1498

This recent review paper presents a detailed overview of the use of lipid-lowering drugs in modern medical practice.

ACKNOWLEDGEMENTS

The author acknowledges financial support from the British Heart Foundation (FS 92001 and FS 94001) and from the SOHHD (K/MRS/ 50/C2310).

Anti-hypertensive therapy

Gordon T. McInnes

11

■ CONTENTS

AIMS OF TREATMENT

The objectives of anti-hypertensive therapy are to prevent the end-organ damage which complicates uncontrolled chronic high blood pressure (myocardial infarction, cerebrovascular incidents, renal failure and heart failure) and to postpone death. There is now conclusive evidence that drug treatment of hypertension, including isolated systolic hypertension, significantly reduces the risk of such events (Collins & MacMahon 1994).

In the vast majority of individuals, hypertension is an asymptomatic condition and the aims of treatment are to prevent future damage. In effect, when we initiate anti-hypertensive management, we act as insurance salesmen: if the patient accepts the lifetime management plan, an event, which may not occur in any case, will be prevented in the distant future and no harm will result from the treatment prescribed. Unfortunately, with our present knowledge, we are unable to determine accurately which hypertensive subject will subsequently suffer an event or experience intolerable adverse effects of treatment. The worst scenario is the patient who is incapacitated by drug side effects but still dies from a heart attack or stroke. All these considerations dictate that drugs used to treat hypertension should be convenient and well tolerated.

LIFESTYLE MODIFICATION

Hypertension is not a disease in itself but is an important risk predictor for vascular events. The aim of treatment is primarily to reduce future morbidity and mortality from cerebrovascular disease and myocardial ischaemia. Therefore, hypertension should not be considered in isolation; its management should form part of a primary prevention package which also addresses other correctable risk factors such as smoking, hyperlipidaemia, diabetes mellitus and obesity.

The first step in anti-hypertensive therapy is non-pharmacological therapy. Weight reduction in obese subjects, moderation of alcohol and salt intake and increased aerobic exercise have all been shown to reduce blood pressure to an extent similar to that of drug monotherapy (Treatment of Mild Hypertension Research Group 1991, Wassertheil-Smoller et al 1992). Discontinuation of cigarette smoking has little long-term effect on resting blood pressure but has an influence on cardiovascular morbidity greater than that of blood pressure. Lifestyle modification is discussed in detail in Chapter 4.

PHARMACOLOGICAL TREATMENT

Long-term trials have demonstrated conclusively the benefit of anti-hypertensive drug therapy in reducing the risk of cerebrovascular events (Collins & MacMahon 1994); a 38% reduction in stroke is exactly that predicted from prospective epidemiological studies, given the average blood pressure change seen. The reduction in coronary heart disease events in these studies was 16%, or about three-quarters of that predicted. However, this deficit is not statistically significant.

The apparent shortfall in protection against heart attack has been emphasized widely and has many hypothetical explanations. Although there is no direct support for any of these, it seems likely that the extent of blood pressure reduction (mean change in diastolic blood pressure of 5 mmHg), the sample size of the study population and the duration of treatment (only 3 years on average) were insufficient to demonstrate benefit. It is important to note that these trials were discontinued on ethical grounds when significant benefit in stroke prevention was demonstrated. There is certainly no valid support for the notion that the drugs used in these trials (thiazides and beta-blockers) had cardiotoxic influences that offset their beneficial effect on blood pressure reduction (McInnes et al 1992).

CHOICE OF ANTI-HYPERTENSIVE DRUGS

In individuals who do not respond adequately to a reasonable trial of non-pharmacological measures, drug therapy is indicated. Several classes of

Box 11.1 Anti-hypertensive drugs

- Diuretics
- Beta-blockers
- Calcium antagonists
- ACE inhibitors
- Angiotensin II receptor antagonists
- Alpha-blockers
- Others

drugs are effective in reducing blood pressure. These drug classes are listed in Box 11.1.

Only diuretics and beta-blockers have been demonstrated to reduce premature stroke and coronary heart disease events in long-term outcome trials (Collins & MacMahon 1994). However, the most recent guidelines from the British Hypertension Society recommend that newer drugs (calcium antagonists, angiotensin-converting enzyme inhibitors or alpha-blockers) may be appropriate options for first-time treatment, at least in some patients (Sever et al 1993).

Diuretics

Diuretics were introduced in the 1950s and are still among the most widely used anti-hypertensive agents. Three classes of diuretics are available.

Classification

• Benzothiadiazine (thiazide) diuretics, such as bendrofluazide, cyclo-penthiazide or hydrochlorothiazide, act at the cortical diluting segment of the distal convoluted tubule in the kidney.
• Loop (high ceiling) diuretics, such as bumetamide, frusemide and tora-semide, act on the thick ascending limb of the loop of Henle (and the proximal tubule).
• Potassium-sparing diuretics, amiloride, triamterene and spironolactone, act at sodium : potassium exchange sites in the distal convoluted tubule and collecting duct.

Thiazide diuretics

Thiazide diuretics are the most useful and by far the most widely used in hypertension. They are fairly weak natriuretic agents with potential to eliminate 5–10% of filtered sodium (potency). However, thiazides have a gradual onset (hours) and prolonged (12 to over 24 hours) duration of action. These properties allow once-daily administration. The dose–response relation is shallow, i.e. there is little increase in sodium excretion at high doses.

In the UK, bendrofluazide is the least expensive thiazide available; more expensive agents offer no advantage. Bendrofluazide is completely absorbed and fairly extensively metabolized; only 30% is excreted unchanged in the urine. It has a plasma half-life of 3–4 hours but a much longer biological half-life. Diuresis starts around 2 hours after drug administration and continues for 12–18 hours. The recommended dose is 2.5 mg daily; larger doses cause more adverse effects without any improvement in blood pressure control.

Loop diuretics

Loop diuretics act more abruptly (30–60 minutes) and tend to have a diuretic effect which persists for only a few (4–6) hours at usual doses. Thus these agents have to be taken at least twice daily to provide 24-hour control of blood pressure. An exception is torasemide which can be used once daily. Loop diuretics have high potency (15–25% of filtered sodium) and steep dose–response curves (high ceiling).

Loop diuretics have a very limited role in hypertension. They are sometimes useful in treatment of resistant hypertension and high doses can also be effective in renal failure, where thiazides are ineffective. Thiazide diuretics become progressively less effective as renal function deteriorates and are not usually useful if serum creatinine exceeds 150 μmol/l (creatinine clearance less than 50 ml/min). Loop diuretics in high doses (e.g. frusemide 80 mg twice daily) retain efficacy.

Potassium-sparing diuretics

Potassium-sparing diuretics have weak natriuretic actions (5% filtered sodium) and, although duration of action is prolonged (12–24 hours), these drugs have a minor role in anti-hypertension therapy. Their main use is in combination with other diuretics to limit disturbances in potassium balance. Spironolactone acts as a specific competitive aldosterone antagonist and this action is utilized in the treatment of rare patients with primary hyperaldosteronism (Conn's syndrome). However, this drug is no longer licensed for the treatment of essential hypertension because of concerns about the carcinogenic potential of a closely related analogue (canrenoate potassium).

Mechanism of action

All diuretics act on the kidneys at renal tubular sites to enhance salt (sodium and chloride ion) and water loss. This results in acute reduction in plasma volume, cardiac output and extracellular fluid volume. However, enhanced sodium excretion persists only for the first few days of chronic administration. In the longer term, homeostatic mechanisms lead to recovery of plasma volume and cardiac output. Lowered blood pressure is sustained by reduction in total peripheral resistance (reverse autoregulation). Although the eventual result is reduced peripheral resistance, probably due to reduction in sodium content in vascular smooth muscle, the prime mover is renal salt and water loss.

Adverse effects

Symptomatic adverse effects of diuretics are rare although frequency, nocturia and prostatism can cause problems particularly in the elderly. Thiazide diuretics cause reversible erectile impotence in about 5% of middle-aged men; accurate assessment of the frequency of this side effect is difficult since the complaint is common in that population. Other uncommon reactions to thiazides include nausea, vomiting, diarrhoea, skin rashes, pancreatitis, agranulocytosis, aplastic anaemia and thrombocytopenia. Thiazides inhibit renal lithium clearance and may precipitate toxicity in patients treated with lithium carbonate.

High doses of loop diuretics can cause ototoxicity particularly in patients with renal impairment. The anti-androgenic action of spironolactone is associated with gynaecomastia in men and mastalgia or menstrual irregularities in women.

The major complications of diuretic therapy are *metabolic disturbances*. The concern is that these changes may predispose to cardiovascular disease and limit their preventive benefit.

As a direct result of their renal action, thiazide and loop diuretics promote urine potassium loss, and a tendency to *reduced serum potassium concentration*. Urine potassium excretion follows that of sodium and returns to baseline within about 1 week but fractional renal clearance of potassium remains increased indefinitely. As a result, serum potassium concentration reaches a new plateau after about 7–10 days and thereafter is unchanged unless clinical conditions alter, e.g. increase in dose. Therefore there is little need for continued monitoring of serum potassium. The average reduction in serum potassium with previously recommended doses of thiazides (e.g. bendrofluazide 10 mg daily) is 0.6 mmol/l. Some 50% of patients become hypokalaemic at this dose but only about 2% have serum potassium levels less than 3.0 mmol/l on long-term therapy.

Although it has been suggested that diuretic-induced hypokalaemia predisposes to serious cardiac arrhythmias, there is little good evidence for this except in patients at particular risk (see Box 11.2). Certainly there is no justification for routine use of potassium supplements or potassium-sparing agents.

If required, potassium replacement is best achieved by the use of potassium-sparing diuretics. Dietary sources of potassium (citrus fruit, bananas, dried fruit, tomatoes) are inadequate except when taken in huge amounts. Slow-release potassium chloride or combined thiazide–potassium formulation similarly contains relatively small amounts of potassium. These preparations are ineffectual since the underlying cause of hypokalaemia (increased fractional renal clearance) is not influenced and much of the absorbed potassium is merely lost in the urine.

As well as being ineffective, potassium supplements can cause serious side effects including oesophageal injury or ulceration. Slow-release formulations simply transfer the damage further down the gastrointestinal tract with risk of small bowel stenosis, ulceration and perforation. Hyperkalaemia is occasionally seen in patients with renal impairment or those prescribed concomitant potassium-sparing agents.

Potassium-sparing diuretics can also precipitate *hyperkalaemia* in patients with renal impairment or where angiotensin-converting enzyme inhibitors are prescribed simultaneously. Hyperkalaemia carries a risk for serious cardiac arrhythmias and sudden death much greater than that due to hypokalaemia.

Box 11.2 Subjects at risk of or from hypokalaemia

Factors increasing risk OF hypokalaemia
- High doses
- Long-acting agents (thiazides more than loops)
- Divided doses
- Women
- Young (more than old)

Factors increasing risk FROM hypokalaemia
- Concomitant digoxin
- Concomitant drugs which prolong QT interval, e.g. amiodarone, disopyramide, flecainide, sotalol
- Chronic liver disease
- Arrhythmias or antiarrhythmic therapy
- Severe or unstable angina
- Post myocardial infarction
- Primary hyperaldosteronism
- Serum potassium less than 3.0 mmol/l

Combined preparations of thiazide or loop diuretics and potassium-sparing agents are difficult to justify since the risk of severe hypokalaemia is generally low. Also such combinations carry a risk of severe *hyponatraemia* which may cause symptomatic neurological consequences including fits and coma. Profound hyponatraemia can arise after only a few doses and is more likely in elderly females. It seems to be particularly associated with use of Moduretic (hydrochlorothiazide and amiloride).

Subjects at risk of or at risk from hypokalaemia are listed in Box 11.2. In such individuals, monitoring of serum potassium and use of potassium-sparing agents as necessary are indicated.

Patients receiving thiazide diuretics have a tendency to develop *hyperglycaemia*, perhaps as a consequence of increased insulin resistance. However, only about 1% of thiazide-treated subjects will develop diabetes mellitus during long-term exposure. There is little evidence that alterations in carbohydrate metabolism short of diabetes is a risk factor for cardiovascular disease.

All diuretics, other than potassium-sparing agents, may cause *hyperuricaemia*. Only about 2% of men and many fewer women go on to develop gout. This is most likely in obese, heavy-drinking males treated with loop diuretics. Increase in serum uric acid does not appear to be an independent risk factor for coronary artery disease.

Short-term (months) treatment with high doses of thiazides causes marked *changes in serum lipoproteins* (increased total cholesterol and low density lipoprotein cholesterol, and reduced high density lipoprotein cholesterol). However, alterations are markedly attenuated in the long term. After 1 year's treatment, the small increase in total cholesterol (1%) is unlikely to be of clinical significance.

Dose

All the metabolic effects of thiazides are dose-related, while the anti-hypertensive effect is not dose-related. Blood pressure reduction is maximal at low doses, e.g. bendrofluazide 2.5 mg daily. At such doses, metabolic changes are trivial. Small reductions in serum potassium are frequent but hypokalaemia is rare.

Outcome studies

A series of long-term outcome trials has demonstrated beyond reasonable doubt that thiazide-based treatment regimens reduce the chances of premature stroke and myocardial infarction in hypertensive subjects (Collins & MacMahon 1994, McInnes et al 1992). Benefits appear to be most marked in the elderly (MRC Working Party 1992).

■ KEY POINTS

- Diuretics should be used in low doses.
- Diuretics need little dose titration.
- Thiazides can be used once daily.
- Diuretics are useful in *pseudotolerance*—resistance to other anti-hypertensive agents (particularly vasodilators) due to fluid retention.
- All diuretics (particularly thiazides) are inexpensive.
- Loop diuretics are useful in renal failure.

Beta-blockers

Beta-adrenoceptor antagonists were discovered by accident to be anti-hypertensive agents in the early 1970s and since then have entered widespread use. Like thiazide diuretics, these agents have been used widely in the trials which have demonstrated the benefits of drug treatment of hypertension (Collins & MacMahon 1994).

Mechanism of action

Beta-blockers are competitive inhibitors of catecholamines at beta-adrenergic receptors. They decrease cardiac activity by inhibiting both the rate and force of cardiac contraction; they also decrease the normal cardiac responses to stress and exercise.

Despite lengthy experience with beta-blockers in hypertension, there remains uncertainty about their mechanism of action. Candidate actions include:

- Cardiac—reduced myocardial contractility, heart rate and cardiac output.
- Central—reduced sympathetic outflow from the brain.
- Renal—reduced renin release from the juxtaglomerular apparatus, and hence inhibition of angiotensin II and aldosterone action. Angiotensin II is a potent vasoconstrictor and aldosterone promotes renal salt and water retention.

Ancillary properties

All beta-blockers inhibit both $beta_1$-receptors, found largely in the heart and in the peripheral vasculature, and $beta_2$-receptors found principally in the bronchi but also in the peripheral vasculature. Some beta-blockers exhibit cardioselectivity and/or partial agonist activity.

Cardioselective drugs have preferential activity at $beta_1$-adrenoceptors located in the heart. Cardioselectivity is relative rather than absolute. Therefore, at high doses, such drugs lose their selectivity. Cardioselective beta-blockers such as atenolol and metoprolol have fewer unwanted effects due to inhibition of $beta_2$-adrenoceptors including less influence on airways resistance.

All beta-blockers act by occupying the beta-receptor and denying access to the natural stimulant (agonist). Drugs with partial agonist activity (PAA), also known as intrinsic sympathomimetic activity (ISA), act as weak agonists in resting conditions. During exercise or arousal, antagonist activity becomes dominant. Beta-blockers with PAA have little demonstrable activity at rest and more marked effects on activity, e.g. little bradycardia at rest but attenuation of tachycardia on activity. In some subjects, such drugs are better tolerated (less bradycardia and coldness of extremities) than other beta-blockers, but they generally have less marked anti-hypertensive activity.

Classification

A pharmacological classification of some commonly used beta-blockers is shown in Table 11.1. In addition to their ancillary properties, beta-blockers differ in their route of elimination and duration of action. Lipid-soluble beta-blockers, e.g. oxprenolol, undergo rapid extensive hepatic metabolism and tend to have relatively short half-lives and durations of action. Water-soluble beta-blockers are slowly eliminated unchanged by the kidney and tend to have longer half-lives and duration of action. Plasma half-life underestimates biological half-life. Atenolol and nadolol are suitable for once-daily administration.

In renal impairment, dosage adjustment may be necessary with drugs which are cleared predominantly by the kidney. Beta-blockers which undergo

Table 11.1 Properties of beta-blockers

Drug name	Beta$_1$-selective	PAA	Water-soluble	Plasma half-life (h)	Duration of action (h)	Elimination
Acebutolol	+	±	±	3	12	Renal/hepatic
Atenolol	+	−	+	6	16	Renal
Bisoprolol	++	−	±	10–12	> 24	Renal/hepatic
Metoprolol	+	−	−	3–4	8	Hepatic
Nadolol	−	−	+	6–24	24	Renal
Oxprenolol	−	+	−	1–2	8	Hepatic
Pindolol	−	++	±	3–4	12	Renal/hepatic
Propranolol	−	−	−	3–6	12	Hepatic

extensive hepatic metabolism should be avoided in severe liver failure and may theoretically be involved in pharmacokinetic interactions with other drugs which undergo similar biotransformation.

Labetalol differs from other beta-blockers in that it also has alpha-receptor blocking properties. As a result, labetalol tends to lower peripheral resistance.

Adverse effects

Beta-blockers are usually well tolerated. Adverse effects are generally due to unwanted blockade of beta-receptors. Thus side effects can be predicted from their pharmacological actions.

- Bronchoconstriction (bronchospasm) is due to blockade of $beta_2$-receptors in bronchial smooth muscle—these receptors modulate bronchodilatation.
- Impaired peripheral circulation and Raynaud's phenomenon are due to blockade of vasodilatory $beta_2$-receptors and/or unopposed alpha-adrenergic stimulation.
- Cardiac failure or cardiac conduction defects (heart block) can arise from excessive $beta_1$-receptor blockade.
- Symptoms of hypoglycaemia (tachycardia, sweating) may be masked since these responses depend on activation of the beta-adrenergic system. $Beta_2$-receptors also mediate the gluconeogenic and glycogenolytic responses to hypoglycaemia. Therefore, non-selective beta-blockers delay the recovery following insulin-induced hypoglycaemia.
- Tiredness and fatigue during beta-blocker therapy probably reflect reduced cardiac output.
- Impairment of quality of life and central nervous system effects (such as nightmares) may represent central effects of beta-blockers and seem more prominent with lipid-soluble agents which more readily cross the blood–brain barrier. Atenolol and nadolol are among the most water-soluble beta-blockers and seem to cause less sleep disturbance. Beta-blockers should be avoided in asthma, cardiac failure, bradycardia and heart block, and used only with caution in diabetes mellitus. Non-selective beta-blockers such as propranolol may have effects on carbohydrate metabolism at least as great as those of thiazides. Use of cardioselective beta-blockers in peripheral vascular disease has been shown to be without ill effects unless drugs which decrease peripheral resistance (e.g. nifedipine) are also prescribed.

New beta-blockers

In recent years, highly cardioselective beta-blockers such as betaxolol and bisoprolol have been introduced. Carvedilol and celiprolol are beta-blockers with vasodilator properties. Carvedilol (like labetalol) probably has weak alpha-blocking properties. Celiprolol is said to be a cardioselective ($beta_1$-) blocker and $beta_2$-agonist with vasodilating activity. In addition, there is evidence that celiprolol actually reduces airways resistance and has favourable effects on serum lipoproteins. The clinical advantage of these agents compared with conventional beta-blockers is yet to be established, although preliminary findings suggest that carvedilol may have overall beneficial effects in patients with heart failure.

■ **KEY POINTS**

• Beta-blockers should be used in low doses to avoid side effects. Anti-hypertensive efficacy is well maintained at low doses.

• Beta-blockers need little dose titration.

• Beta-blockers can be administered once or twice daily.

• Cardioselective beta-blockers are preferred since some adverse effects are less marked.

• Other pharmacological differences between beta-blockers have marginal clinical significance.

• All beta-blockers are contraindicated in patients with asthma (or severe irreversible airways disease) or heart failure.

Calcium antagonists

The calcium antagonist class embraces three groups of drugs with distinct actions:

• dihydropyridines, e.g. amlodipine, felodipine, lacidipine, nifedipine
• phenylalkylamines, e.g. verapamil
• benzothiazepines, e.g. diltiazem.

Mechanism of action

Calcium antagonists inhibit transmembrane calcium influx through so-called slow calcium channels during membrane depolarization. Therefore, they lower intracellular free calcium, the final common mediator of all vaso-constrictor mechanisms. Although all calcium antagonists reduce blood pressure, they have variable affinities for calcium channels at different sites in the cardiovascular system (Table 11.2).

Dihydropyridines have the most potent action at vascular smooth muscle sites, while only verapamil and diltiazem have measurable direct cardiac effects in man. These two drugs suppress electrical conduction in cardiac conductive tissue and hence have a role in the management of tachyarrhythmias.

All three types of calcium antagonist tend to depress myocardial contractility. However, the direct cardiac effects are offset by reflex cardiac stimulation secondary to vasodilatation. Thus, with dihydropyridines, because of their particularly potent vasodilatory effect, the net result is a tendency to increase heart rate while verapamil and diltiazem tend to reduce heart rate (rate-limiting calcium antagonists).

Adverse effects

The adverse effects of calcium antagonists are predictable from their sites and mechanisms of action (Table 11.3). Side effects due to vasodilatation (e.g. flushing, headache and dizziness) and reflex cardiac stimulation (palpitation) are more likely with dihydropyridines. Cardiac conduction delays (heart block and bradyarrhythmias) are seen only with verapamil and diltiazem. Heart failure is also slightly more common with rate-limiting calcium

Table 11.2 Sites of activity and pharmacokinetics of first-generation calcium antagonists

Drug name	Classification	Site of activity			Pharmacokinetics		
		Vascular smooth muscle	Myocardium	Conducting tissue	Bioavailability	Elimination	Half-life (h)
Nifedipine	Dihydropyridine	+++	±	–	30–60%	Hepatic	2–6
Diltiazem	Benzothiazepine	++	+	++	30–60%	Hepatic	2–5
Verapamil	Phenylalkylamine	++	+	+++	1–20%	Hepatic	3–7

Table 11.3 Adverse effects of calcium antagonists

Drug name	Vasodilatation (flushing, headache, dizziness)	Palpitation	Ankle oedema	Constipation	Heart block	Heart failure
Nifedipine	+++	++	++	+	–	±
Diltiazem	+	+	+	++	++	+
Verapamil	+	+	+	+++	++	++

antagonists. Ankle oedema, which appears to be due to local small vessel leakiness and is not a reflection of fluid retention, appears to be more frequent with dihydropyridines, particularly longer-acting agents. Calcium antagonist-induced ankle swelling does not respond to diuretic treatment. Verapamil causes constipation in a relatively high proportion of patients because of its direct action on gastrointestinal smooth muscle, although this symptom is not usually particularly troublesome.

The incidence of symptomatic side effects with calcium antagonists is high relative to earlier agents. Original formulations of nifedipine (capsules) were associated with a withdrawal rate due to intolerable side effects of 20%. Newer long-acting drugs (e.g. amlodipine) or long-acting formulations of older agents (e.g. Adalat LA) are better tolerated, with the exception of ankle oedema.

Pharmacokinetics

The first generation calcium antagonists (nifedipine, verapamil and diltiazem) are well absorbed but undergo extensive first-pass hepatic elimination and are readily eliminated from the body (Table 11.2). As a consequence, oral bioavailability is low and plasma levels show considerable interindividual variability; elimination half-lives are short. In their original formulations, these drugs have to be administered in divided daily doses to provide 24-hour control of blood pressure.

Thus, there was a requirement for longer-acting calcium antagonists. Two approaches were adopted: naturally occurring long-acting agents and sustained-release preparations of earlier drugs.

Several new dihydropyridines have appeared in recent years (Table 11.4). The second generation dihydropyridine, amlodipine, does not undergo significant first-pass metabolism. Therefore it has consistently high oral bioavailability and prolonged elimination half-life. Once-daily amlodipine appears to provide smooth blood pressure control throughout the dosage interval. Other new agents in this class, such as isradipine and lacidipine probably should be administered twice daily to ensure 24-hour control.

Sustained-release formulations of otherwise short-acting drugs have inconsistent durations of action. The more reliable of these preparations include Adalat LA (nifedipine), Plendil (felodipine), Securon SR (verapamil)

Table 11.4 Critical pharmacokinetics of second generation dihydropyridines (compared with nifedipine)

Drug name	Bioavailability (%)	Time to max. serum conc (h)	Half-life (h)
Nifedipine	30–60	1–2	2–6
Amlodipine	52–88	6–12	34–50
Felodipine	12–16	1–2	10–25
Isradipine	16–18	1	5–9
Lacidipine	2–52	1–2	2–10
Nicardipine	15–45	< 1	1–7

and Tildiem LA (diltiazem). Because of the variability between different sustained-release formulations of the same drug, these should be prescribed by proprietary rather than generic name, and substitution should be avoided.

Drug interactions

Because of their complex bioavailability and high degree of hepatic metabolism, there is potential for interaction with drugs which undergo similar biotransformation. Pharmacokinetic interactions between calcium antagonists and carbamazepine, cimetidine, cyclosporin, quinidine and theophylline have been demonstrated but are of uncertain clinical significance. Co-administration of verapamil increases steady state serum digoxin levels by about 100%. This can cause problems in susceptible individuals.

The most clinically relevant drug interaction with calcium antagonists is that between rate-limiting agents (verapamil and diltiazem) and other drugs with direct cardiac actions, notably beta-blockers. Combined cardiodepressant effects can result in life-threatening bradyarrhythmias and heart failure.

Outcome trials

Unlike diuretics and beta-blockers, calcium antagonists have not been demonstrated to have beneficial effects on cardiovascular events in long-term outcome trials. Calcium antagonists have neutral metabolic effects and animal studies suggest that these agents may have anti-atherogenic properties. These potential advantages have yet to be translated into clinical benefit in hypertension. Indeed, recent analyses (Psaty et al 1995) have suggested that short-acting dihydropyridines given in large doses may increase mortality. As yet, the evidence against calcium antagonists is not strong enough to influence clinical practice.

■ KEY POINTS

• Calcium antagonists should be started at low doses to minimize the risk of side effects.

• Some dose titration is usually necessary.

• Once- or twice-daily dosing depends on drug or formulation.

• Relatively poor tolerability.

• Major differences between drugs.

• Adverse drug interactions may cause complications. Verapamil and diltiazem should not be administered with beta-blockers except under close hospital supervision.

ACE inhibitors

Theoretical findings suggest that the renin–angiotensin system may be involved in the pathogenesis of hypertension and its complications (McInnes 1995). Drugs which inhibit this axis, such as angiotensin-converting enzyme (ACE) inhibitors, may have an important role in the management of hypertension.

Mechanism of action

Renin produced by the juxtaglomerular apparatus in the kidney acts on angiotensinogen produced by the liver to generate angiotensin I. The primary action of ACE inhibitors is inhibition of ACE which converts the inactive decapeptide, angiotensin I, to the active octapeptide, angiotensin II, one of the most potent endogenous vasoconstrictors. Angiotensin II also stimulates the synthesis and release of aldosterone in the adrenal cortex; aldosterone acts on the kidneys to promote salt and water retention. Thus ACE inhibitors have dual effects to reduce blood pressure; inhibition of angiotensin II-induced vasoconstriction and aldosterone-mediated homeostasis.

Other non-specific actions may also contribute to the anti-hypertensive effect of ACE inhibitors. ACE modulates the breakdown of vasodilator peptides such as bradykinin; thus ACE inhibitors potentiate the kallikrein–kinin system. Indirect stimulation of vasodilator prostaglandins and inhibition of the sympathetic nervous system are other potential mechanisms.

The conversion of angiotensin I to angiotensin II occurs in the circulation but also within many tissues. Such local systems may have a critical role in the development of hypertension or its complications. ACE inhibitors block some but not all of the pathways of angiotensin II production within tissues.

Classification

ACE inhibitors can be classified according to their chemical structure and pharmacokinetic properties (Table 11.5).

The main structural difference between the available ACE inhibitors is the presence or absence of a sulphur-containing moiety in the molecule. Only captopril has such a grouping. It has been claimed that this may be responsible for some of the drug's adverse effects and beneficial properties. However, there is little evidence that the presence of sulphur in the molecule has a clinically significant influence on the action of ACE inhibitors.

Most ACE inhibitors are prodrugs, i.e. the drug is administered as a relatively inactive molecule which is metabolized during or after absorption to the active diacid, e.g. enalapril to enalaprilat. Initially, there was concern that the dependence on hepatic or pre-hepatic metabolism would expose these drugs to interference from other drugs similarly metabolized and reduce efficacy in patients with impaired liver function. These concerns have proved unfounded. The main consequence of using the prodrug is delay in onset of action. Prodrug ACE inhibitors take longer to demonstrate activity after administration compared with non-prodrug ACE inhibitors.

ACE inhibitors are mainly eliminated by the kidneys and the rate of elimination determines their half-lives and durations of action. Thus captopril must be administered twice or three times daily to provide 24-hour control of blood pressure. In contrast, lisinopril has 24-hour duration of action at most doses and trandolapril at all doses. Most other ACE inhibitors have intermediate half-lives and durations of action.

Duration of action of ACE inhibitors is highly dependent on dose. For instance, at low doses enalapril should be administered twice daily and is a once-daily preparation only at the highest dose.

Table 11.5 Properties of ACE inhibitors

Drug name	Sulphydryl group	Prodrug	Onset of action (h)	Peak action (h)	Duration of action (h)	Elimination
Captopril	+	−	0.5	1–4	3–12	Renal
Cilazapril	−	+	1–2	4–6	≤ 24	Renal
Enalapril	−	+	1–4	4–8	12–30	Renal
Fosinopril	−	+	1–2	3–4	≤ 24	Renal/hepatic
Lisinopril	−	−	1–2	2–8	18–30	Renal
Perindopril	−	+	1–2	4–8	≤ 24	Renal
Quinapril	−	+	1–2	2–6	≤ 24	Renal
Ramipril	−	+	0.5–2	3–8	24	Renal
Trandolapril	−	+	1–2	2–4	> 24	Renal/hepatic

Some drugs have dual routes of elimination (fosinopril and trandolapril). This offers theoretical advantages in renal and hepatic impairment. There is little evidence that this property is of clinical significance.

Adverse effects

ACE inhibitors are well tolerated but growing clinical experience indicates that significant side effects do occur.

A dry irritating cough or other upper respiratory tract symptoms are seen in 15% of patients (10% of men and 20% of women). This adverse effect tends to accumulate with time; it may be seen after only a few days of treatment but may take several months to develop. It is independent of dose and is class specific rather than drug specific. Therefore changing ACE inhibitor is not helpful. However, the symptom is unpredictable; only about two-thirds of patients with well-established ACE inhibitor-induced cough will experience cough on rechallenge.

An abrupt fall in blood pressure after introduction of ACE inhibitors (first-dose hypotension) is a recognized complication. This side effect is only likely if blood pressure is highly dependent on activation of the renin–angiotensin system, e.g. subjects who are sodium depleted as a result of high-dose diuretic therapy or patients with bilateral renal artery stenosis (or obstruction of the renal artery to a single functioning kidney). Such circumstances are uncommon in hypertension but, if suspected, a low test dose of ACE inhibitor should be prescribed under hospital supervision. Otherwise, ACE inhibition can safely be introduced in outpatients at usual doses. The time to onset of first-dose hypotension depends on the ACE inhibitor administered (early with captopril, late with prodrugs) but the magnitude of the fall is similar.

ACE inhibitors can cause renal impairment by two mechanisms. During first-dose hypotension, perfusion of vital organs including the kidneys may be impaired. With short-acting agents, the duration of hypotension is brief and renal ischaemia is less likely. This complication is uncommon in essential hypertension.

In bilateral renal artery stenosis (or renal artery stenosis in a single functioning kidney), glomerular perfusion is highly dependent on angiotensin II. ACE inhibition can result in sudden renal impairment reflected by a rapid rise in serum creatinine. Thus, renal function should be monitored 1–2 weeks after the introduction of an ACE inhibitor since renal artery stenosis may be unsuspected. A marked fall in blood pressure after introduction of an ACE inhibitor may be an indication that renal artery stenosis is present. Particular caution is necessary in patients with clinical evidence of peripheral vascular disease, which is a useful marker for atheromatous renal artery stenosis. Renal impairment may be severe but is usually reversible on stopping treatment.

Theoretically, elderly patients and those with renal impairment may be at particular risk of such adverse events but there is little sound evidence for this. In these patient groups, the duration of effect rather than the magnitude of the effect is likely to increase. ACE is inhibited almost completely at low doses and increasing plasma drug concentrations merely prolongs the action.

Normal renal elimination of potassium is highly dependent on aldosterone. Therefore, inhibition of the renin–angiotensin–aldosterone axis is associated with a tendency to increased serum potassium. The effect of ACE inhibitors is usually trivial but may attenuate diuretic-induced hypokalaemia. However, in patients with pre-existing renal impairment or who are receiving concomitant potassium-sparing diuretics or potassium supplements, dangerous hyperkalaemia can arise. Cyclosporin, indomethacin and probably other non-steroidal anti-inflammatory drugs also increase the risk of hyperkalaemia with ACE inhibitors. ACE inhibitors should not be administered with such drugs.

Uncommon side effects of ACE inhibitors include rash, angioedema, neutropenia and dysgeuesia.

Some side effects of ACE inhibitors (cough, angioedema) are likely to reflect the non-specific action of these drugs. In particular, accumulation of tissue bradykinin or other peptides is implicated.

Although ACE inhibitors are widely promoted for their favourable influence on quality of life, there is little evidence that these drugs have an advantage over currently used agents (Fletcher et al 1993, Hjendahl & Wikland 1992).

Outcome trials

It is often speculated that ACE inhibitors may have advantages beyond blood pressure reduction. ACE inhibitors are at least as effective as other anti-hypertensive agents in regressing left ventricular mass in patients with left ventricular hypertrophy, and anti-atherogenic effects have been demonstrated in animal models. These drugs have no adverse metabolic effects and may have a beneficial influence on insulin resistance, although well-controlled studies have failed to confirm this property. Whether or not these features have clinical significance in the management of hypertension requires to be established in large, long-term outcome trials.

■ **KEY POINTS**

- A low starting dose is usually recommended to avoid rare dose-dependent side effects.
- Dose titration is needed to ensure duration of action throughout the dose interval.
- ACE inhibitors can be used once or twice daily.
- ACE inhibitors are generally well tolerated.
- ACE inhibitors have beneficial effects on surrogate markers of risk but outcome trials are required.
- ACE inhibitors are expensive compared with diuretics and beta-blockers.

Angiotensin II receptor antagonists

Because of the presumed importance of the renin–angiotensin–aldosterone system in the pathogenesis of hypertension and the lack of specificity of the action of ACE inhibitors, attention has been diverted towards drugs which inhibit the axis at other sites. To date, renin inhibitors have not been successful clinically because of low oral bioavailability and poor adverse reaction profile. In contrast, the first specific angiotensin II receptor antagonist, losartan, has recently been launched in this country.

Mechanism of action

Angiotensin II receptors exist in two forms (AT1 and AT2). The AT1 receptor modulates all the cardiovascular effects of angiotensin II derived from all sources including local renin–angiotensin systems. The AT2 receptor serves no known physiological function.

Losartan denies access of angiotensin II to the AT1 receptor. It has high affinity for the AT1 receptor and exhibits little or no action at the AT2 receptor. Thus, losartan is a potent, specific angiotensin II antagonist with selectivity for the AT1 receptor (Brunner et al 1993).

Losartan undergoes biotransformation in the liver with creation of an active metabolite, EXP 3174. This metabolic product has stronger receptor-binding characteristics and a longer duration of action than the parent drug.

Losartan has anti-hypertensive efficacy similar to that of other drugs from the main therapeutic classes. Its duration of action is at least 24 hours even at low doses. Higher doses have no additional peak anti-hypertensive effect but prolong duration of action even further. The active metabolite, EXP 3174, is likely to be responsible for losartan's prolonged action.

Adverse reactions

Losartan appears to be very well tolerated. In contrast to ACE inhibitors, it does not cause the side effects due to the non-specific action of these drugs.

Dry cough during ACE inhibition is probably due to potentiation of a peptide substrate of ACE, such as bradykinin or neurokinin. ACE is identical to kinase II, the enzyme responsible for the degradation of bradykinin and other vasoactive peptides, accumulation of which is associated with the development of cough.

Since angiotensin II receptor antagonists lack the bradykinin potentiation of ACE inhibitors, these drugs should also be devoid of other rare side effects of ACE inhibition, such as urticaria and angioedema, which are mediated by this mechanism.

No detrimental biochemical disturbances have been noted and losartan appears to counteract some unwanted metabolic effects of diuretics, particularly changes in plasma potassium, uric acid and blood sugar. Losartan has a significant uricosuric action which may be an important adjunctive effect when used in combination with a diuretic.

Losartan causes changes in renal haemodynamics similar to those of ACE inhibitors. Thus, angiotensin II blockade carries the same risk in patients with renal artery stenosis.

Clinical experience with losartan is limited and it is uncertain whether the favourable side effect profile will be maintained when the drug has been exposed to widespread clinical use.

Outcome trials

Whether these drugs will have an advantage over other agents, including ACE inhibitors, in relation to end-organ damage, such as reversal of the long-term effects of angiotensin II on cardiac hypertrophy, remains to be tested in adequate clinical trials.

■ **KEY POINTS**

- Specific inhibition of the renin–angiotensin axis.
- Little need for dose titration.
- Once-daily dosing.
- Well tolerated.
- Putative beneficial cardiovascular effects as with ACE inhibitors.
- Expensive.

Alpha-blockers

Stimulation of the alpha-adrenergic system causes vasoconstriction and increased arterial pressure. Thus, inhibition of vascular alpha-receptors is a logical approach to lowering blood pressure.

Classification

Non-selective alpha-adrenoceptor antagonists (inhibition of $alpha_1$- and $alpha_2$-receptors) have been available for many years. However, a high incidence of side effects and the rapid development of tolerance make them unsuitable for general use. Oral phenoxybenzamine and intravenous phentolamine are now obsolete except in the management of phaeochromocytoma, where there is dramatic excess of circulating catecholamines.

More recently, selective post-junctional $alpha_1$-adrenoceptor antagonists have become available—doxazosin, indoramin, prazosin and terazosin. Indoramin is the least selective of these agents and is associated with the least favourable side effect profile.

Mechanism of action

The selective post-junctional $alpha_1$-adrenoceptor blockers reduce blood pressure by vasodilatation. Prazosin has relatively abrupt onset and short duration of action, necessitating multiple daily dosing. Doxazosin and terazosin have more gradual and prolonged actions, and are suitable for once-daily dosing.

Adverse effects

Postural hypotension, particularly after the initial dose, is a commonly experienced problem. The alpha-adrenergic system is activated with adoption of the upright posture. Thus, alpha-blockers are most effective with the patient erect. Indeed, these drugs have relatively little activity in the supine posture.

Other major side effects—headache and palpitation (due to reflex tachy-cardia)—are predictable from the vasodilator properties of alpha-blockers. Fatigue, sedation and sexual dysfunction have also been reported. With doxazosin and prazosin, problems with sexual dysfunction are probably no more common than in the general population.

Avoidance of orthostatic hypotension

Because of the frequency of postural hypotension, precautions are required during the initiation of alpha blockade. A low starting dose before the patient retires to bed at night is recommended; an abrupt fall in blood pressure is then unlikely. Diuretics should be withheld for 24–48 hours before dosing since the magnitude of postural blood pressure reduction is greater if the patient is sodium depleted. If tolerated, the dose of alpha-blocker is then gradually increased over several weeks.

Doxazosin and terazosin are absorbed slowly and therefore have a gradual onset of action, making postural hypotension less likely. Even with newer drugs, however, postural symptoms are still troublesome.

The inconvenience of the dosing schedule greatly reduces the attraction of alpha-blockers. These drugs are not popular as first-line agents in the UK.

Outcome trials

Long-term outcome trials with alpha-blockers have not been conducted. Alpha-blockers have beneficial effects on serum lipid profiles. About 5% reduction in total cholesterol and low density lipoprotein cholesterol, and a similar increase in high density lipoprotein cholesterol can be expected during long-term therapy. Whether the potential advantage in cardiovascular protection of such small changes in hypertensive patients overcomes the poor adverse effect profile is uncertain. The benefit in reducing coronary heart disease risk is likely to be slight.

■ **KEY POINTS**

- Low starting dose recommended.
- Lengthy period of dose titration necessary.
- Once- or twice-daily dosing.
- Poorly tolerated compared with other first-line agents.
- Reduce atherogenic lipid fractions.
- Expensive.

Other anti-hypertensive drugs

Drugs occasionally used in the management of hypertension include:

- direct vasodilators, e.g. hydralazine, minoxidil, diazoxide and sodium nitroprusside are sometimes used in hypertensive emergencies
- centrally acting agents, e.g. clonidine, methyldopa, reserpine are now very rarely used in this country

- adrenergic neurone blockers, e.g. bethanidine, debrisoquine, guanethidine are largely of historical interest
- ganglion blockers, e.g. trimetaphan may be used in hypertensive crises
- tyrosine hydroxylase inhibitors, e.g. metirosine may be useful in patients with severe hypertension due to phaeochromocytoma.

Adverse effects

Direct vasodilators are powerful anti-hypertensive agents but cause predictable side effects. The most common are tachycardia and fluid retention. Therefore, these drugs are best used in combination with beta-blockers and diuretics.

Centrally-acting anti-hypertensive drugs cause predictable unwanted actions, e.g. somnolence and lethargy. Such drugs also commonly cause dry mouth and nasal stuffiness.

In addition drug-specific side effects are seen.

Hydralazine. The principal drawback with use of hydralazine is a systemic lupus erythematosis (SLE)-like syndrome which arises more commonly in females and is dose-dependent. Hydralazine undergoes onward metabolism by acetylation in the liver. The extent of acetylation is under genetic control; the SLE-like syndrome is more common in slow acetylators where hydralazine levels are higher. The daily dose of hydralazine should be limited to 50 mg in women and 100 mg in men. The development of malaise, weight loss or arthritis should raise suspicion of the SLE-like syndrome.

Minoxidil. This potent vasodilator causes particularly marked fluid retention. A loop diuretic is usually required to compensate for this. Minoxidil frequently causes unsightly hair growth (hypertrichosis). As a result, this drug is not popular with women and, even in men, the site of hair growth can cause cosmetic problems. Hair growth across the forehead is common in patients taking minoxidil.

Clonidine. The main complication of clonidine use is the rapid offset of its action if a dose is missed. Blood pressure returns quickly to pretreatment levels but rarely to higher levels. Therefore the usual appellation of 'rebound hypertension' is not entirely accurate.

Methyldopa. Long-term treatment with methyldopa may be associated with increases in hepatic enzyme activity as assessed in serum samples. In affected patients, methyldopa induces a mild hepatitis. Since this may go on to cirrhosis in a few patients, liver enzymes should be monitored during methyldopa therapy and the drug discontinued if abnormalities appear.

■ KEY POINTS

- These drugs are potent anti-hypertensive agents with steep dose–response curves, i.e. increasing doses lead to marked increases in efficacy.

- Treatment is complicated by many subjective side effects which also tend to be dose-related.
- These drugs are reserved for refractory patients, i.e. failure to respond adequately to first-line drugs in combination, or patients with particular problems, for example:
  —hypertensive crises—diazoxide, sodium nitroprusside or trimetaphan
  —phaeochromocytoma—metirosine.
- There is little need to institute these drugs in general practice.

GENERAL COMMENTS

Efficacy

The major anti-hypertensive agents (thiazides, beta-blockers, calcium antagonists, ACE inhibitors, angiotensin II receptor antagonists and alpha-blockers) have similar efficacy (Treatment of Mild Hypertension Research Group 1991). Between 30 and 40% of patients with mild hypertension are likely to respond adequately to monotherapy. The response rate depends on the initial level of blood pressure and the level accepted as adequate control (usually diastolic blood pressure less than 90 mmHg).

Much higher response rates (80–90%) are often quoted in promotional literature. These rates refer to patients with very mild hypertension observed without adequate controls. Thus, such response rates include placebo responders (usually about 30%) and are hugely optimistic.

Dose

Dose–response curves are relatively shallow. By employing low doses, side effects are much less likely, but it must be remembered that duration of action is dependent on dose. Therefore, at low starting doses, efficacy should be assessed at the end of the dosage interval to avoid undertreatment.

Factors influencing responsiveness

Response rate is not influenced importantly by patient characteristics. Age, sex and plasma renin concentrations have been used to predict responses to particular drugs but results have usually been unconvincing. Elderly hypertensives appear to respond better to thiazide diuretics than to beta-blockers but few other differences have been noted. Black patients of Afro-Caribbean origin respond well to diuretics and calcium antagonists and less well to beta-blockers and ACE inhibitors. This response pattern may reflect the usual low renin status of such patients.

Drug choice in coexistent disease

There are marked differences between drugs in side effect profiles. Drug tolerability may be influenced by patient characteristics. The presence of coexistent diseases may determine the appropriate choice of drug (Table 11.6).

Thus, in a patient with *airways disease*, a beta-blocker is contraindicated because of the risk of provoking bronchospasm. Even cardioselective agents should be avoided.

Table 11.6 Anti-hypertensive drugs in coexistent diseases

	Thiazide	Beta-blocker	Calcium antagonist	ACE inhibitor	AII antagonist	Alpha-blocker
Airways disease	+	−	+	+	+	+
Angina	+	++	++	+	+	+
Heart failure	++	−	−	++	++	+
Diabetes mellitus	−	(+)	+	+	+	−
Claudication	+	(+)	+	(+)	(+)	+
Renal impairment	−	+	+	(+)	(+)	+

Key: ++ positive indication; + no contraindication; (+) caution; − contraindication

In *angina,* a beta-blocker or a calcium antagonist would be a good choice because these drugs have anti-anginal properties. A combination of beta-blocker plus dihydropyridine calcium antagonist may be particularly useful.

Patients with overt *heart failure* should be given a diuretic and ACE inhibitor regardless of whether there is hypertension. Beta-blockers should usually be avoided, although some patients may respond well to beta-blockade particularly with carvedilol. This is best undertaken under hospital supervision. Although theoretically advantageous due to their vasodilatory action (cardiac offloading), calcium antagonists generally cause a deterioration in ventricular function. There is some evidence that amlodipine may be beneficial but confirmation is needed before such treatment can be recommended.

Diabetes mellitus may be worsened or precipitated by thiazide diuretics. Non-selective beta-blockers appear to have at least as marked diabetogenic effects and all beta-blockers tend to mask subjective sensations of hypoglycaemia. Alpha-blockers do not influence carbohydrate metabolism to an important extent but the tendency to postural hypotension may exacerbate orthostatic hypotension in diabetic patients with autonomic neuropathy.

Intermittent claudication may be worsened by treatment with beta-blockers which reduce cardiac output. However, controlled studies suggest that cardioselective agents have little adverse effect, unless combined with dihydropyridine calcium antagonists which may divert blood flow to non-ischaemic tissue. ACE inhibitors should be used with caution in patients with clinically overt peripheral vascular disease because of the high risk of bilateral renal artery stenosis.

In significant *renal impairment,* thiazides have little effect. A loop diuretic should be preferred. It is usually recommended that ACE inhibitors should be used in low doses but there is little evidence that this is necessary.

DRUG INTERACTIONS

Anti-hypertensive drugs are often used in combination or along with drugs prescribed for other conditions. Therefore, it is important that significant drug interactions are not encountered.

Other anti-hypertensives

The anti-hypertensive effects of most agents are additive. This means that low doses of more than one drug can be combined to improve blood pressure control without necessarily imposing a greater burden of adverse effects.

Beta-blockers and ACE inhibitors have less than additive effects since both drug types interfere with the renin–angiotensin system. Part of the anti-hypertensive effect of calcium antagonists appears to be mediated by renal sodium loss; dihydropyridine calcium antagonists and thiazide diuretics have a less than additive anti-hypertensive effect.

There is little evidence that any anti-hypertensive drug combination has a greater than additive effect. However, thiazides and ACE inhibitors appear to be particularly effective in combination. ACE inhibitors block the activation of the renin–angiotensin system secondary to diuretics; stimulation of this system may offset the blood-pressure-lowering effect of thiazides.

Adverse interactions between anti-hypertensive agents are uncommon. However, concomitant use of beta-blockers with verapamil or diltiazem may cause profound bradycardia and heart block, and precipitate heart failure. This combination should be avoided. ACE inhibitors and potassium-sparing diuretics both increase serum potassium concentrations and combined use is associated with the risk of life-threatening hyperkalaemia. Potassium-sparing diuretics should be discontinued if an ACE inhibitor is prescribed.

Other drugs

Some drugs can attenuate the effect of anti-hypertensive drugs and lead to loss of blood pressure control. Non-steroidal anti-inflammatory drugs (NSAIDs) cause sodium retention and are often implicated in such inter-actions. These agents are often used in elderly patients and blood pressure should be carefully monitored when NSAIDs are introduced to older patients with hypertension.

NSAIDs can also cause hyperkalaemia and renal impairment when used with ACE inhibitors and potassium-sparing agents. Again this is a particular problem in the elderly and in those with pre-existing renal impairment.

Diuretic-induced hypokalaemia rarely leads to problems but even mild hypokalaemia can be dangerous in patients receiving drugs which prolong the QT interval (Box 11.2). The major risk is the dimorphic ventricular arrhythmia, torsade de pointes, which can result in sudden death.

FACTORS INFLUENCING CHOICE OF DRUGS

Drugs used to treat hypertension should satisfy certain criteria:

- efficacy in reducing blood pressure
- convenience for the patient (i.e. once- or twice-daily administration) and the prescribing physician (no need for prolonged dose titration)
- tolerability
- safety
- compatibility with other drugs
- modification of outcome (reduction of morbid events).

Most first-line anti-hypertensive agents satisfy most of these criteria. However, only thiazide diuretics and beta-blockers have been demonstrated to favourably influence outcome. These drugs also have the enormous advantage of good safety records during long-term, widespread experience. The potential of the more expensive newer agents remains to be established.

If all other factors are equal, consideration should be given to cost. Thiazides are by far the least expensive agents. Bendrofluazide 2.5 mg daily costs only a little over £1 per year. Newer agents (calcium antagonists, ACE inhibitors, angiotensin II receptor antagonists and alpha-blockers) are more than 100 times more expensive at equivalent doses.

USE OF ANTI-HYPERTENSIVE DRUGS

Most patients with sustained hypertension require more than one drug in combination to achieve adequate control. The conventional approach is stepped care.

Stepped care

The principles of stepped care are:

- drugs have additive anti-hypertensive effects
- use of drugs at submaximal doses results in side effects which are less than additive
- addition of some drugs attenuates the side effects of others, e.g. ACE inhibitors lessen diuretic-induced hypokalaemia.

In this approach, drugs are added in a stepwise manner until control is achieved. If side effects supervene, other drugs can be tried. Although usually described as restrictive, the policy is infinitely flexible.

An example of stepped care:

Step 1: Bendrofluazide or beta-blocker
Step 2: Bendrofluazide plus beta-blocker
Step 3: Add ACE inhibitor *or* dihydropyridine calcium antagonist *or* alpha-blocker.

There is little to choose between thiazides and beta-blockers as first choice in the absence of specific contraindications. Thiazides are less expensive and appear to be better tolerated in women. Beta-blockers may have a marginal advantage in tolerability in men.

Other options might be employed in specific patients, e.g. non-insulin-dependent diabetes mellitus:

Step 1: ACE inhibitor
Step 2: Add calcium antagonist
Step 3: Add alpha-blocker.

Very rarely, a fourth drug from another therapeutic class may have to be added. If there is a risk of pseudotolerance due to vasodilator therapy, a loop diuretic as fourth drug may be very useful. In these circumstances, serum bio-chemistry must be monitored closely because hyponatraemia, hypokalaemia and increased serum creatinine can be troublesome.

In refractory hypertension, diuretics should be considered even in patients in whom such drugs are normally contraindicated, e.g. diabetes where oral hypoglycaemic drugs can be given in increased doses if necessary. In patients with a history of gout, the risk from diuretic-induced hyperuricaemia can be avoided by coadministration of allopurinol.

Limitations of stepped care

Compliance may deteriorate with multiple drugs. Although compliance is mainly influenced by the frequency with which drugs have to be taken, many patients find multiple drugs inconvenient, particularly if dosing times differ.

When patients are taking multiple drugs, it is often difficult to be certain of the contribution to blood pressure control made by individual drugs. Therefore, a patient may be taking one or more drug which is having little beneficial effect but nonetheless be exposed to the risk of side effects from that drug.

Even if all drugs are contributing to blood pressure control, side effects may accumulate. Side effects from submaximal doses of drugs are usually less than additive but the frequency is generally greater than that attributable to one drug alone.

The costs of multiple drugs are additive. To ensure economic prescribing, it is imperative that individual drugs are contributing to control.

Adverse drug interactions are uncommon with anti-hypertensive agents. However, in refractory patients, unusual combinations may have to be tried, e.g. verapamil and beta-blockers. In such cases, careful monitoring is essential.

Stepped care is subject to the law of diminishing returns. About 40% of truly hypertensive patients will respond to step 1; 65% to step 2 (i.e. 40% responding to step 1 and 40% of remaining 60% to step 2) and 75–80% to step 3. Thus, fewer and fewer patients (in absolute numbers) respond to each additional drug.

New approaches
Because of the perceived shortcomings of stepped care, other approaches have been advocated. These treatment plans are termed individualization and substitution.

Individualization
In individualization, drugs are matched to the requirements of individual patients. The attempt is to gain specific benefit and/or to avoid adverse effects. Unfortunately, other than in the examples listed in Table 11.6, our ability to achieve this is limited.

Substitution
The aim of substitution is to control blood pressure with the minimum number of drugs. Drugs are administered in series to identify the most suitable agent(s) in terms of efficacy and tolerability. If there is an inadequate response or an adverse reaction to a particular drug, that agent is withdrawn and replaced with another. Substitution depends on the untested assumption that patients who fail to respond to one drug will eventually respond to another. This policy is time-consuming, unpopular with the patient and usually unsuccessful.

Limitations of individualization and substitution
It is difficult and may be impossible to identify patients who will respond particularly well to a given drug. Despite popular misconceptions, factors such as age, sex and plasma renin activity are poor predictors of responsiveness. In any case, multiple drug therapy is usually required.

Modern stepped care takes account of many individual characteristics and is an essential aid to management. In the view of practising physicians in this country, it remains the most practical approach to the treatment of hypertension (Waller et al 1990).

BEYOND BLOOD PRESSURE REDUCTION

Anti-hypertensive therapy reduces the risk of the main complications of hypertension, stroke and myocardial infarction. In preventive medicine, it is often assumed that a successful preventive measure will eliminate entirely the risk of an event. In fact, it can only hope to prevent that proportion of events attributable directly to the risk factor. For stroke, anti-hypertensive treatment reduces risk by 35–40%, exactly the proportional change predicted from epidemiological data. For coronary heart disease, blood pressure lowering reduces events by about 16% compared with the expected reduction of 20–25%.

These estimates are based on the results of trials with diuretics or beta-blockers and there is speculation that with newer drugs the full reduction in coronary heart disease risk attributable to blood pressure might be achieved (i.e. 22.5% instead of 16%). This small improvement in protection will be very difficult to establish unless a very large outcome trial is completed. Even if the results were positive, over 75% of the risk of coronary events would be unaffected.

To make inroads into this requires a strategy beyond blood pressure reduction alone. Attention to the risk factors such as smoking and cholesterol would be beneficial. However, more aggressive blood pressure control using existing drugs would also contribute. Epidemiological data suggest a 'doubling effect', i.e. twice the reduction in blood pressure twice the reduction in risk (Collins & MacMahon 1994). Alternatively, newer drugs with properties which interfere with the pathogenesis of the complications of hypertension independently of blood pressure reduction might allow greater benefit. There is preliminary evidence that ACE inhibitors and calcium antagonist may have antiatherogenic effects and interrupt directly the vascular and cardiac muscle complications of hypertension. At present, the clinical relevance of such speculation is uncertain. Long-term trials are required urgently (Yusuf et al 1984).

CONCLUSIONS

We now have many, effective, convenient and well-tolerated anti-hypertensive drugs. Choice should be based on these properties but also on the results of long-term experience, prospective trials to evaluate the influence on outcome (events), and on cost. Conventional bendrofluazide-based stepped care remains the most logical approach to the management of hypertension.

Case Study 11.1

A 59-year-old female is found to be hypertensive while attending a well-woman clinic. There is no relevant history and physical examination is unremarkable other than raised blood pressure and obesity. Blood pressure remains high on repeated measurements. Routine investigations are negative except for a random blood sugar of 12 mmol/l. Calorie restriction results in satisfactory reduction in weight and normalization of non-fasting blood sugar, but blood pressure remains elevated after 3 months' observation.

Questions
1. What anti-hypertensive drugs would you consider appropriate?
2. If blood pressure does not settle on monotherapy, what would be your preferred treatment option?

Answers
1. Calcium antagonist or ACE inhibitor (angiotensin II receptor antagonist). Thiazide diuretics and non-selective beta-blockers should be avoided.
2. Calcium antagonist plus ACE inhibitor. If calcium antagonist was first choice, you might try an ACE inhibitor (or vice versa) but usually more than one drug will be necessary.

PRACTICAL EXERCISE

Carry out an audit of anti-hypertensive drug therapy in all patients in your practice.

- What drugs are being used?
- Are the drugs appropriate for the individual patients, i.e. have they been selected after consideration of coexistent diseases?
- Are the doses optimal?
- How many patients are taking more than one anti-hypertensive drug?
- Are the drug combinations logical?
- Is there a clearly defined policy for drug treatment of hypertension?

REFERENCES

Brunner H R, Nussberger J, Burnier M et al 1993 Angiotensin II antagonists. Clinical and Experimental Hypertension 15: 1221–1238
Collins R, MacMahon S 1994 Blood pressure antihypertensive drug treatment and the risks of stroke and coronary heart disease. British Medical Bulletin 50: 272–298
Fletcher A E, Bulpitt C J, Chase D M et al 1993 Quality of life with three antihypertensive treatments—cilazapril, atenolol, nifedipine. Hypertension 19: 499–507
Hjendahl P, Wikland I K 1992 Quality of life on antihypertensive therapy: scientific end point or marketing exercise? Journal of Hypertension 10: 1437–1446
McInnes G T 1995 Hypertension and coronary artery disease: cause and effect. Journal of Hypertension 13 (Suppl. 2): S49–S56
McInnes G T, Yeo W W, Ramsay L E, Moser M 1992 Cardiotoxicity of diuretics: much speculation—little substance. Journal of Hypertension 10: 317–335
MRC Working Party 1992 Medical Research Council trial on treatment of hypertension in older adults: principal results. British Medical Journal 304: 405–412

Psaty B M, Heckbert S R, Koepsell T D et al 1995 The risk of myocardial infarction associated with antihypertensive drug therapies. Journal of the American Medical Association 274: 620–625

Sever P, Beevers G, Bulpitt C et al 1993 Management guidelines in essential hypertension. Report of the Second Working Party of the British Hypertension Society. British Medical Journal 306: 983–987

Treatment of Mild Hypertension Research Group 1991 The Treatment of Mild Hypertension Study: a randomized, placebo-controlled trial of a nutritional hygienic regimen along with various drug monotherapies. Archives of Internal Medicine 151: 1413–1423

Waller P C, McInnes G T, Reid J L 1990 Policies for managing hypertensive patients: a survey of the opinions of British specialists. Journal of Human Hypertension 4: 509–515

Wassertheil-Smoller S, Blaufox M D, Oberman A S, Langford H G, Davis B R, Wylie-Rosett J 1992 The Trial of Antihypertensive Interventions and Managements (TAIM) study: adequate weight loss, alone and combined with drug therapy in the treatment of mild hypertension. Archives of Internal Medicine; 152: 131–136

Yusuf S, Collins R, Peto R 1984 Why do we need some large, simple randomized trials? Statistics in Medicine 3: 409–420

FURTHER READING

Carlsen J E, Kober L, Torp-Pedersen C, Johansen P 1990 Relation between dose of bendrofluazide, antihypertensive effect, and adverse biochemical effects. British Medical Journal 300: 975–978

Dahlof D 1992 Reversal of left ventricular hypertrophy in hypertensive patients: a meta-analysis of 109 treatment studies. American Journal of Hypertension 5: 95–110

Jackson R, Barham P, Billo J et al 1993 Management of raised blood pressure in New Zealand: a discussion document. British Medical Journal 307: 107–110

Joint National Committee on Detection, Evaluation and Treatment of High Blood Pressure 1993 Fifth report. Archives of Internal Medicine 153: 154–183

Materson B J, Reda D J, Cushman W C et al 1993 Single-drug therapy for hypertension in men: a comparison of six antihypertensive agents with placebo. New England Journal of Medicine 328: 914–921

McInnes G T, McGhee S M 1993 Delivery of care for hypertension. Journal of Human Hypertension 9: 429–433

Neaton J D, Grimm R H, Prineas R J et al 1993 Treatment of Mild Hypertension Study: final results. TOMHS Research Group. Journal of the American Medical Association 270: 713–724

Rosman J, Weidmann P, Ferrari P 1990 Antihypertensive drugs and serum lipoproteins. Journal of Drug Development 3 (Suppl. 1): 129–139

Smith W C S, Lee A J, Crombie I K, Tunstall-Pedoe H 1990 Control of blood pressure in Scotland: the rule of halves. British Medical Journal 300: 981–983

Stamler R, Grimm R, Gosch F C et al 1987 Control of high blood pressure by nutritional therapy: final report of a 4-year randomised controlled trial. The Hypertension Control Program. Journal of the American Medical Association 257: 1484–1491

Swales J D, Ramsay L E, Coope J R et al 1989 Treating mild hypertension. British Medical Journal 298: 694–698

WHO/ISH Guidelines Subcommittee 1993 Guidelines for the management of mild hypertension: memorandum from a WHO/ISH meeting. Journal of Hypertension 11: 905–918

Cardiac rehabilitation

Elizabeth M. Keith

■ CONTENTS

INTRODUCTION

This chapter is devoted to the mechanism by which individuals who have suffered an acute coronary event as a consequence of coronary heart disease (CHD) are restored to optimal health. This process is known as cardiac rehabilitation; the following definitions of rehabilitation are helpful in understanding its wider objectives:

> to make fit, after disablement or illness, for earning a living or playing a part in the world (Chambers Twentieth Century Dictionary 1972)

> helping to restore someone after illness, to readjust to society (Collins English Dictionary 1992).

In other words, rehabilitation is a method of supporting someone to adjust to changes in their health in order that they achieve the optimum level of recovery. Rehabilitation is recognized as an essential service required in many areas. Amongst the most commonly recognized forms of rehabilitation is that dealing with victims of stroke, neurological trauma, spinal injury and acute cardiac events.

Cardiac rehabilitation was recognized more than 20 years ago as being of value to the patient with CHD but it is only recently that the setting up of programmes of rehabilitation has become more widespread. It has been recognized widely that many patients are surviving longer yet many lead miserable and unproductive lives after the diagnosis of CHD is made. In addition, 'cardiac rehabilitation and secondary prevention measures which might improve this situation have not become part of routine care: many patients are receiving less than optimal care'(WHO 1993).

In 1992 the British Cardiac Society made the following recommendations in their Working Party Report on cardiac rehabilitation (Horgan et al 1992):

• Every major district hospital that treats patients with heart disease should provide a cardiac rehabilitation service.
• The programme should be multidisciplinary and usually exercised-based, depending on the resources available.
• The expertise available for a comprehensive programme is available in most district and major cardiothoracic centres, but requires consultant leadership, most appropriately by a cardiologist.
• There is a continued need for research into the evaluation of not only the physiological response, but also the social and psychological aspects of rehabilitation.
• The role of vocational rehabilitation in recovery needs greater recognition.
• The special problems of women and children and certain ethnic groups need to be addressed. Rehabilitation should be tailored to the individual needs of patients and special group requirements.
• Arrhythmia monitoring is necessary for high-risk patients.
• Individual programmes should evaluate their outcome, and a standard format of audit could be agreed nationally to allow comparison.

In the Autumn of 1995, the British Association of Cardiac Rehabilitation (BACR) produced national guidelines for rehabilitation of the cardiac patient, including an overview of research findings as well as information on exercise testing and motivating adults to exercise.

Many rehabilitation groups have started through British Heart Foundation start-up grants and with support from The Chest Heart & Stroke Association. Although cardiac rehabilitation has been shown to reduce cardiac mortality, anxiety and depression, and increase the ability to return to work, many physicians, cardiac surgeons and cardiologists remain unconvinced of the benefits. A 10-year study into cardiac rehabilitation carried out in Sweden reported a reduction in non-fatal reinfarctions during the first 5 years after myocardial infarction followed by a significant reduction in total and cardiac mortality in the later part of the observation period (Hedback et al 1993).

The support and education of patients following myocardial infarction or coronary bypass graft surgery are essential elements of the overall care and long-term strategy when dealing with CHD. It has been advocated that secondary prevention should be included in national health policies and appropriate resources allocated (WHO 1993). The level of education and exercise available to patients and families is generally dictated by the resources within the hospital or community and there is a wide variety of programmes available (Horgan et al 1992). The aim of cardiac rehabilitation is to return patients to optimum health within the confines of their disease, to highlight individual risk factors and encourage patients to initiate long-term changes where indicated. It is also an opportunity to educate relatives and particularly those with a positive family history of CHD, and for this reason families and friends should be encouraged to participate in the education programme. It is an opportunity for patients and families to acknowledge their role in accepting responsibility for their health and to emphasize the necessity of dealing with a progressive disease. The balance within cardiac rehabilitation has to be between preventing recurrence of coronary events (secondary prevention) and helping patients to come to terms realistically with the experience of myocardial infarction and to overcome their memories and fears which may be impeding their recovery.

CORONARY CARE UNIT

The coronary care unit exists for the care of the patient in acute cardiac crisis and to provide immediate resuscitation when required. The unit is staffed by nurses and physicians with specific training in the management of acute coronary events. Most patients experiencing an acute myocardial infarction are aware of the life-threatening nature of their illness. Severe pain, breathlessness and vomiting must all be dealt with as soon as possible with the use of analgesia, oxygen therapy, anti-emetics and any other therapy or intervention deemed necessary to stabilize the patient's condition. For many patients the coronary care unit can be both reassuring and alarming. The attachment to technical equipment to monitor and control the condition may feel intrusive and also alerts patients to the seriousness of their condition. Knowing what the equipment is for, what purpose the medication has, and the importance of communicating their needs to the nursing and medical staff should help to reduce the patients' fear. The knowledge that they are being cared for by highly skilled and experienced staff can give them a great feeling of security, though it may be tempered by the fact that patients do not always readily understand the language used amongst the staff. It is therefore crucial for patients to be spoken to in terms that are easily understood. Many patients are unable to communicate effectively in the first few days following their heart attack because of the psychological trauma they may have experienced.

Dealing with the relatives

In many ways the relatives may find the admission of patients to hospital far more alarming than the patients who may be too ill to be aware of their surroundings. Cardiac arrest is a common event during acute myocardial infarction and is not necessarily an indicator of the severity of the event, but for the relative who witnesses a cardiac arrest either within or out of the hospital it is an experience not easily dealt with. Listening to and dealing with the fears of the relatives is essential. When relatives say, 'What will I do if he arrests at home?' it is not good enough to pat them on the shoulder and tell them reassuringly that it is unlikely to happen again. Their fears remain and have not been addressed. Unless dealt with effectively, the recovery and progress of patients may be restricted by the terror of their relatives. Informing the relatives each step of the way about medication, tests and the patients' progress will lessen their anxiety. Offering them the opportunity to go through basic life-support skills may be an option to consider.

The close relationship between the nurse and the patient in a coronary care unit allows an ideal opportunity for the nurse to gently introduce to the patient the concept that certain lifestyle changes may be advisable, e.g. smoking cessation. The nurse acts as translator, converting medical terminology into easily understood language, explaining what drugs are being used, what tests are being done and why, and what the next stage in the recovery process is likely to be. Explaining simply and clearly the diagnosis to both patient and relative may need to be done repeatedly as the powers of concentration and comprehension are often reduced at moments of stress. The normal stay in a coronary care ward for an uncomplicated acute myocardial infarction is 24 hours and the overall length of stay in hospital between 5 and 7 days.

Framework of knowledge

What does the patient require to know following an acute myocardial infarction? The initial diagnosis of heart attack will be given to the patient as soon as possible, usually within 24 hours of admission to hospital following confirmation by raised serum cardiac enzyme levels. On occasions it is safe to make the diagnosis of acute myocardial infarction from the electrocardiograph alone.

For the first 24 hours the majority of patients are too unwell to absorb much in the way of information. The aware nurse working with the patient should be ready to answer any questions the patient may have concerning the cause of his heart attack and encourage the patient to begin thinking about lifestyle changes which may need to be addressed, in particular smoking. It is interesting to note that the majority of patients, although familiar with the term 'heart attack' do not understand what it means. As with all diagnoses, it behoves the nurse to sit with the patient for only a few minutes to ensure that the patient has interpreted correctly the discussion with the doctor. Patients frequently feel vulnerable, ignorant and lacking in understanding of their illness and the terminology used either directly or indirectly to them or between staff, e.g. 'let's arrange an ETT' or 'his CK is well up', and feel unable to admit to their confusion. Clarifying gently with patients their level of understanding and building from that level reduces the likelihood of cardiac misconceptions. It is also worth noting that patients from all social classes may require the same level of educational input and it would be a mistake to assume that the patient from social class 1 has more awareness of myocardial infarction than the patient from social class 5. Most patients are vaguely aware of the position and function of their heart but many are confused on the difference between stroke and heart attack. A simple drawing or explanation of myocardial infarction can be helpful to the patient and relative. For some patients it may be acceptable to use a model of the heart as a means of explanation but this should be agreed with the patient rather than produced without permission. If the basic concept of acute myocardial infarction is grasped, then the possibility of the patient making essential lifestyle changes is increased. It is worth letting patients know as soon as possible after admission how long they will be hospitalized, with emphasis on this being a general guideline which may vary depending on their day-to-day recovery and the results of any tests.

Mobilization

Transfer from coronary care to the general wards brings mixed reactions from patients. For some there is a feeling of relief that they are no longer deemed to be critically ill, but others feel vulnerable to be leaving somewhere with a high ratio of nurses to patients. The former patient may need to be encouraged to slow down and increase mobilization gradually whereas the latter may lie rigid with terror in bed, unwilling to mobilize at all. The role of the cardiac rehabilitation nurse in the medical ward is to expand and bring together the information given to patients by the many people responsible for their care prior to discharge. The specialist nurse must take care not to de-skill the ward staff but encourage them to develop their rehabilitative role as they work with patients, for example enabling them to answer patients' questions about cardiac status and risk factors as they arise.

Ward nurses should be encouraged specifically to ask the patient about definitive symptoms of angina rather than relying on the patient to inform the nurse. Many patients 'don't want to bother the nurse', so incorporating gentle questioning during the administration of medication or during any other interaction between nurse and patient should be considered. Inconsistency of advice from shift to shift is confusing for the patient. Unless there is a reason for slowing down the mobilization of the patient due to the onset of complications, there should be a smooth link between shifts. The patient who has been walking to the toilet in the morning without problems but who is taken by wheelchair to the toilet in the afternoon will be confused and mistrustful of the staff unless given a logical explanation.

Guidelines for mobilizing the *uncomplicated* myocardial infarction patient are given in Box 12.1. The uncomplicated myocardial infarction patient is one who has *no* symptoms of angina on transfer to the medical wards from the coronary care unit.

On a busy ward there is rarely time for the ward nurse to sit down and spend 10 uninterrupted minutes with a patient. This is where the rehabilitation nurse has the advantage of being a 'visitor' to the ward and can therefore usually give undivided attention to that patient and identify social and domestic problems of which the ward staff may have been unaware. Many patients, particularly the more elderly, have been the main supporter in the household, perhaps looking after a relative or spouse who is in poor health. These patients should be referred to the social services department for both financial and physical support.

It is important to identify these issues as early as is possible in the patient's care in order, where necessary, to arrange help for the domestic situation prior to discharge.

The identification of risk factors such as hyperlipidaemia or obesity will require referral to the dietitian as would the diagnosis of diabetes. A referral to a diabetic sister if available should be considered.

Box 12.1 Guidelines for mobilizing the uncomplicated myocardial infarction patient

Days after myocardial infarction

Day 3
The patient may sit beside the bed for 1 hour in the morning and afternoon and if symptom-free may walk to the toilet with a nurse in attendance. The patient may carry out gentle self-hygiene at the bedside, i.e. bathing above the waist, shaving and combing the hair.

Day 4
If still symptom-free, the patient may take a sitting shower with a nurse in attendance. Patients should not wash their own hair at this point as working above the head increases the output demand of the heart. The patient can begin gentle walking around the ward. It should be emphasized to patients that they are not to move any of the ward furniture such as bedside chairs.

Day 5
If still symptom-free, the patient can take a standing shower and can continue walking around the ward. From day 5 onwards an exercise tolerance ECG test pre-discharge may be carried out if the medical staff require one.

Day 6
The patient may be taken up and down one flight of stairs under supervision.

Day 7
The patient may be discharged having been given clear guidelines concerning increasing activity and instructions concerning medication. If possible, patients should be able to tell the nurse what medication they are taking, why it has been prescribed and when it has to be taken. It is worth checking that the patient has been given a card indicating that he/she has been given streptokinase and that patients understand the importance of carrying it with them at all times. (The use of streptokinase is discussed in detail in Ch. 9.)

CORONARY ARTERY BYPASS GRAFT SURGERY

Intervention in the form of coronary artery bypass graft (CABG) surgery is carried out in patients who have severe symptoms of angina limiting their mobility and in those patients found to have a severe life-threatening stenosis of the coronary arteries. Patients with diffuse coronary artery disease are unlikely to be offered revascularization in the form of bypass grafting. Revascularization is most commonly carried out in one of two ways:

• by diverting the left internal mammary artery from the muscle of the chest wall and attaching it to the affected coronary artery beyond the area of stenosis
• by removing a segment of saphenous vein, reversing it and attaching one end to the aorta and the other beyond the affected portion of the coronary artery, thus providing a new source of arterial blood.

It is necessary to provide basic information about postoperative recovery for those who have undergone such surgery. The following issues can be discussed with patients either in a pre-discharge group talk or individually.

• Hallucinations both visual and auditory are common in the first few postoperative days. Flashing and coloured lights may be experienced and patients who wear spectacles may complain that their glasses are not 'right'.
• Taste and appetite are disrupted for several days and many surgeons will prescribe drugs such as ranitidine to protect the patient gastrointestinally for the first few weeks.
• Memory loss and difficulty in concentrating may last for 2–3 weeks.
• Depression and emotional frailty can occur anywhere from 2 days to 3 months postoperatively.
• Sleep disturbance is common and may take many weeks to resolve.
• Irritability with relatives is common in the first few weeks but usually resolves as the patient's condition improves.

The sternum, which is divided to allow access to the heart, is wired together following completion of the operation. Any patient complaining of a 'clicking' sensation in the sternum should be referred back to the surgeons as it may indicate separation of the bone. It is wise to warn patients with dissolving sutures that, as weeks pass, they may find that slivers of suture commonly make their way out through the wounds. Patients should be encouraged to contact their GP if there is any sign of redness, tenderness, leaking or swelling on or around the wound in case a wound infection has arisen.

Elastic stockings are prescribed for all CABG patients postoperatively. The circulation of the leg used for vein retrieval is compromised for several weeks causing reduced venous flow, swelling and the risk of deep venous thrombosis occurring. It is possible that both legs will be used.

The normal length of hospitalization for CABG is 7 days including the first 24 hours spent in the intensive care unit.

All the risk factors described for the myocardial infarction patient also apply to the bypass graft patient.

Risk factors

The identification of risk factors is an integral part of the rehabilitation process. The main and modifiable risk factors of smoking, hypertension and hyperlipidaemia are considered briefly in the context of cardiac rehabilitation and are discussed in more detail in Chapters 3, 4 and 5.

Smoking

Despite the warnings on cigarette packets, billboards and by health promotion generally, many patients deny the connection between cigarettes and CHD. One of the first questions asked of patients with acute myocardial infarction, either during or immediately after admission, concerns their smoking habits. If the answer is in the affirmative they are recommended strongly to stop. Most patients are stunned that a heart attack could have happened to them. It is perhaps an appropriate time to move in with support and a positive message as regards smoking cessation. It is important that the nurse is seen as a supporter of the patient in his/her effort to quit rather than as a disciplinarian. So the key is to remember to support patients not to judge them. It is wise to involve the key members of the family so that they too understand that nagging is counterproductive.

The fact that smoking cessation halves the likelihood of further infarction (WHO 1993) should be emphasized. It is worth noting that mortality in smokers from CHD was increased fivefold between 35 and 44 years of age and nearly fourfold between 45 and 54 years of age compared to age-matched non-smokers (Julian & Marley 1991). Patients who continue to smoke after myocardial infarction have a greatly increased chance of developing angina and of having a second myocardial infarction. Time should be spent discussing with patients how to tackle the problem in their own individual ways and what difficulties they believe will be encountered. While in hospital the majority of patients cope well with not smoking. Visualizing and planning for difficult situations on discharge can be helpful to some patients; however, talking about smoking cessation can in some cases rekindle the desire to smoke, so always check with patients whether or not it would be helpful for them to discuss the subject. Encouraging a belief in their own ability to tackle the challenge and succeed is crucial. Recognizing that patients, and women in particular, have a problem accepting weight gain as a result of smoking cessation means that they need a great deal of support and reassurance.

On returning to the outpatient cardiac rehabilitation programme, the current situation needs to be evaluated and change re-instigated if necessary. Identifying where the patient is in the cycle of change is essential otherwise both the patient's time and your own time will be wasted. More guidelines on behavioural change can be found in the chapter dealing with this (Ch. 8). Some patients may request support through hypnosis. This should always be done through a referral by the GP to a recognized practitioner. Nicotine patches are contraindicated in individuals who have had a myocardial infarction.

Cholesterol

Particularly in the younger patient who is admitted with acute myocardial infarction, it is highly desirable to obtain even a random lipid measurement. If the lipids are not able to be measured on admission, then the rehabilitation nurse should be active in arranging a full lipid screen for the patient if this has not already been dealt with by the GP or practice nurse.

Hypertension

A number of patients suffering acute myocardial infarction will have a confirmed diagnosis of hypertension and may have been on prescribed treatment. A further number will not have visited their general practitioner for many years, so will be unaware of their level of blood pressure. Of those diagnosed hypertensive and prescribed medication, many will have failed to comply with their drug therapy because of the lack of symptoms. Poor compliance may also be caused by the side effects of certain drugs. Time spent defining the term hypertension and its effect on health if not controlled is useful to the patient but must be done with care if the 'white coat syndrome' is to be avoided. Patients should be encourage to discuss with their doctor any side effects which they feel may be linked to their medication so that the medication may be altered if appropriate.

During the outpatient phase of cardiac rehabilitation it is crucial to monitor a patient's blood pressure for both hypotension and hypertension. Good communication between the general practitioner and consultant cardiologist or physician is essential to avoid doubling up of procedures or indeed to ensure no-one is slipping through the net. A patient blood pressure record card is useful to chart the level of blood pressure over a few weeks.

The referral of the diabetic patient to a nurse specialist in diabetes, if available, should be considered.

Patients who have undergone CABG surgery require special attention, since most pre-operative medications are prescribed to relieve the symptoms of angina and will normally be discontinued following surgery. For patients who are unaware of any history of hypertension, it is wise to monitor their blood pressure over the next few months in order to detect any hitherto undiagnosed hypertension masked by the dual effect of anti-anginal medication. It is also common for patients who have previously been treated for hypertension to be restarted on anti-hypertensive therapy some weeks after surgery. It should be borne in mind that CABG surgery is not a cure for hypertension or any other underlying risk factor.

Exercise to some degree will help to reduce blood pressure, especially if there is a period of relaxation built in to the exercise class, but care should be taken with those who have uncontrolled hypertension taking part in fairly vigorous exercise. Including relaxation within rehabilitation is essential, as many patients feel that there are great sources of stress within their lives and appreciate being able to use components of relaxation techniques easily. Exercises that should be encouraged are ones that can be done in traffic jams or waiting in supermarket checkout queues as well as sitting at home watching television.

Diet

Eating is a fundamental nutritional need, a social occasion, a demonstration of caring for someone and for some a way of coping with stress or unhappiness. Many patients are overweight which aggravates their hypertension, causes them to be dyspnoeic and listless and may precipitate diabetes. The average intake of fruit and vegetables falls far short of the daily recommended levels and indeed many patients eat no fruit, and vegetables only in the shape of potatoes, frequently fried. Because eating is something that is a basic requirement of life and is carried out several times a day, it requires great perseverance and motivation on the part of the patient and constant encouragement from the rehabilitation nurse. The patient who is attempting to stop smoking and lose weight is more than likely to fail. The two issues are very hard to deal with together so the emphasis must be put on smoking cessation. When recording a patient's weight it is essential to use the body mass index (BMI). When reading a case sheet or letter without seeing the patient it is impossible to know if 70 kg is a reasonable weight. Therefore the height at least should be recorded alongside the weight to allow calculation of BMI. For patients who may not require referral to a dietitian, the nurse can help by discussing with them which changes the patients feel can be introduced to their diet. You may wish to consider referring patients to a dietitian if they are defined as overweight or have a total cholesterol > 5.5 mmol/l.

For the patient who has an elevated serum lipid profile and who smokes, it is a massive change to previous lifestyle and can be difficult to maintain.

Patients attending cardiac rehabilitation can have their weight monitored regularly. If there is no change in weight, you would discuss in a non-judgemental way whether patients are complying and if not, why not? Perhaps they have no real interest in improving their health or have too many demands on them within the family or from the peer group.

Many problems arise within families when patients are trying to restrict their intake of fat but are regularly presented with food by caring partners who feel hurt and rejected when the patients refuse to eat it, e.g. home-baked cakes, rich sauces. In most cases it is advantageous to include the person who does the cooking within the house when discussing the need for dietary change. Simple charts to pin up in the kitchen of guidelines on which foods to increase or decrease intake are useful. A small credit-card-sized fold-up list which can be carried in a purse or pocket and taken to the supermarket helps to ease the confusion felt when learning a new way of shopping.

Stress

At some point in the discussion with patients about myocardial infarction, it is worth probing gently and asking them what they feel may have contributed to their heart attack. Despite general health warnings and health education promotions, patients are more likely to blame overwork, family relationships, bereavement and general anxieties than their use of tobacco or alcohol. Some patients will not identify with the word stress as relating to themselves, as exemplified by the following case.

A lady was asked if she felt that she had any stress in her life and commented that she did not feel she had any more than the next person. On being asked what she felt may have contributed towards her heart attack, she then lost control of herself, describing how she had been caring for her husband with Parkinson's disease until she felt she could cope no longer. He had been taken into a nursing home and she had eventually received a bill for several hundreds of pounds, which she could not pay. This lady did not identify with the word stress.

Many patients require to be referred to social services for advice on benefits or for home help assessment. Those unable to afford a phone and other benefits may qualify for assistance from social services and The Chest Heart & Stroke Association may also be of help.

Being given time to discuss their anxieties and fears and indeed being allowed to voice openly their feelings which perhaps they have previously denied is crucial for some patients. Knowing how to listen is a skill which increases the effectiveness in dealing with the patient who finds it difficult to communicate. Listening has been described by Burley-Allen (1982) as a highly selective, subjective experience where information that conflicts with the listener's present ideas may simply be tuned out when we expect to hear certain things; we do not listen to what is really said. Present in each situation are attention, reception and perception.

Allowing themselves to admit to feelings of fear, anger and sadness may be something the patients have never experienced and they will need to be reassured that such feelings are normal for all of us, both men and women. Allowing patients to express their feelings without judgement can provide a release for long-held feelings. It is of paramount importance that patients are ensured privacy when discussing emotional issues. When arranging to spend time discussing sensitive areas with patients, it is wise to agree a fixed time span so that your time is focused and the patients understand what length of time is theirs. This allows you to focus your time and use it constructively. At the end of the agreed time a further appointment can be made if patients feel that they need it. The issue of confidentiality is important and should be outlined to patients before starting any session. Discussing with patients that you would like to reserve the right to notify their doctor if you felt they were a danger to themselves or someone else and whether they are willing to go ahead under this agreement is important. In other respects, patients should be assured of total confidentiality.

The self-image of many patients is greatly altered following acute myocardial infarction. For example a 36-year-old man may feel that he has an 'old man's disease'. A woman who has always been the organizer and pivot of the family for husband, children and grandchildren may find it hard to relinquish the reins of the family. Women frequently experience a loss of control, especially over domestic issues such as cleaning, and are very likely to get up and do the task themselves out of sheer frustration. Encouraging them to accept a less than perfect house can be difficult as they may have been taught that a woman is judged by the state of her windows!

Driving

The Driver and Vehicle Licensing Authority (DVLA) recommend no driving for 4 weeks following uncomplicated myocardial infarction (DVLA 1993). Patients must inform their insurance company that they have had a heart attack. The insurance company will probably ask them to contact the DVLA. This can be done by letter or phone. If patients have still had no reply from the DVLA after the 4 weeks have passed, they should ask their insurance company if they can drive. Many companies agree to this. Patients should not drive if they experience light-headedness or angina while driving.

HGV and PCV drivers require an exercise-tolerance test to be carried out with the patient off medication for 24 hours. Patients should have no symptoms and no electrocardiograph changes. Coronary angiography is not required.

For CABG surgery patients it would be more advisable to wait a minimum of 6 weeks before driving to allow the sternum adequate time to heal. Unless patients have an exemption certificate they are still obliged by law to wear seat belts regardless of their sternotomy wound.

Back to work

Generally a patient will be told to expect to be away from work for 12 weeks following myocardial infarction or CABG surgery but this obviously varies from person to person and what type of employment the patient has. The rehabilitation nurse needs to discuss in full with patients what their employment entails, e.g. if it involves shift work, driving a great deal, travelling abroad, heavy labouring. It is important to discourage patients from making any long-term decisions too early in their recovery but at the same time bringing in an edge of reality. All patients should be encouraged to discuss their situation fully with their hospital consultant at their outpatient clinic visit and also their GP.

Resuming sexual relations

Ensure that the patient is comfortable discussing sex before embarking on the do's and don'ts! Most (but not all) patients are reluctant to initiate the conversation concerning sexual relations so it is wise to check with patients whether this is an area that they would like to discuss. Never assume that an elderly patient will not be having a sexual relationship.

As a general guideline it can be suggested that it is wise to wait about 5 weeks before resuming sexual habits. It should be pointed out to patients that their partner may very well be concerned about participating in sexual intercourse so it should be discussed between them both. Patients who are prescribed beta-blockers will have been told that impotence can be a side effect of the drug but it is also wise to point out that the impotence may be because of fear of causing chest pain or heart attack. If the patient feels that he needs some sort of indicator it can be suggested that if he can go up a flight of 20 stairs rapidly without chest pain or breathlessness, then that would indicate that there should be no problem having sexual intercourse. The areas of warning for myocardial infarction patients are as follows:

- patients who have uncontrolled hypertension—because of the rapid rise in blood pressure during sex.
- extra-marital affairs or 'one night stands'—because of the stress involved.
- anal sex—causing vasovagal episodes.

Drugs

If patients are to comply with medication, they must understand the effect of the drug on their body and why they need to be given it. They need to know how long they are likely to be advised to take it and what side effects may occur. The fact that they must never stop taking their medication without their doctor's agreement must be emphasized. They should be encouraged to discuss with their pharmacist any worries they may have.

Many patients are on multiple medication and have difficulty in remembering the names of their drugs and the times at which they should

Thrombolytic therapy – Yes/No	Drug used	Date given		
Drug name	Morning	Midday	Evening	Night
Aspirin 75 mg dissolved in water	*			
Frusemide 40 mg	*			
Captopril 25 mg	*	*		*
Comment e.g. 'Take aspirin after food.' Date of exercise test.................... Date of cholesterol check..........				

Figure 12.1 Example of a drug record card.

be taken. A card listing their drugs and any other relevant information is useful although it is only of benefit if kept up to date (Fig. 12.1).

Before being discharged from hospital the patient should be given guidelines on how to deal with chest pain, e.g. if experiencing angina that may present as chest pain, arm pain or heaviness, pain in the throat, jaw or ears, choking sensation in the throat, extreme breathlessness (see Box 12.2).

OUTPATIENT CARDIAC REHABILITATION

Outpatient cardiac rehabilitation exists in many different forms, depending usually on the resources available or the geographical area served. The rehabilitation service provided by an inner city hospital will differ from that offered by a district general hospital in that the latter will be required to meet the needs of a rural and widespread community. The resources provided by trusts and local health authorities differ according to the perceived

---

Box 12.2 Guidelines for dealing with chest pain

- Ask patient to stop and rest, with the legs propped up if possible.
- Ensure that the patient knows how to use glyceryl trinitrate (GTN) spray.
- If symptoms have not resolved within a few minutes, use two puffs of GTN spray.
- If the pain has not resolved within another 5 minutes, repeat the spray.
- If pain has not resolved in another 5 minutes (10 minutes from onset), call the GP.
- If the symptoms worsen while awaiting GP, dial 999.
- If patients experience dizziness or light-headedness they are advised to lie down.

importance of the service and funds available. Indeed, many rehabilitation services have grown and improved through the fund-raising efforts of patients and staff involved in the service.

For most rehabilitation programmes, exercise is a core requirement and is dealt with in Chapter 7.

The length of programmes varies from 6–12 weeks with an average duration of 10 weeks. Ideally, a programme providing both exercise and education for both patients and relatives is to be aimed for. However, in order to include a greater number of relatives it may require an evening service which then has implications for staffing resources.

The educational input should be multidisciplinary.

A postmyocardial infarction cardiac rehabilitation programme could be run along the following lines:

- The programme starts 3 weeks after discharge from hospital and is of 12 weeks' duration.
- Ask patients to bring a relative along with them; this gives you another perspective on any potential or actual problems within the domestic arena.
- Ask patients to bring their drugs with them as they may have misunderstood the instructions given on discharge from hospital.
- On their first visit:
  —assess blood pressure, heart rate and rhythm, symptoms of angina, breathlessness
  —emphasize drug compliance and identify any side effects
  —try to define their psychological status, e.g. depression, anxiety
  —establish their smoking status, i.e. stopped, considering stopping, restarted smoking
  —weigh if necessary.

An example of a multidisciplinary education programme could be as follows:

- Diet and the heart—dietitian
- Cholesterol and heart disease—clinical biochemist
- Exercise and the heart—physiotherapist
- Drugs for the heart—pharmacist
- Blood pressure—cardiologist or physician
- Stress—rehabilitation nurse
- Risk factors—rehabilitation nurse.

The selection of videos dealing with heart disease is increasing all the time and they are enjoyed by the patients. The Chest Heart & Stroke Association and the British Heart Foundation provide reasonably priced videos as do many local area health authorities.

A relatives-only session could be considered to offer the opportunity for the relatives to discuss their fears openly without being in the presence of the patients. A group session may be useful so that others are able to hear how common their fears are and thus feel less isolated.

A programme following CABG surgery would run along the same lines as the one described but would start approximately 4 weeks after discharge. This would be dependent on patients being contacted within the first 2 weeks after discharge to identify any problems that may exist, e.g. wound infections, excessive pain or breathlessness, or anything which would exclude them from early entry to the programme and would suggest they should be seen by their surgeon before participating in any exercise.

Rural cardiac rehabilitation

Patients who live some distance from a rehabilitation service or who are unable to travel may be encouraged to use a self-help manual devised for home use with input from a community nurse trained in the use of the manual. *The Heart Manual* (Lothian Health Board 1993), dealing with both exercise and the psychological impact of myocardial infarction on the patient, comes with audio cassette tapes dealing with some of the normal questions patients may ask as well as a relaxation tape. 'The cost effectiveness of the home based programme has yet to be compared with that of a hospital based programme, but the findings of this study indicate that it might be worth offering such a package to all patients with acute myocardial infarction' (Lewin et al 1992).

Documentation

It is crucial that the health care team involved in providing rehabilitation keep individualized records on each patient. All meetings with the patient should be kept on record and documentation completed at the time or as soon after as possible. On busy days it is easy to forget what you have said to whom, so it is wise to have some kind of check list to remind you of where you are with each individual. A cardiac rehabilitation patient profile (Fig. 12.2) will help to guide you and can be handed over to another health care worker who can see at a glance what still requires to be dealt with. Below are examples of documentation which may be of help.

Baseline information should be gathered on admission to the rehabilitation programme and updated regularly. This can be used to reassure the patient of progress even if he feels there is none! In the same way, any deterioration in the patient's condition will be easily identified. Crucially, the risk factors of each patient should be highlighted and prioritized. Any risk factors still outstanding at the end of the programme should be communicated to the patient's GP. Photocopies of any letters sent out should be filed for future reference.

It is recommended that once patients have completed the hospital-based rehabilitation programme they should be encouraged to continue to exercise thereafter and many areas have community-based groups which meet for this purpose. Other groups meet to continue support and friendships forged during their rehabilitation programme.

Patients and their relatives who attend the cardiac rehabilitation programme are an ideal group to whom basic life-support skills could be taught. The British Heart Foundation recommend the teaching of basic life-support

Acute Myocardial Infarction

Date of admission ☐☐☐☐☐☐
Date of discharge ☐☐☐☐☐☐
Name: Phone No:
Address: Next of kin:
                                Phone No:
Hosp. No ☐☐☐☐☐☐
DOB
Ward ☐   GP:
consultant: Address:

Diagnosis:
Cardiac enzymes:
Thrombolytic therapy   Reperfused?
Streptokinase card given?
Investigations:
ETT/thallium
Result:
Echo:
Result:
Other:
Issues discussed pre-discharge:
☐ Structure and function of the heart   ☐ Smoking cessation
☐ Dealing with chest pain   ☐ Alcohol reduction
☐ Reducing the risk of CHD   ☐ Resuming sexual relations
☐ Relaxation   ☐ Medication
☐ Return to fitness and activity   ☐ Home exercise
☐ Return to work   ☐ Return to driving
☐ Healthy eating
Medication on discharge from hospital:

Figure 12.2 Cardiac rehabilitation: (A) post-MI patient record file.

skills to these people, and information, advice and guidance can be obtained from Heart Start, a project funded by the British Heart Foundation. It may be worth considering inviting paramedics to participate as they bring with them the experience of dealing regularly with cardiac arrest in the community, which is a very different situation from a cardiac arrest within the hospital.

THE FUTURE

Cardiac rehabilitation in the UK lags well behind other countries, for example the USA and Canada. The Toronto Rehabilitation Center is a public hospital

Post-Coronary Artery Bypass Graft Surgery

Date of admission ☐☐☐☐☐☐
Date of discharge ☐☐☐☐☐☐
Name: Phone No:
Address: Next of kin:
                                         Phone No:

Hosp. No ☐☐☐☐☐☐
DOB
Ward ☐   GP:
consultant: Address:

Diagnosis:
Complications:
Investigations:
ETT/thallium
Result:
Echo:
Result:
Other:
Issues discussed pre-discharge:
☐ Structure and function of the heart   ☐ Smoking cessation
☐ How revascularisation is achieved   ☐ Alcohol reduction
☐ Reducing the risk of CHD   ☐ Resuming sexual relations
☐ Relaxation   ☐ Medication
☐ Return to fitness and activity   ☐ Home exercise
☐ Return to work   ☐ Return to driving
☐ Healthy eating   ☐ Care of wounds
Medication on discharge from hospital:

Comments:

Figure 12.2 Cardiac rehabilitation: (B) post-CABG surgery patient record file.

whose operating funds are provided by the Ontario Ministry of Health. Nevertheless, when it comes to expansion this centre of excellence like many of the smaller services in Britain relies on charitable funding. In 1980, a new wing including a 120-seat lecture theatre for patients and their spouses, a

Risk Factors

☐ Significant family history
☐ Smoking   No of cigarettes per day ☐☐☐
☐ Ex-smoker   How long? ☐☐ years
☐ Weekly units of alcohol
☐ Diabetes
☐ High blood pressure
☐☐ Body mass index
☐ High levels of stress
☐ Low level of physical activity?

Chol.   LDL   HDL
Trig.   VLDL
Date of sample ☐☐☐☐☐☐

Previous medical history:

Social circumstances:

Exercise functional capacity:

Occupation:

Hobbies:

Comments:

Figure 12.2 Cardiac rehabilitation: (C) risk factor file for post-MI and post-CABG patients.

Initial Assessment at Outpatient Cardiac Rehabilitation

Date ☐☐☐☐☐☐

Blood pressure:

Heart rate: Rhythm:
                              (if irregular carry out resting ECG)
Breathlessness?

Symptoms of angina?
If yes, describe frequency, intensity and how the patient deals with it.

Pre-exercise class walking test carried out?

Amount of activity managed:

Complying with medication?
(detail any problems patient may be experiencing)

Other:

Figure 12.2 Cardiac rehabilitation: (D) initial outpatient assessment form.

	Outpatient progress report		
Date	Comment	BP	HR and rhythm

Figure 12.2 Cardiac rehabilitation: (E) outpatient progress report form.

Discharge from Cardiac Rehabilitation Outpatient Programme

Date of discharge from rehabilitation ☐☐☐☐☐☐

☐ Cholesterol check done?
☐ Risk factors emphasized?
☐ Walking test repeated?
☐ Exercise guidelines given?
☐ Community exercise group membership form given?
☐ Discharge letter sent to consultant/GP?

Other:

Figure 12.2 Cardiac rehabilitation: (F) discharge from outpatient programme form.

large gymnasium, two exercise test laboratories and a 200-meter indoor walking/jogging track was opened. A 200-meter indoor track with additional space for seminar rooms and patient monitoring was added 12 years later. To have such facilities available to the majority of patients should be our aim and is an enormous target to aim for. Nevertheless, there was a time when cardiac rehabilitation did not exist at all. With this in mind we need to believe in the power of rehabilitation to improve the quality of life of the cardiac patient and continue to cajole, persuade and prove that such a service deserves major government funding.

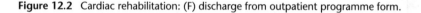

■ KEY POINTS

- A 10-year Swedish study into cardiac rehabilitation reported a reduction in non-fatal reinfarctions during the first 5 years followed by significant reduction in total and cardiac mortality in the later part of the study.
- The aim of cardiac rehabilitation is to return patients to optimum health within the confines of their disease.
- Risk factors need to be identified early in admission and referred to appropriate services, e.g. dietitian, diabetic service.
- Serum lipids should be measured within the first 12–24 hours as cholesterol levels drop following trauma or major illness. It is then necessary to wait 3 months for the serum lipids to return to their normal levels.

- The myocardial infarction patient should be given clear advice on dealing with symptoms of angina before leaving the hospital.
- Individual records on each patient should be kept.
- Cardiac patients should have their domestic situation identified as early as possible following admission in order to prepare their discharge home into a safe and supportive environment with the help of social services if necessary.
- Cardiac rehabilitation should be multidisciplinary.
- It is an opportunity to educate relatives, family and friends about the meaning of heart disease and risk factors.
- Many patients misunderstand their medication instructions and those with hypertension fail to comply with their medication.
- Patients are more likely to blame their illness on stress than on smoking.
- MI patients should not drive for 4 weeks following their infarction and should not drive if they experience light-headedness or angina while driving.
- CABG surgery patients should wait a minimum of 6 weeks before driving. They should not drive if they have light-headedness or their wounds are painful causing them to be unable to brake suddenly or turn the steering wheel quickly.
- Following either MI or CABG surgery, patients must inform their insurance company before resuming driving.
- Return to work is generally 12 weeks after both myocardial infarction and CABG surgery but this must be discussed with the consultant cardiologist/surgeon and the general practitioner.
- Sexual relations may be resumed after 4–5 weeks providing the patient has made an uncomplicated recovery.
- Basic life-support skills should be taught to relatives and when appropriate to patients.
- Any risk factors still outstanding at the end of the rehabilitation programme should be communicated to the patient's GP.

PRACTICAL EXERCISE

To ensure continuity of the cardiac rehabilitation programme in primary care, find out about local cardiac rehabilitation programmes in your area. Find out:

- where and when these programmes are held
- what form the programmes take
- how you can refer patients on to them
- what advice is given to the patients at the rehabilitation programmes and how you can ensure continuity of information in the community.

Case Study 12.1

Mrs B is admitted to a medical ward suffering an acute inferior myocardial infarction and with a history of hypertension. Her recovery is unremarkable and prior to discharge she is seen by the rehabilitation nurse and the physiotherapist. As she has stairs at home, she is supervised on a flight of stairs outside the ward by the physiotherapist and manages without any problems. Discussing her home circumstances with the rehabilitation nurse, she discloses that she never goes anywhere without her husband and that he does all of the shopping and all of the housework. Knowing that she was going home to full support, she was discharged and asked to return for exercise tolerance testing 1 week later.

The ECG technician was surprised to see Mrs B return for her exercise test in a wheelchair, which according to the husband was on the instructions of the GP. Mr B was very angry that Mrs B had been asked to undergo an exercise test so soon after her heart attack. Such was the situation that the doctor decided that he would postpone the exercise test until she had recuperated further.

How would the rehabilitation nurse resolve this problem?

Answer

Mrs B had been contacted on discharge and there had been no developments or complications since discharge. She had been mobilizing well around the ward and the only reason she had not been exercise-tested prior to discharge was that there was no appointment slot available. Mrs B and her husband were invited to come up to the hospital for a check on her blood pressure and to attend the series of talks available to patients after myocardial infarction. Mrs B's blood pressure was within the normal parameters, she had no symptoms of angina and was complying with her medication. The nurse noticed how frequently Mr B answered questions asked of Mrs B and how involved in her care he was. He was completely responsible for her drug administration. The nurse praised Mr B for taking such good care of Mrs B but gently pointed out that all patients unless physically or mentally disabled must assume responsibility for their own care at some point.

A few weeks later the nurse managed to see Mrs B on her own and discussed her domestic relationship with her husband. Mrs B admitted that she would love to be allowed out on her own to visit friends or go shopping for an hour. It was agreed that the nurse would invite Mr and Mrs B for joint counselling to try to find options that would suit both of them. When they arrived for the counselling session, the nurse took great care to praise Mr B and asked him if it had been hard for him when his wife had been diagnosed as having had a heart attack. At this point Mr B started to weep. His mother had died when he was 18 years old as a result of 'heart disease'. He had had to shoulder the burden of responsibility for himself and his father and had never had the opportunity to grieve fully. Since his marriage, he had lived in fear of losing his wife and was terror-stricken when the diagnosis of heart attack was made. After hearing an explanation of how the care of the cardiac patient has progressed so dramatically, Mr B was able to understand the source of his fears and to acknowledge the restriction he was putting on his wife's recovery. Mrs B went on to have an exercise test and to participate in the exercise class. Her physical and psychological health improved by leaps and bounds.

REFERENCES

Burley-Allen M 1982 Listening—the forgotten skill. John Wiley & Sons, Chichester, p 40

Driver and Vehicle Licensing Authority (DVLA) 1993 For medical practitioners: at a glance guide to the current medical standards of fitness to drive. DVLA, Swansea, p 10

Hedback B, Perk J, Wolden P 1993 Long term reduction of cardiac mortality after MI: 10 year study of a comprehsive rehab programme. European Heart Journal 14: 831–835

Horgan J, Bethell H, Carson P, Davidson C, Julian D, Mayou R A, Nagl R 1992 Working party report on cardiac rehabilitation. British Heart Journal 67: 412–418

Julian D, Marley C 1991 Coronary heart disease: the facts. Oxford University Press, Oxford, pp 22–23

Lewin B, Robertson I H, Cay E L, Irving J B, Campbell M 1992 Effects of self-help post-myocardial infarction rehabilitation on psychological adjustment and use of health services. Lancet 339: 1036–1040

Lothian Health Board 1993 The heart manual. HMSO, Edinburgh

World Health Organization 1993 Cardiac rehabilitation and secondary prevention: long-term care for patients with ischaemic heart disease. WHO, Regional Office for Europe, pp 1–5

FURTHER READING

Ashworth P, Clark C 1992 Cardiovascular intensive care nursing. Churchill Livingstone, Edinburgh
A comprehensive textbook covering a wide aspect of caring for the cardiac patient in the acute phase.

Burley-Allen M 1982 Listening—the forgotten skill. John Wiley & Sons, Chichester
An excellent guide to improving listening using exercises and developing self-awareness.

Coronary Prevention Group 1989 Guidelines for setting up & running a cardiac rehabilitation programme. Coronary Prevention Group, London
A superb and humorous book with cartoon illustrations—a must for anyone setting up a programme from scratch.

Hampton J R 1992 The ECG made easy, 4th edn. Churchill Livingstone, Edinburgh
A step-by-step to reading and understanding the basic ECG.

Horne E M, Cowan T 1992 Effective communication, 2nd edn. Professional Nurse, Professional Development Series, Wolfe Publishing, London
A series of articles previously published in Professional Nurse providing useful guidelines on communicating.

Julian D, Marley C 1991 Coronary heart disease: the facts. Oxford University Press, Oxford
An easily understood guide to the facts of heart disease written for the lay person.

Stewart I, Vann Joines 1993 TA today: a new introduction to transactional analysis. Lifespace Publishing, Nottingham
Transactional analysis presented in an easily understood format.

Women and coronary heart disease

Grace M. Lindsay   Elizabeth Farish

13

■ CONTENTS

INTRODUCTION

It is important to explain why we believe a chapter specifically devoted to coronary heart disease (CHD) in women should be included in this book. CHD has been well recognized as a major cause of mortality and disability in males but as a less important threat to the health of women. Yet, in all the developed countries CHD is the leading cause of death in women past the age of the menopause, accounting for more deaths than all the cancers combined. One in four women die from CHD (Registrar General for Scotland 1994). In addition, in Scotland, inpatient hospital stay for CHD-related admissions is the same for both men and women; so in terms of health need and resource utilization the demand is just as high for women as it is for men.

Most epidemiological studies and intervention trials conducted to investigate the cause of CHD involved only male subjects. The results from such studies have been used as a basis for CHD prevention practice for both men and women. This may or may not be appropriate.

The natural course of CHD is different in males and females. Analysis of the limited data collected in women has been undertaken in an effort to improve our understanding of the nature of CHD risk in women.

This chapter aims to discuss the CHD risk factors that are particularly important or unique to women. It will include a detailed examination of the use of postmenopausal hormone replacement therapy (HRT) in CHD prevention in women.

PROFILE OF CHD IN WOMEN

CHD risk in women

For the purpose of the clinical evaluation of CHD risk in women it is important to understand the differences that occur among women and not only the differences between women and men. The traditional CHD risk factors that have been shown to be operative in men are also important in women (Manson et al 1992). These include smoking, hypercholesterolaemia, and hypertension. However, their effect on CHD risk is different and they have been shown to be less predictive of subsequent CHD in women than in men (Wilhelmsen et al 1977). These CHD risk factors are discussed in more detail in Chapters 3, 4 and 5.

Age

Since the early decades of this century it has been noted that there is a marked gender difference in risk of CHD with a significant age disparity in males and females who succumb to CHD (Glendy et al 1937). Although many disease patterns have changed since that early work, the natural course of CHD with increasing age still differs in males and females today. Premenopausal women appear to be protected from CHD when compared to men. However, with advancing age this gender difference in CHD risk diminishes and in all developed countries CHD is the leading cause of death and disability in women past the age of the menopause. CHD accounts for more deaths than all cancers combined (Fig. 13.1).

It can be clearly seen in Tables 13.1 and 13.2 that the incidence of CHD death in females before the age of 54 is comparatively low and much lower than in males. Beyond this age, however, incidence rises markedly and in females over 75 years old approaches levels observed in males (Fig. 13.2). It should be noted that CHD mortality figures are only one index of the impact of CHD on health, but are readily accessible from Government statistics. Morbidity information is not available to the same extent but would add further to our recognition of CHD as a major health problem.

Socioeconomic class

The detrimental effects of deprivation on the health of both sexes have been clearly documented (Black 1980), but it appears that in areas of high deprivation, women are particularly disadvantaged in terms of increased CHD risk when compared with their better-off counterparts.

A comparison of standardized mortality rates for CHD among women living in the West of Scotland, an area of high CHD incidence, reveals a large gradient in CHD mortality. There is a twofold increment in deaths from

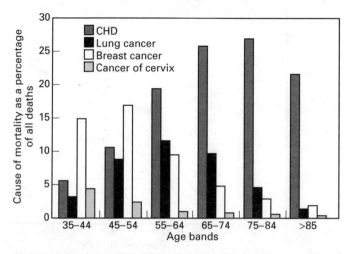

Figure 13.1 Mortality due to CHD (ICD codes 410–414), lung cancer (ICD code 101), breast cancer (ICD code 113) and cervical cancer (ICD code 120) as a percentage of all deaths by age bands in females (adapted from the Report of the Registrar General for Scotland 1994).

Table 13.1 Age and gender distribution of deaths from CHD, (ICD codes 410–414) in England and Wales in 1993, OPCS 1993

	Age range (years)				
	< 44	45–54	55–64	65–74	> 75
Males	1.4%	5.1%	14.6%	32.4%	46.5%
Females	0.3%	1.2%	5.4%	20.5%	72.6%

Table 13.2 Age and gender distribution of deaths from CHD, (ICD codes 410–414) in Scotland, 1993

	Age range (years)				
	< 44	45–54	55–64	65–74	> 75
Males	1.5%	6.0%	16.8%	35.8%	39.8%
Females	0.4%	1.6%	7.4%	24.1%	66.4%

CHD between the areas of lowest and highest incidence. Table 13.3 shows CHD mortality rates in six standard areas with the most affluent area at the top of the table and the least affluent area at the bottom. The areas of high incidence of CHD are those associated with high levels of deprivation. This variation in incidence of CHD in women from areas of high deprivation compared to more affluent areas is greater than the difference observed in

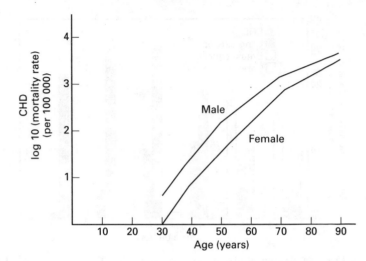

Figure 13.2 Trends in CHD mortality (ICD codes 410–414) with increasing age for males and females (adapted from the Report of the Registrar General for Scotland 1994).

Table 13.3 CHD (ICD codes 410–414) mortality, standard areas 1993

	Females (rate per 1000)	Males (rate per 1000)
Bearsden & Milngavie	1.74	2.83
Eastwood	2.30	2.80
Monklands	3.05	4.14
Renfrew	3.13	3.52
Cunningham	3.23	3.98
Glasgow City	3.48	4.21

males from the same areas. The difference in CHD incidence cannot be accounted for by differing age distributions in the six areas. The age distributions in these areas are similar as outlined in Tables 13.4 and 13.5.

Smoking

Smoking has an additional effect on CHD risk in women. Women who smoke become menopausal on average 1–2 years earlier than non-smokers (Department of Health and Human Resources 1989). Studies have reported lower plasma oestrogen levels in women smokers when compared to age-matched non-smokers (Mattison & Thorgeirsson 1978). The mechanism for this is not well understood with two main theories postulated; that of an anti-oestrogen effect of smoking, or an ageing effect on the oocyte causing a decline in oestrogen production. Since oestrogen is believed to protect against CHD, it is clear that smoking, a well-documented major contributor to CHD risk in both sexes, has an additional adverse effect that is specific to women.

Table 13.4 Age distribution of females as a percentage of total female population

	Age bands				
	≤ 24	25–44	45–64	65–74	≥ 75
Bearsden & Milngavie	30.6	26.2	25.8	9.7	7.6
Eastwood	30.4	28.3	24.1	8.8	8.3
Monklands	33.9	28.6	22.1	8.9	6.5
Renfrew	30.9	29.3	23.4	9.2	7.2
Cunningham	31.5	28.2	22.9	9.4	8.0
Glasgow City	31.4	29.0	20.6	9.2	6.6

Table 13.5 Age distribution of males as a percentage of total male population

	Age bands				
	≤ 24	25–44	45–64	65–74	≥ 75
Bearsden & Milngavie	37.4	26.1	26.4	8.5	4.1
Eastwood	34.3	29.8	24.1	7.5	4.3
Monklands	37.1	30.3	21.8	7.3	3.4
Renfrew	34.8	30.6	23.5	7.5	3.7
Cunningham	35.7	29.4	23.0	7.7	4.3
Glasgow City	35.1	31.9	20.7	8.1	4.2

Hypertension

In young adults, systolic and diastolic blood pressures tend to be higher in men than women (Table 13.6). Throughout adulthood blood pressure gradually rises in both sexes (Whelton et al 1994). However, the gradient of increase is slightly steeper in women. The resultant effect is that by the fifth to sixth decade blood pressure levels are similar in males and females. With advancing years, systolic blood pressure continues to rise in women. Isolated systolic hypertension is more prevalent in females than males and is estimated to affect about one-third of women over 65 years of age. The higher incidence of elevated blood pressure levels observed in older women has been attributed to the fact that the average life expectancy for a women is longer and males with the highest levels of blood pressure may have died

Table 13.6 Average blood pressure levels in young adults

	Females	Males
Systolic pressure (mmHg)	110–120	120–130
Diastolic pressure (mmHg)	70–75	75–80

already. However, the observed discrepancy in systolic blood pressure between men and women in later life cannot be explained by the fact that women live longer (Silagy & McNeil 1992). Isolated systolic hypertension is a problem for older women as it is associated with increased risk of both stroke and CHD (Saltzberg et al 1988). Health care practitioners should therefore be vigilant in identifying this common modifiable CHD risk factor in women.

Hypertension during pregnancy

Hypertension has been documented to occur in between 5 and 10% of pregnancies. Not all hypertensive states during pregnancy are the result of the same underlying process, which in turn has important implications for subsequent CHD risk. There are three broad classes of hypertension in pregnancy:

- coexisting hypertension
- 'pregnancy-induced' hypertension
- 'pre-eclampsia'.

Coexisting hypertension or essential hypertension is present prior to the pregnancy and continues throughout. The impact on future CHD risk is similar to that observed in the general population with similar blood pressure levels. This is discussed in more detail in Chapter 4.

Specific to pregnancy, there are two main classes of hypertension: 'pregnancy induced' and 'pre-eclampsia'. The former hypertensive state tends to arise in the third trimester and is characterized by moderate elevations in both systolic and diastolic blood pressure that may require treatment. Blood pressure returns to normal after delivery and is thought not to be linked to an increased likelihood of hypertension or risk of CHD in the future. The latter, 'pre-eclampsia', is a specific disorder of pregnancy that is dangerous and poorly understood. It is rare before the 20th week of gestation but can occur at any time beyond, and is characterized by the presence of hypertension, proteinuria and oedema; earlier onset is associated with greater severity of the condition. Follow-up work has reported an association between pre-eclampsia and subsequent CHD (Croft & Hannaford 1989, Rosenberg et al 1983).

In practice, particularly when reviewing case records retrospectively, the potential for confusion regarding diagnosis of hypertensive states during pregnancy is significant and the ability to target appropriate individuals lost. However, during pregnancy may be the first time that a woman has a blood pressure check and any woman who has a record of hypertension during pregnancy warrants follow-up to ensure that blood pressure levels remain within the normotensive range postpartum. Such women are therefore targets for early monitoring and prevention strategies.

Oral contraceptives

The use of the older high-dose contraceptive pill increased risk of CHD, in particular risk of myocardial infarction. This was shown to be mediated through increasing levels of LDL-cholesterol, lowering HDL-cholesterol, raising blood pressure and promoting clotting mechanisms (Stadel 1981). Because younger women are at lower absolute risk of CHD, the additional risk was only small in women who were non-smokers. However, there was a greatly increased risk of myocardial infarction when the combination of high-dose oral contraceptives and cigarette smoking was present (Hennekens et al 1979). In a meta-analysis of 13 studies of health outcome in past users it was shown that the deleterious effects of these preparations applied to current users and that duration of use did not affect risk (Stampfer et al 1990). The authors concluded that there was a rapid return to baseline CHD risk following discontinuation of therapy and that increased risk of thrombosis, a short-term mechanism, explained most, if not all, of the increased risk in current users.

There is insufficient evidence to comment on whether the risk of CHD is increased with the use of the modern lower-dose contraceptive pill although work is currently in progress.

Diabetes mellitus

Diabetes is an even stronger risk factor for CHD in women than in men. Mortality rates for CHD in diabetic women are three- to sevenfold higher than in non-diabetic women. This is in comparison to a two- to fourfold increase in risk in male diabetics over male non-diabetics (Barrett-Connor & Wingard 1983, Manson et al 1991). The mechanism for this observation is not clear although it has been hypothesized that diabetes exacerbates the effects of other risk factors and impairs oestrogen-binding thus negating the protective effects that oestrogens confer on premenopausal women (Ruderman & Haudenschild 1984).

Gestational diabetes, which occurs in 3% of pregnancies in the UK, may be a marker for increased CHD risk. Long-term follow-up studies reviewed by Rich-Edwards and colleagues (1995), have shown an increased incidence of hypertension, insulin resistance and adverse lipid profiles in women who had gestational diabetes compared to women who had normal pregnancies. More than one-third of women who had gestational diabetes subsequently developed non-insulin-dependent diabetes compared to a rate of 5% in women who had normal pregnancies (Mestman 1988). Postnatal follow-up usually involves an oral glucose tolerance test to exclude the presence of diabetes mellitus. Longer-term follow-up could help to identify earlier those women who develop diabetes mellitus and would provide the opportunity for more comprehensive CHD risk factor assessment and intervention.

Lipid profile

The lipid profile of total cholesterol, triglyceride, LDL-cholesterol and HDL-cholesterol measurements is important in both genders in risk factor assessment. In the Framingham study (Castelli 1984), CHD risk factors and events were observed over a 6-year period. It was shown that at *any* cholesterol level the risk of CHD over that time period in women was only one-third of that observed in men, irrespective of smoking and blood pressure status. The lack of predictive power of total cholesterol in CHD risk assessment in women has been documented by others (Isles 1993).

It has been suggested that in females, more emphasis should be placed on levels of the other lipid parameters, namely triglyceride, LDL-cholesterol and HDL-cholesterol, rather than relying on a total cholesterol measurement alone. Elevated triglyceride levels have been identified as posing a greater threat to women than men (Castelli 1986). The independent nature of their effect in women remains in debate with some studies (Castelli 1986) demonstrating an independent association with increased CHD risk (after adjusting for the effect of other key risk factors) while other work does not (Bush et al 1987).

HDL-cholesterol levels in the population are higher in females than males and it has been postulated that this effect may account for at least some of the CHD protection observed in younger females (Kannel & Brand 1985). A low HDL-cholesterol is a particularly strong indicator of increased CHD risk (Jacobs et al 1990).

In conclusion, both elevated triglyceride and lower HDL-cholesterol levels, themselves metabolically inversely linked, have an important role in assessing risk of CHD in women.

Obesity

In the Nurses' Health Study, Manson et al (1990) studied over 120 000 females, aged between 30 and 55 years old. The risk of CHD was over three times higher in women with a body mass index (BMI) (calculated as weight in kilograms divided by the square of height in metres) of 29 and above compared to those women with a BMI of less than 21. A large proportion of the excess risk could be attributed to effects of obesity on blood pressure, glucose intolerance and lipid levels. However, after adjustment for these factors, an effect of obesity per se on CHD risk was still discernible.

Localization of adipose tissue may be even more important than degree of adiposity with an increased waist : hip ratio significantly predictive of both myocardial infarction and total mortality. The risk of CHD rises steeply with increasing waist : hip ratios above 0.80 (Bjorntorp 1985).

Parity

Studies of CHD risk and its relationship to number of pregnancies have produced differing results; some studies show a positive correlation, some a negative and others no association at all. The subject is reviewed by Barrett-Connor & Bush (1991) who conclude that women with five or more pregnancies have a 1.8-fold increase of myocardial infarction before taking into account smoking status and social class. Most studies have failed to take into account the confounding variable of social class. Lower social class is associated with earlier first pregnancy which in turn is related to number of pregnancies. It is also postulated that it is the number of miscarriages, not the number of live births, that increases CHD risk. This suggests that it may not be the hormonal changes during and after pregnancy that increase risk but the possible presence of an adverse hormonal status that is also responsible for the poor reproductive history. Pregnancy, childbirth and parenthood obviously involve many fundamental changes with lasting consequences that further complicate the interpretation of any effect multiparity may impose on future risk of CHD.

Menopause

Inextricably linked with the CHD risk associated with increasing age in females is that associated with the menopause. The dramatic increase of CHD in middle-aged females has led to the belief that the menopause and its accompanying decline in ovarian hormones underpins the apparent loss of protection against CHD. This theory is further supported by the observation that women who had an early sudden menopause as a result of bilateral oophorectomy and who did not receive oestrogen replacement therapy were at a significantly higher risk of CHD than premenopausal women of similar age (Colditz et al 1987). There is considerable evidence that premature menopause increases CHD risk, which is thought to be due at least in part to changes in lipid levels, principally an increase in LDL-cholesterol, resulting in a more atherogenic profile (Jensen 1991). However, because the natural menopause occurs at different ages in different individuals and marks an arbitrary time point in a variable and gradual decline in ovarian function it is very difficult to establish a clear association with increased CHD risk.

The term 'menopause' is used to describe the state that follows the permanent cessation of menstruation. By necessity this diagnosis can only be made in retrospect, and the convention is amenorrhoea for a minimum period of 12 months. The menopausal transition is characterized from a hormonal and endocrine perspective by decreasing ovarian activity, decreased levels of circulating oestrogens, increased levels of follicle stimulating hormone and luteinizing hormone and decreased fertility. The median age at menopause in most western industrialized societies is around 50 years of age, although there is wide variation between 35 and 59 years of age. A large number of the conditions associated with the peri- and postmenopausal period can be largely attributed to oestrogen loss. The increased risk in CHD in postmenopausal women has also been linked to oestrogen loss. This provides an important opportunity for therapeutic manipulation via the use of hormone replacement therapy (HRT) to improve CHD risk.

HORMONE REPLACEMENT THERAPY

For many years HRT has been used to treat women suffering from the distressing symptoms of the menopause, such as hot flushes and psychological disturbances, and long-term oestrogen use is acknowledged to be the only well-established prophylactic measure that reduces the incidence of osteoporotic fractures. The cardiovascular benefits of postmenopausal oestrogen are less well recognized in spite of the large and increasing body of epidemiological data which indicates that postmenopausal oestrogen use significantly reduces a woman's risk of CHD (Stampfer & Colditz 1991).

Given that CHD is the commonest cause of death in postmenopausal women it is important that awareness of the benefits of HRT to the cardiovascular system and its potential role in CHD prevention is increased.

Epidemiology

Oestrogen-only HRT

Results from a number of large studies carried out in the USA have indicated that postmenopausal oestrogen use is associated with a significant reduction in CHD risk. Meta-analyses of observational studies suggest a reduction in CHD risk of about 50% in oral oestrogen users compared with non-users (Stampfer & Colditz 1991). Treatment with oestrogen-only HRT is referred to as 'unopposed', i.e. without the addition of a progestogen.

. One of the most important studies is the Lipid Research Clinics follow-up study, which compared oestrogen users with non-users over an 8-year period and found that users had about one-third of the risk of fatal CHD compared with non-users (Bush et al 1987). Both groups had a similar distribution of most risk factors (age, blood pressure, smoking, etc.), but users had higher triglyceride levels, lower LDL-cholesterol and higher HDL-cholesterol levels. Statistical analysis of the data suggested that about half of the protective effect could be accounted for by the lipid changes, particularly the increase in HDL-cholesterol. No correlation was found between triglyceride levels and CHD risk. The Nurses' Health Study involved over 120 000 women, almost 50 000 of whom were postmenopausal. These postmenopausal women were followed for 10 years, and oestrogen-treated women had half the incidence of CHD observed in untreated women (Stampfer et al 1991).

The protective effect of oestrogen applies also to women with CHD. One of the larger trials followed over 2000 women with established CHD for a 10-year period and found that oestrogen users had a significantly better overall survival than non-users (Sullivan et al 1990).

Combined therapy

In almost all of the large epidemiological studies, oral unopposed oestrogen was used exclusively. There are no epidemiological data available for parenteral oestrogen and very little for oestrogen/progestogen therapy, although the little there is suggests that combined preparations also have a protective effect. A Swedish study followed over 20 000 women who had been prescribed HRT, two-thirds of which was oestrogen only and one-third cyclical combined therapy, for 6 years (Falkeborn et al 1992). The group treated with combined therapy had approximately half the incidence of myocardial infarction of that expected from the incidence rates for the population of the region (relative risk = 0.53). Those treated with oestrogen alone also had a significantly lower relative risk (0.69). These results are very encouraging, particularly as the most commonly used combined preparation was one containing a high-dose androgenic progestogen, which would be expected to reduce HDL-cholesterol levels.

An American group compared the use of HRT in over 500 postmenopausal women who had sustained a myocardial infarction with that of over 1000 age-matched controls. One-third of those on HRT were taking oestrogen combined with the non-androgenic progestogen medroxyprogesterone acetate (MPA) while the rest had an oestrogen-only preparation. The relative risk of myocardial infarction for those on HRT compared with those not on treatment was 0.69 for those on oestrogen alone and 0.68 for those on combined therapy, indicating that the reduced risk associated with oestrogen use was not compromised by addition of MPA (Psaty et al 1994). Additionally, 3-year data from the Postmenopausal Estrogen/Progestogen Interventions (PEPI) trial, a large American multicentre randomized placebo-controlled study designed to assess the effects of unopposed oestrogen and three different oestrogen/ non-androgenic progestogen regimens on cardiovascular risk factors have recently been published. It indicated that all the regimens improved lipid profile and coagulation factors without adversely affecting blood pressure or insulin levels (Writing Group for the PEPI Trial 1995).

Unfortunately many of the trials to date have been observational, and can be criticized on the grounds of selection bias, although the consistency and magnitude of the decrease in CHD risk observed make it unlikely that all the apparent protection could be due to this factor. Large randomized controlled clinical trials are now underway in the USA to determine whether HRT does reduce the risk of heart disease in healthy women (Women's Health Initiative) or the risk of new cardiovascular events in women who already have CHD (Estrogen/Progestin Replacement Study), but neither of these studies is expected to provide results for at least 5 years.

Effects of oestrogens on risk markers for CHD

The most commonly prescribed postmenopausal oestrogens in the UK are conjugated equine oestrogens and human oestrogens (17β-oestradiol, oestradiol valerate). Treatment with 0.625 mg/day conjugated equine oestrogens, which is the minimum dose recommended for prevention of bone loss, results in a small increase in triglyceride levels, a reduction in LDL levels and an increase in HDL levels (Fig. 13.3). The increase in HDL is most marked in the HDL2 subfraction, which is believed to be the important fraction in relation to improving CHD risk. 17β-oestradiol or oestradiol valerate in the minimum recommended dose for bone protection (2 mg/day) has also been shown to decrease LDL-cholesterol and increase HDL-cholesterol but to have little or no effect on triglycerides. Thus oestrogen has a beneficial effect on the main lipoprotein risk factors for CHD (Jensen 1991).

Lipoprotein changes are dose-related and depend on the pretreatment lipid status of the patient. On average, in the normolipidaemic woman, the above-mentioned standard doses of postmenopausal oestrogen would effect a decrease in LDL-cholesterol of between 4 and 10% and an increase in HDL of around 10–15%. The rise in HDL is very consistent, being almost invariably seen, whereas there is sometimes no change in LDL, particularly in women with low pretreatment levels.

Oestrogen as a treatment for hyperlipidaemia

Hyperlipidaemic women are likely to experience much greater lipid changes

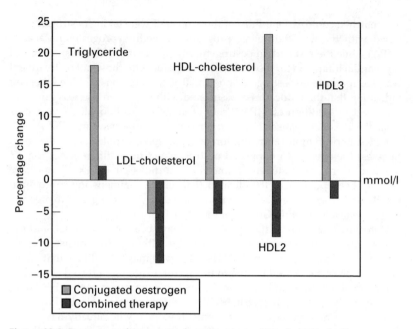

Figure 13.3 Percentage change in triglyceride, plasma LDL-cholesterol, plasma HDL-cholesterol and HDL subfractions HDL2 and HDL3 on conjugated equine oestrogens and combined therapy of conjugated equine oestrogens alone and norgestrel (adapted from Farish et al 1991).

than normolipidaemic women. In 1978 a Swedish group published a study in which oestrogen was used as a treatment for type II hyperlipidaemia in postmenopausal women (Tikkanen 1978). The women had an average cholesterol of 8.7 mmol/l. After 6 months' treatment with 2 mg oestradiol valerate, LDL-cholesterol was reduced by 18%, HDL-cholesterol increased by 30% and triglyceride levels were unchanged. The magnitude of the decrease in LDL was positively correlated with the initial level. The authors suggested that hyperlipidaemia should be regarded as an additional indication for oestrogen therapy in postmenopausal women. The Expert Panel on Detection, Evaluation and Treatment of High Blood Cholesterol in Adults (1993) recommended that oestrogen should be considered as a first-line treatment for hyperlipidaemic postmenopausal women. In spite of this, dyslipidaemia has remained in the datasheets as a contraindication for oestrogen therapies and practitioners considering HRT as a treatment option for hyperlipidaemia in their postmenopausal patients are in the minority.

Oestrogen effects on non-lipid risk markers
In addition to its beneficial effects on lipids, oestrogen induces favourable changes in other cardiovascular risk markers. These effects have been less well investigated as yet, but there is increasing evidence that postmenopausal oestrogen exerts positive effects on blood flow and fibrinolysis (Winkler

1992). It can inhibit vasoconstrictor agents, has a calcium channel blocking effect and tends to reduce blood pressure. There is also evidence that it acts as an antioxidant. Ongoing research suggests that oestrogen may have beneficial effects on carbohydrate metabolism and body fat distribution, both of which are associated with CHD risk. Again, in spite of these findings, it is widely believed that women with hypertension, CHD or thrombotic disease should not be prescribed HRT.

Hormone replacement regimens

The traditional route of oestrogen administration is the oral one, but in recent years there has been increasing interest in parenteral administration mainly by means of oestradiol-releasing skin patches or subcutaneous implants. Replacement by these methods avoids 'first-pass' effects on the liver and is often well tolerated in women who experience gastrointestinal side effects on oral therapy. The lipid changes exerted by these forms of therapy are much less marked than those induced by oral oestrogens. In particular, there is no rise in HDL-cholesterol, which has led to concern that replacement by the non-oral route may not be as advantageous with regards to reduction in CHD risk (Jensen 1991).

Combination therapy

Unopposed oestrogen therapy (without a progestogen) has been associated with an increased risk of endometrial cancer. Therefore, for women who have not had a hysterectomy a progestogen is added to the regimen. This is usually given cyclically for 10–12 days out of each 28-day period to induce a withdrawal bleed. This prevents oestrogen-induced hyperplasia of the endometrium and eliminates the potential increased risk of carcinoma.

Progestogen

The progestogens used in combined HRT fall into two main categories, namely derivatives of 19-nortestosterone such as norethisterone or norgestrel, and 17-hydroxyprogesterone derivatives such as medroxyprogesterone acetate or dydrogesterone. Most of the combined therapies currently available in the UK contain progestogens of the 19-nortestosterone series. These progestogens have androgenic as well as progestogenic activity and tend to counteract the beneficial effects of oestrogen on lipid metabolism. Most importantly, both norethisterone and norgestrel markedly reduce HDL-cholesterol levels. However, they also induce a small decrease in triglyceride levels and reduce levels of lipoprotein(a) (Farish et al 1991), one of the newer lipoprotein predictors, elevated levels of which are associated with increased risk of CHD and stroke. Reports on the effects of these progestogens on LDL-cholesterol are inconsistent. Progesterone-related compounds are less androgenic and have much less marked effects on lipids (Jensen 1991).

Combined HRT preparations

The effects of combined preparations vary according to the relative doses and potencies of the oestrogens and progestogens which they contain. Ideally the dose of progestogen should be sufficient for adequate endometrial protection while exerting as little an influence as possible on favourable changes induced by the oestrogen component on lipid levels. In most oral cyclical preparations which employ norethisterone or norgestrel the balance is such that the oestrogen-induced rise in HDL is negated (Fig. 13.3), although there is generally no reduction from pretreatment levels, while in preparations where these progestogens are given continuously there may be a small net decrease in HDL. Triglyceride levels are unchanged or reduced, and lipoprotein(a) levels are decreased. In regimens which include MPA the oestrogen-induced rise in HDL may be blunted, while those with dydrogesterone appear to affect lipids in a similar manner to oestrogen monotherapy. There are very little data to date concerning the effects of the addition of progestogens on the non-lipid mechanisms by which oestrogen is thought to protect against CHD, but from the limited evidence it would appear that progestogens do not counteract the oestrogen effects.

TREATMENT STRATEGIES

Prior to prescribing HRT, the benefits and risks have to be weighed up for each individual patient and discussed with the patient herself. This is particularly important when HRT is being considered for prevention of CHD, since treatment will be long term. This section is designed to help with this process.

Benefits

While the preceding sections have been devoted to the potential benefits of oestrogen on the cardiovascular system, it should be noted that menopausal women may derive many other benefits, both short- and long-term, from oestrogen replacement. HRT is the most effective treatment for the relief of the acute symptoms of the menopause, principally flushing and sweating and insomnia. It is also effective in reducing psychological symptoms such as irritability, anxiety and depression. In the medium- to longer-term it can bring relief from lower urogenital tract problems, for example vaginal dryness and atrophy, help prevent skin thinning and may help to alleviate aches and pains in the joints. One of the most important long-term benefits of HRT is the prevention of osteoporosis, a major cause of disability and death in elderly women. There is also limited evidence to suggest that HRT may reduce the incidence of stroke.

Risks

Some doctors and patients are reluctant to embark upon long-term therapy due to concerns about safety. Many of the fears associated with HRT use are unfounded since they are based on data derived from high-dose oral contraceptive use. However, as with any form of drug treatment, there are some risks, and for a few women HRT is contraindicated.

Cautions and contraindications

There are some pre-existing medical conditions which, although not contraindications to oestrogen therapy, may require that the patient be more carefully assessed than is usual and may make her suitable for only certain types of regimen. These include the following:

- previous deep vein thrombosis
- previous pulmonary embolism or stroke
- diabetes
- gallstones
- mild or previous liver disease
- endometriosis
- fibroids.

It should be emphasized that these are not absolute contraindications to HRT and in most instances a suitable regimen which will benefit the patient can be worked out. However, it may be advisable to refer such cases to a specialist menopause clinic.

Absolute contraindications to HRT:

- Active endometrial or breast cancer
- Undiagnosed abnormal vaginal bleeding or breast lump
- Known or suspected pregnancy
- Severe active liver disease with abnormal liver function tests
- Acute-phase myocardial infarction, pulmonary embolism or deep vein thrombosis.

The most commonly voiced worries about HRT

Does HRT increase the risk of breast cancer?

Around 40 epidemiological studies have been carried out since 1970 in an attempt to answer this question. The results have been inconsistent, some studies reporting a small increase in risk and others failing to show any effect. Taken together, the results from the majority of the better-designed studies indicate that there is no increase in risk for at least up to 5 years' use of HRT, but there may be a small increase in incidence with more than 10 years' therapy, although there is no excess mortality (Hunt & Vessey 1991).

Women with family histories of breast cancer are usually particularly worried about this aspect of HRT. These women are already at increased risk but it is not clear from the small amount of data available whether HRT further increases the risk. Similarly, women with benign breast disease carry a small increased risk of breast cancer and it is unclear whether HRT adds to the risk. As in the case of CHD, most of the epidemiological data refer to oestrogen-only preparations and it is uncertain whether adding a progestogen increases or decreases breast cancer risk.

What about endometrial cancer?

It is well established that unopposed oestrogen increases the risk of endometrial cancer. However, for this reason combination therapies are nowadays always prescribed for women with an intact uterus, which eliminates this increased risk.

Does HRT cause hypertension?

The natural oestrogens used in HRT preparations do not normally increase blood pressure and in fact tend to reduce it. On very rare occasions conjugated oestrogens can cause severe hypertension which returns to normal when the therapy is stopped. This is regarded as an idiosyncratic response. Patients who already have hypertension should have it controlled before HRT is started and blood pressure should be checked regularly.

Will I put on weight?

Many studies have shown that HRT does not cause weight gain in most women. There may be a tendency for weight to be increased during the first few months of therapy, but this is usually lost over the next few months and most studies have indicated that women on oestrogen are on average lighter than those who are not. The majority of studies carried out on women on combined oestrogen/progestogen therapy have also indicated that there is usually no increase in weight. However, occasionally the progestogen can cause fluid retention and weight gain. These problems arise only during the combined phase of treatment and appear to be more likely to occur in women who have previously experienced similar problems premenstrually.

The 'risk/benefit equation'

On average, a 50-year-old woman's baseline lifetime risk of CHD is 45%, hip fracture 15% and breast cancer 8%. Therefore for the majority of women, the major long-term benefits associated with oestrogen replacement therapy, namely an approximately 50% reduction in the risk of CHD combined with an estimated 25% reduction in the risk of hip fractures and a reduction of at least 50% in the risk of vertebral fractures, add up to an increased life expectancy. Obviously, the greater the risk of osteoporosis and/or heart disease the greater the benefit obtainable from oestrogen replacement. The situation is not quite so clear cut for oestrogen/progestogen combination therapy. While this treatment is as good as or even better than oestrogen for prevention of osteoporosis, it has not yet been established whether it is as effective as unopposed oestrogen for heart disease prevention. Therefore for women requiring combined therapy, particularly if they are at high risk for breast cancer and have few risk factors for osteoporosis and heart disease, the risk/benefit balance may not be so favourable.

Several expert bodies have recently published recommendations concerning the use of HRT in CHD prevention. In 1992, the American College of Physicians published guidelines for counselling postmenopausal women about preventive hormone therapy (American College of Physicians 1992). They recommended that it should be considered by all women. Women who have had a hysterectomy and did not require the addition of a progestogen were likely to benefit as were women who had CHD or were at increased risk for coronary heart disease. The International Consensus Conference on Hormone Replacement Therapy and the Cardiovascular System, held in 1993, sponsored by The American Fertility Society and the American Heart Association, concluded that 'because of the magnitude of cardiovascular disease as a cause of morbidity and mortality, the beneficial role of oral oestrogen in the primary prevention of cardiovascular disease in most women outweighs its potential risks' (Lobo & Speroff 1994). It was considered that there were insufficient data available on the effects of combined and non-oral therapy and further clinical investigation was required before definite conclusions about the benefits of these therapies relative to those of oral oestrogen could be drawn. It was also noted that there is consistent evidence to support a beneficial effect of oestrogen in postmenopausal women with existing cardiovascular disease and limited evidence to indicate that therapy is even more effective in reducing mortality in those with severe disease.

When should treatment be started and for how long should it be continued?

From the evidence to date it would appear that the maximum reductions in risk for coronary heart disease and osteoporotic fractures are most likely to be achieved with long-term therapy, i.e. 10–20 years or more. Generally, treatment should be considered at the time of the menopause, since it is at this time that the risk of these diseases begins to increase. However, there is no reason to believe that beginning treatment later in life will not be beneficial.

HRT preparations and their indications for use

Treatment should be tailored to suit the individual, bearing in mind that it should be kept as simple, problem-free and cost effective as possible. Where cardioprotection is the prime objective, attention should be paid to obtaining as favourable a lipid profile as possible and a pretreatment profile will help in the choice of preparation.

Hysterectomized women

The vast majority of the long-term data on the benefits and safety of HRT relate to unopposed oral oestrogens (principally conjugated equine oestrogens) and therefore for a woman who has had a hysterectomy oral conjugated equine oestrogens or oestradiol should be the first choice. Since oestradiol is less likely to increase triglyceride levels, in a woman with a tendency to high triglyceride, oestradiol may be the better choice. If the treatment causes unacceptably high levels of triglyceride or if there are side effects such as nausea or dyspepsia which persist and cannot be averted by taking the tablet with food or at night rather than in the morning, transdermal therapy (oestradiol skin patches) can be tried. This type of therapy will reduce triglycerides but will have less of an impact on LDL-cholesterol than oral therapy and will not increase HDL-cholesterol. The patches can sometimes cause skin irritation and in these cases implants may be considered. Implant insertion requires a minor surgical procedure, although the technique is simple and can easily be performed at outpatient clinics under local anaesthetic. However, tachyphylaxis can occur (i.e. as plasma oestradiol levels begin to fall several weeks after implant, patients experience recurrence of symptoms, even though the actual oestradiol levels are well within the premenopausal range). This can lead to replacement implants being needed sooner and sooner and very high levels of oestradiol being reached.

Non-hysterectomized women

In patients with an intact uterus, a combined oestrogen/progestogen preparation should be prescribed. Again, an oral preparation should be first choice. Although it is possible to prescribe the oestrogen and progestogen separately, it is preferable where possible to use a commercially available combination pack. These are 'user friendly' and the progestogen component, which is essential for endometrial protection, is less likely to be omitted. The majority of the combined preparations available in the UK incorporate an androgenic progestogen for 10 or 12 days in each 28. All of these preparations will probably decrease LDL-cholesterol but the effect on HDL-cholesterol will vary according to the oestrogen/progestogen balance. To avoid decreasing HDL, preparations with high-dose (500 μg) norgestrel should be avoided. One of the new combined preparations on the market has the progesterone derivative, dydrogesterone, as the progestogen and affects lipid profile in a manner similar to unopposed oestrogen. However, if hypertriglyceridaemia is present, a preparation with an androgenic progestogen may give a better profile. Additionally, if the lipoprotein(a) level is high, the androgenic progestogen-containing preparations will be most likely to reduce it.

Side effects. If there are side effects with oral preparations which are thought to be due to the oestrogen component, combination oestradiol/norethisterone patches or oestradiol patches with oral norethisterone may be used, although these preparations will have less favourable effects on lipoproteins than the oral oestrogen/progestogen preparations. The majority of side effects which occur on cyclical combined preparations are associated with the progestogen component. These tend to be PMS-like symptoms such as breast tenderness, headaches, water retention, etc. The best course of action is to change the preparation to one incorporating a different progestogen.

Many women, especially those who have been amenorrhoeic for several years, find the return to monthly bleeds unacceptable, and this is one of the commonest reasons for discontinuing therapy. There are two new combined preparations which may be useful for these women. One incorporates MPA to induce bleeds only once every 3 months and will have only a minor influence on the oestrogen effects on lipids; the other incorporates continuous norethisterone and bleeding is avoided altogether. However, this preparation, while decreasing LDL-cholesterol, may cause a small decrease in HDL-cholesterol. Another 'no-bleed' preparation which has recently been licensed for use in the UK and is being prescribed widely is tibolone, which is a synthetic steroid with weak oestrogenic, progestogenic and androgenic activity. This preparation decreases triglycerides, HDL-cholesterol and lipoprotein(a) and does not affect LDL-cholesterol. Its effects on cardiovascular risk are not known.

CONCLUSIONS

In summary, most of the risk factors for CHD and the preventive strategies advocated in men are applicable to women. For several of these risk factors the magnitude of their effect on prevalence rate differs from that observed in males and warrants particular attention in women. These include diabetes mellitus, triglyceride and HDL-cholesterol levels, isolated systolic hypertension in the elderly and central obesity, and should be considered in association with the factors that are unique to women, namely menopausal status, oral contraceptive use and pre-eclampsia and gestational diabetes in pregnancy.

The data from a large number of studies of HRT use, both in healthy women and those with established CHD, are very consistent and suggest that oral oestrogen replacement therapy reduces the risk of cardiovascular mortality by between 40 and 60%. Changes in risk factors, such as lipoproteins, blood flow and fibrinolysis help to provide a biologically plausible explanation for these findings. There is also evidence that oestrogen causes a reduction in all-cause mortality. The possible cardioprotective effects of non-oral oestrogen or combined oestrogen/progestogen regimens are less clear, although the data which are available at present are encouraging. It will be several years before results of randomized controlled trials of therapy, including non-oral and combined oestrogen/progestogen therapy, become available. Until then the decision to use HRT for prevention of heart disease has to be made on an individual basis.

■ KEY POINTS

- CHD is the leading cause of death in women.
- The traditional risk factors for CHD and the preventive strategies advocated in men are applicable to women.
- Diabetes mellitus, triglyceride and HDL-cholesterol levels, pre-eclampsia, isolated systolic hypertension in the elderly and central obesity warrant particular attention in women.
- Consistent clinical data suggest that oral oestrogen replacement therapy reduces the risk of cardiovascular mortality by between 40 and 60%.
- Changes in risk factors, such as lipoproteins, blood flow and fibrinolysis help to provide a biologically plausible explanation for these findings.
- There are insufficient data to draw definitive conclusions about the benefits of non-oral and combined HRT preparations, although the data so far are encouraging.
- Women with or at increased risk of CHD are likely to benefit from HRT.
- HRT should be considered as a first-line treatment for hyperlipidaemic postmenopausal women.
- New HRT preparations are available for women with an intact uterus which do not necessitate a return to monthly bleeds.

Case Study 13.1

A 56-year-old women is undergoing CHD risk factor assessment at the end of the cardiac rehabilitation programme. She has suffered a myocardial infarction 4 months previously.

Her fasting lipids are: total cholesterol 7.2 mmol/l; triglyceride 1.7 mmol/l; and HDL-cholesterol 1.0 mmol/l. Her blood pressure is 140/85, and her BMI is 27. She is non-diabetic but continues to smoke 10 cigarettes a day. How would you interpret these results? How would you proceed with the management of this case and what advice would you offer to this woman?

Answers
She should be strongly advised to stop smoking; the most important modifiable CHD risk factor.

Lipids. Elevated total cholesterol and a low HDL-cholesterol. Reinforce lipid-lowering diet. Consider HRT if there are no contraindications. Discuss this treatment option with the patient. Explain to her the benefits she is likely to gain and encourage her to ask questions and voice concerns she may have about HRT.

If the woman has previously undergone hysterectomy, oestrogen-only therapy (conjugated equine oestrogens or oestradiol) should be prescribed as this has the most beneficial effect on lipids. If her uterus is intact, consider a combined oral preparation of oestrogen and a non-androgenic progestogen (dydrogesterone) which affects lipids in a similar manner to oestrogen alone. HRT also provides additional non-lipid benefits to CHD risk through favourable changes in thrombotic factors and vascular tone. Review in 3 months. If lipid levels remain at levels greater than 5.5 mmol/l consider also lipid-lowering therapy.

PRACTICAL EXERCISE

Find out how many female patients you have on the practice list between the ages of 50 and 60. How many of them would be eligible for HRT? How many are actually taking HRT? Ensure that you have information on HRT easily available in the waiting room and in health promotion clinics.

REFERENCES

American College of Physicians 1992 Guidelines for counseling postmenopausal women about preventive hormone therapy. Annals of Internal Medicine 117: 1038–1041

Barrett-Connor E, Wingard D L 1983 Sex differential in ischaemic heart disease mortality in diabetics: A prospective population-based study. American Journal of Epidemiology 118: 489–496

Barrett-Connor E, Bush T L 1991 Estrogen and coronary heart disease in women. Journal of the American Medical Association 265: 1861–1867

Bierman E L, Hazzard W R (eds) 1994 Principles of geriatric medicine. McGraw-Hill, New York, p 109

Bjorntorp P 1985 Regional patterns of fat distribution. Annals of Internal Medicine 103: 994–995

Black D 1980 Inequalities in health: report of a Research Working Group chaired by Sir Douglas Black. DHSS, London

Bush T L, Barrett-Connor E, Cowan L D et al 1987 Cardiovascular mortality and non contraceptive use of estrogen in women: results from the Lipid Research Clinics Program Follow-up Study. Circulation 75: 1002–1009

Castelli W P 1984 Epidemiology of coronary heart disease: the Framingham Study. American Journal of Medicine 76(2A): 4–12

Castelli W P 1986 The triglyceride issue: a view from Framingham. American Heart Journal 112: 432–437

Colditz G A, Willett W C, Stampfer M J, Rosner B, Speizer F E, Hennekens C H 1987 Menopause and the risk of coronary heart disease in women. New England Journal of Medicine 316: 1105–1110

Croft P, Hannaford P C 1989 Risk factors for acute myocardial infarction in women: evidence from the Royal College of General Practitioners' Oral Contraception Study. British Medical Journal 298: 165–168

Department of Health and Human Resources 1989 Reducing the consequences of smoking: 25 years of progress: a report of the Surgeon General. HHS Publication No. (CDC 89-8411), Rockville, Md

Expert Panel on Detection, Evaluation and Treatment of High Blood Cholesterol in Adults (Adult Treatment Panel II) 1993 Summary of the second report of the National Cholesterol Education Program. Journal of the American Medical Association 269: 3015–3023

Falkeborn M, Persson I, Adami H I et al 1992 The risk of acute myocardial infarction after oestrogen and oestrogen–progestogen replacement. British Journal of Obstetrics and Gynaecology 99: 821–828

Farish E, Rolton H A, Barnes J F, Hart D M 1991 Lipoprotein(a) concentrations in postmenopausal women taking norethisterone. British Medical Journal 303: 694

Glendy R E, Levine S A, White S A, White P D 1937 Coronary disease in youth: comparison of 100 patients under 40 with 300 persons past 80. Journal of the American Medical Association 109: 1775–1778

Hennekens C H, Evans D, Peto R 1979 Oral contraceptive use, cigarette smoking and myocardial infarction. British Journal of Family Planning 5: 66–67

Hunt K, Vessey M 1991 The use of hormone replacement therapy and breast cancer risk. In: Sitruk-Ware R (ed) The menopause and hormone replacement therapy: facts and controversies. Marcel Dekker, New York

Isles C 1993 Prevention of coronary disease in women. Scottish Medical Journal 38(4): 103–106

Jacobs D R, Meban I L, Bangdiwala S I, Criqui M H, Tyroler H A 1990 High density lipoprotein cholesterol as a predictor of cardiovascular disease mortality in men and women: the follow-up study of the Lipid Research Clinics Prevalence Study. American Journal of Epidemiology 131: 32–47

Jensen J 1991 Effects of sex steroids on serum lipids and lipoproteins. Baillière's Clinical Obstetrics and Gynaecology 5: 867–887

Kannel W B, Brand F N 1985 Cardiovascular risk factors in the elderly. In: Andres R, Lobo R A, Speroff L (eds) 1994 Summary: International Consensus Conference on Postmenopausal Hormone Therapy and the Cardiovascular System. Fertility and Sterility 6 (Suppl. 2): 176S–179S

Manson J E, Colditz G A, Stampfer M J et al 1990 A prospective study of obesity and risk of coronary disease in women. New England Journal of Medicine 322: 882–889

Manson J E, Colditz G A, Stampfer M J et al 1991 A prospective study of maturity-onset diabetes and risk of coronary heart disease and stroke in women. Archives of Internal Medicine 151: 1141–1147

Manson J E, Tosteson H, Ridker P M et al 1992 The primary prevention of myocardial infarction. New England Journal of Medicine 326: 1406–1416

Mattison D R, Thorgeirsson S S 1978 Smoking and industrial pollution, and their effects on menopause and ovarian cancer. Lancet I: 187–188

Mestman J H 1988 Follow-up studies in women with gestational diabetes mellitus: the experience at Los Angeles County / University of Southern California Medical Center. In: Weiss P A M, Coustan D R (eds) Gestational diabetes. Springer-Verlag, Vienna, pp 191–198

Office of Population Censuses and Surveys (OPCS) 1995 Series OH2 No 20 HMSO, London

Psaty B M, Heckbert S R, Atkins D et al 1994 The risk of myocardial infarction associated with the combined use of estrogens and progestogens in postmenopausal women. Archives of Internal Medicine 154: 1333–1339

Registrar General for Scotland 1994 Report of the Registrar General for Scotland. HMSO, Edinburgh

Rich-Edwards J W, Manson J E, Hennekens C H, Buring J E 1995 The primary prevention of coronary heart disease in women. New England Journal of Medicine 333: 1758–1766

Rosenberg L, Miller D R, Kaufman D W 1983 Myocardial infarction in women under 50 years of age. Journal of the American Medical Association 250: 2801–2806

Ruderman N B, Haudenschild C 1984 Diabetes as an atherogenic factor. Progress in Cardiovascular Diseases 26: 373–412

Saltzberg S, Stroh J A, Frishman W H 1988 Isolated systolic hypertension in the elderly: pathophysiology and treatment. Medical Clinics of North America 72: 523–547

Silagy C A, McNeil J H 1992 Epidemiologic aspects of isolated systolic hypertension and implications for future research. American Journal of Cardiology 69: 213–218

Stadel B V 1981 Oral contraceptives and cardiovascular disease. New England Journal of Medicine 305: 672–677

Stampfer M J, Colditz G A 1991 Estrogen replacement therapy and coronary heart disease: a quantitative assessment of the epidemiological evidence. Preventive Medicine 20: 47–63

Stampfer M J, Willett W C, Colditz G A, Speizer F E, Hennekens C H 1990 Past use of oral contraceptives and cardiovascular disease: a meta-analysis in the context of the Nurses' Health Study. American Journal of Obstetrics and Gynecology 163: 285–291

Stampfer M J, Colditz G A, Willett W C et al 1991 Postmenopausal estrogen therapy and coronary heart disease: ten year follow-up from the Nurses' Health Study. New England Journal of Medicine 325: 756–762

Sullivan J M, Van Der Swaag R, Hughes J P, Maddock V, Croetz F W, Ramanathan K B, Mirvis D M 1990 Estrogen replacement and coronary heart disease: effect on survival in post menopausal women. Archives of Internal Medicine 150: 2557–2562

Tikkanen M J, Nikkila E A, Vartiainen E 1978 Natural oestrogen as an effective treatment for type II hyperlipoproteinaemia in post menopausal women. Lancet 2: 490–492

Whelton P K, He J, Klag M J 1994 Blood pressure in westernized populations. In: Swales J D (ed) Textbook of hypertension. Blackwell Scientific Publications, Oxford, ch 1: 11–21

Wilhelmsen L, Bengtsson C, Elmfeldt D et al 1977 Multiple risk prediction of myocardial infarction in women as compared to men. British Heart Journal 39: 1179–1185

Winkler U H 1992 Menopause, hormone replacement therapy and cardiovascular disease: a review of haemostaseological findings. Fibrinolysis 6 (Suppl. 3): 5–10

Writing Group for the PEPI Trial 1995 Effects of estrogen and estrogen / progestin regimens on heart disease risk factors in postmenopausal women. Journal of the American Medical Association 273: 199–208

FURTHER READING

Burger H G (ed) 1993 The menopause. Clinical endocrinology and metabolism. Baillière Tindall, London, vol 7(1)

Three chapters in this book are devoted to issues of cardiovascular disease and its

relationship to the menopause. Other chapters deal with osteoporosis, cancer and the practicalities of HRT. Detailed and extensively referenced.

Edwards R W (Chairman) 1993 Hormone replacement therapy—a critical review of current practice and the way ahead. Consensus statement. Clinical Resource and Audit Group (CRAG), National Health Service in Scotland, The Scottish Office, Edinburgh

Clearly written, easy to read report of CRAG consensus conference. Consensus statement and four key review papers presented at the conference provide guidance on which women should be targeted for HRT, discuss therapies, review risks and benefits and deal with practical aspects of treatment.

Grady D, Rubin S M, Pettiti D B et al 1992 Hormone therapy to prolong life in postmenopausal women. Annals of Internal Medicine 117: 1016–1037

A review of the risks and benefits of hormone therapy which presents the supporting evidence for the American College of Physicians' (1992) Guidelines.

Whitehead M, Godfrey V 1992 Hormone replacement therapy. Your questions answered. Churchill Livingstone, Edinburgh

A comprehensive, easily readable guide for health care specialists containing theoretical information and practical advice on all aspects of the menopause and HRT.

Prevention in practice: the role of the nurse in risk assessment

Margaret Clubb

■ CONTENTS

INTRODUCTION

Increasing emphasis in health care is placed on health promotion and disease prevention. In recent years, the professional role of the nurse has extended to meet these changing priorities and provide a leading role in their implementation. This has occurred in practice through successful teamwork and use of agreed protocols. The health care team includes all general practice staff members as well as district nurses, health visitors, community psychiatric nurses and pharmacists along with outside agencies such as dietitians and many hospital-based services such as the cardiac rehabilitation programme (Box 14.1).

Nurses in all areas of patient care have the opportunity to assess and advise on CHD risk factors. Nurses based in primary care have a large practice list and may be able to offer support to a large number of patients and their families over a long period of time in less-formal surroundings. Patients often view the nurse as the first line of contact as he or she may appear to have more time, be more approachable and less-threatening or be known to the patient through previous contact. In contrast, doctors may be perceived to be available for consultation only when the patient has symptoms.

THE MULTIDISCIPLINARY TEAM

It is essential for health care professionals involved in the assessment of CHD

> **Box 14.1** Members of the multidisciplinary health care team involved in CHD prevention
>
> **Hospital-based**
> Cardiologist/physician
> Cardiac surgeon
> Dietitian
> Diabetic specialist nurse
> Cardiac specialist nurse
> Pharmacist
> Clinical biochemist
> Physiotherapist
> Occupational therapist
>
> **Community-based**
> General practitioner
> Practice nurse
> District nurse
> Health visitor
> District staff nurse
> Treatment room nurse
> Community psychiatric nurse
> Receptionist/clerical staff
>
> **Other**
> Outside agencies
> Smoking cessation groups
> Slimming clubs
> Sports clubs
> Alcohol advice centres
> National charities, e.g. BHF

risk factors and health promotion to work together as a cohesive team. All members of this team have something to offer and should be involved in the service and consulted on developments. Within the 'practice team', agreed aims and objectives for patient care should be identified. A care plan is then developed in partnership with the patient. The key elements of successful care management are good communication channels and the identification of a pathway of care, key events, individual responsibilities and standards of care. Teamwork can be more enjoyable, constructive and supportive than working in isolation; it encourages role development and increases the standard of care offered to the patients. Care provision should draw on contributions of all relevant members of the team, utilizing their variety of skills and expertise to produce a 'shared-care' programme of care.

Goals in shared care

One of the perceived hurdles in planning shared care is the continuation of care across the primary, secondary and even tertiary care settings. Guidance to facilitate this process is reviewed and practical advice provided elsewhere

(NHS Management Executive 1991). Integrated multidisciplinary care planning provides a comprehensive approach to care planning that has been shown to be both cost-effective and provide better outcomes (Badenhausen 1993, Buchanan & Smith 1993).

Patients must be involved from the outset in the planning of their care. Without their cooperation it is difficult to identify lifestyle risk factors accurately and to plan appropriate healthy lifestyle programmes to achieve targets. Representatives from all health care professions should contribute to the planning process and, preferably, they should include those at the point of care delivery. Key events, such as assessments and tests, in the care pathway should be decided upon on the basis of research-based practice. Clinical guidelines are presently being developed in order to ensure standardization and consistency of fundamental aspects of health care practice. These guidelines should be drawn upon where available.

An appropriate timescale in which items of care are delivered and the sequence in which events should take place should be documented throughout the care pathway.

Intermediate and final outcomes are identified within the care pathway, e.g. whether the patient has reached his or her target body weight at a certain time. By referral to the case record it will be clear if this outcome has been achieved, and if it has not, reasons for variance from the pathway recorded. This process can help to identify problem areas or areas where practice should be altered. Information that is collected and documented in such a systematic and comprehensive way also facilitates the audit process resource management, and promotes good practice.

Improving communication: multidisciplinary records

Documentation of care is the responsibility of all health care professionals. However, instead of multiple records, this approach lends itself to a single record to which all contribute. One document, with a patient-held card, is practical and easy to use, avoids duplication of effort and facilitates monitoring of care delivery. This documentation is provided for an individual area of care delivery with key areas of care outlined as a proforma. It provides the means of integrating protocols of care with case record documentation. The end result is a comprehensive planned care pathway that is owned by the local team, based on professional knowledge or 'evidence-based medicine', and promotes equity and systematic delivery of care.

HEALTH PROMOTION BANDING

Patient screening and assessment of CHD risk factors had already been underway in general practice and through other agencies prior to the publication of *The Health of the Nation* by the British Government (DoH 1992). This white paper was implemented on 1 July 1993 and is aimed at structuring and defining health promotional activities in the primary care setting. A summary of the main directives and targets that a practice must meet are shown in Box 14.2.

Box 14.2 The main directives and targets that a practice must meet to comply with the new health promotion package

1. Development of an age/sex register.
2. Recording patients' smoking habits.
3. Recording patients' blood pressure, so identifying previously undiscovered raised blood pressure.
4. Keeping a register of patients who have had either a stroke, hypertension or CHD.
5. Recording information on diet, physical activity, BMI, alcohol consumption and family history of CHD. Offering lifestyle advice to patients, as necessary.

Health promotion activities have been classed in three levels or 'bands' which are summarized in *The New Health Promotion Package* (General Medical Services Committee 1993). The target population is all individuals between the ages of 15 and 74 years on the practice list.

With reference to Box 14.2:

- band one health promotion covers programmes to reduce smoking and meets the requirements of items (1) and (2)
- band two involves programmes to minimize mortality and morbidity of patients at risk of hypertension, or with established CHD or stroke, and meets the requirements of items (1), (2), (3) and (4)
- band three involves programmes offering a full range of primary prevention services of CHD and stroke and meets the requirements of all items, i.e. (1)–(5).

Band three is therefore the most comprehensive health promotional category and aims to reduce the incidence of CHD and stroke through primary prevention. During each of the following years there should be an increase in the percentage of the practice population screened of at least 15%, up to a maximum of 80% for smoking status, 90% for blood pressure and 75% for body mass index, alcohol and family history as recorded information available in the practice records. Ellis & Chisholm (1993) have produced a guide to implementation of the recommendations into practice.

These British Government guidelines for health promotion activities provide GPs and nurses with the opportunity to offer an even more comprehensive level of care to patients, by:

- increasing patients' knowledge of their own health and well-being both physically and psychologically, so enabling informed decisions to be made about their future health
- providing a greater understanding of the nature of CHD and how preventive measures can be effective
- monitoring of patient care to ensure appropriate treatment through lifestyle intervention and medication and so improving the quality and length of life

- targeting future generations through education in schools, general practice and sports clubs, for example. This would involve all health professionals working in partnership with other agencies and professions to promote healthy eating and enjoyable exercise, and discourage smoking.

The health care team have a clear mandate to improve CHD mortality and morbidity rates through these screening and health promotional activities. In general, advice should be tailored to the individual and his or her family and be both realistic and achievable. This is an important undertaking and, with careful planning, joint organization and commitment, a realizable achievement.

HEALTH PROMOTION SERVICE

This service is aimed at healthy individuals, high-risk patients and those with established CHD. The practice may want to start various 'clinics' which would be available to patients, e.g. a well-person clinic. The success of these initiatives may depend on the area in which the practice is based. Areas of high unemployment and poverty may find that health promotion does not rate very highly on the patients' agenda, resulting in a disappointing uptake of this service. Furthermore, CHD risk factor screening in primary care may be effective but the cost of providing the service may not be justified (OXCHECK 1995). This charge warrants further investigation including a detailed evaluation of clinical practice. However, it should be noted that such investigations only yield applicable findings if the practice studied is consistent with current practice.

Opportunistic screening sessions and completion of new patient medicals are instances where the nurse can collect information on the patients' health and assess CHD risk factors. This can be useful, though lack of time and the amount of information the patient may absorb can be disappointing. The patient, however, will be aware of the service and will know how to contact the nurse at a later date. The length of time allocated to these appointments should also be discussed, as a practice nurse may usually only have a 10-minute appointment slot in surgery time but may need to offer 40-minute appointments for well-person checks. Allowing a longer time for an appointment may appear useful on paper, but in practice the patient may only retain 2 or 3 minutes of discussion and may benefit from a succession of shorter appointments over a period of time. Throughout all the patient contacts the 'holistic' approach should be adopted, as patients often attend with their own agendas and can only concentrate on that one topic. An example may be in the case of a patient who has lost his licence through drunk-driving. The assessment highlights obesity, smoking and drinking risks. As the patient has been prompted to come along because of losing his licence, drinking would appear to be the risk factor worth tackling first. Another example may be when teenagers attend for their diphtheria, tetanus and polio booster at 15-years old. These individuals can be offered information on healthy eating, smoking, etc., although by that age many will already be smoking and using alcohol and may not be prepared to review their lifestyle at that point. As nurses are also available to offer contraception advice, the consultations must be left open for teenagers to feel that they can attend at a later date without thinking they are going to be criticized for smoking and drinking.

The early identification of individuals with CHD or those at a high risk of CHD is a priority, as these patients are the most likely to suffer a CHD event in the future. The patients should be encouraged to have a greater understanding of the disease and its complications and how these may be reduced by modifying lifestyle or through the use of medication. Relatives of patients with a known family history of heart disease can also be included within the service.

Service location

This may be dictated by the availability of space at the surgery. Support groups may be held outside the surgery premises by health visitors or dietitians for example, while other agencies may hold smoking cessation classes which may require an attendance fee. The patient's employer may also offer screening privately or through the workplace. The results of the screening service may be followed up by occupational health services in the place of work or the patient may attend the practice for advice. Health education programmes at school may enable the school nurse to identify risk factors amongst pupils. Practice nurses will, in the main part, provide risk assessment within the practice population. The appointment times offered to patients will vary but evening and Saturday morning appointments can be popular as these do not interfere with the patients' working hours. Screening at the time of routine appointments may provide a means of seeing patients who are unlikely to attend health promotional clinics.

THE HEALTH CARE TEAM IN PRACTICE

Even within the practice there are a number of different individuals who are involved directly or indirectly with health promotion activities. At the initial meeting to plan the service it is important to involve everyone and to identify the most appropriate members of the health care team to provide individual elements of the health promotion activities, e.g. if one of the team has completed a course in smoking cessation, has some experience and is comfortable using this skill, he or she will lead this aspect of lifestyle counselling. This may be the practice nurse, health visitor or GP. The patient will therefore be meeting a health professional with a genuine interest in that area.

Two important groups of people that are often overlooked in this process are the practice clerical staff and the local pharmacists.

The clerical staff have an important and varied role, ranging from running computer searches, identifying the various groups to be targeted and sending out appointments, to being at reception to direct patients towards the service. The clerical staff are therefore aware of the objectives of the service and can answer basic enquiries from patients.

The local pharmacists should be informed of the services offered by the practice and will then be able to direct patients towards the practice. Pharmacists can also provide a supportive role to their clients through the provision of health education leaflets and direct patient advice.

Contacting patients

The age / sex register is useful at this stage to provide the names and addresses of patients aged between 15 and 74 years, while the practice computer can be used to identify the details of patients on specific medications. Patients may be contacted by telephone but some patients object to this method while others may agree to attend and then fail to do so. Personalized letters of invitation or practice multipurpose postcards can also be considered while bright, eye-catching posters and leaflets freely available in the waiting room, or even attached to a prescription to be collected, may also attract the patient's attention. Other clinic screening opportunities should not be missed. All women are regularly contacted for cervical screening. This appointment will allow assessment and discussion of CHD prevention as well as other issues. As previously mentioned, all teenagers attending for school-leaving booster vaccinations can be interviewed. Patients attending disease-management clinics within the surgery can also be assessed within that clinic.

It is important to extend this CHD prevention service to patients with learning disabilities and psychiatric illnesses who have been discharged into the community and registered with the practice. These patients can often be more comfortable with their care support workers or community psychiatric nurses, and assessment or intervention may be completed within the patient's familiar home surroundings.

Information storage and audit

The information required for audit purposes can be collected and stored in various ways, either recorded in the patients' notes in an agreed format, which can be transcribed into the computer later, or entered directly into the computer in the first instance. Other practices may collect the information on the patient appointment sheet and transfer the data to the computer, so allowing notes to be filed at the end of a surgery. Noting the non-attendance of patients in their notes may prompt the person who sees them next to complete the assessment.

Educational support

From the patient's point of view, the service will be poor if the personnel involved do not have a sound knowledge of the service being offered. Very few practice nurses come into the general practice setting knowing all medical disorders in great depth. Nurses may find it quite unnerving to discover how much a patient assumes that they know, and very quickly spend time reading or attending as many lectures or courses as possible to try to match their own and the patients' expectations. What works with one individual may not work with another, so the nurse must be able to adapt from one consultation to another. Good interview techniques need to be acquired to gain the maximum information and to discover the patient's real concerns and reasons for attending, as they may not be what the nurse is assuming or expects.

Nurses may feel that they would like to update their knowledge on particular areas, and their employer should be prepared to offer study leave to facilitate this. This will also promote a feeling of 'worth' in the practice as their professional needs have been recognized by their employer.

Equipment

The environment that the patient encounters is one of the most important factors in an interview. The atmosphere within the surgery premises should appear warm and friendly while the consultation room should be light. This can be a stressful time for the patients, who are having their whole way of life examined. Although nurses think they are providing helpful advice and discussion, patients may see this advice as criticism or even condemnation of both themselves and their health beliefs. Even the placing of the furniture in the consulting room can influence the interview. A desk can give the impression of being a 'barrier' between nurse and patient, so it is often advantageous to position the chair to the side of the desk so that the nurse can keep the patient records to the side but continue to sit opposite the patient and, therefore, appear more approachable and allow free-flowing dialogue. The equipment required may include items such as a regularly calibrated sphygmomanometer with standard and obese cuffs and a lipid desk-top analyser. It is important to inform patients about the tests that you are about to perform even for what may appear routine assessments. The nurse may also decide to use risk-assessment aids such as the Dundee Coronary Risk-Disk. Such tools are discussed in more detail in Chapter 2.

Protocols

Through discussion with the team members, the best way of integrating protocols or guidelines into clinical practice may be reached. All nurses are accountable for their own actions within the United Kingdom Central Council Code of professional conduct (UKCC 1994). Protocols may be requested by the health board for their inspection while the medical defence societies also expect practices to hold protocols for all actions within the practice. Protocols identify the standard of care to be provided for the patient, define areas of responsibility and recognize the training needs. In addition, they provide a structured and comprehensive framework to ensure that all appropriate elements of care are addressed. Protocols should be reviewed and amended at least annually. By dating them when they come into operation and when they are updated, they will have medico-legal value (Parker 1994). In practice the considerations that must underpin any new service development are summarized in Box 14.3.

Having established the format which will be most suitable to a particular environment, the nurse can then start to implement and manage the proposed service, the content of which will vary slightly between the needs of primary and secondary prevention.

> **Box 14.3** Points to consider in planning a new service development
>
> - Purpose of service
> - Patient characteristics
> - Practitioners identified for all elements of care
> - Location and time
> - Numbers of patients at each session
> - Frequency of service
> - Method of contacting patients
> - Screening and clinical procedures to be performed
> - Mechanism of follow-up and recall
> - Evaluation and audit
> - Educational updates for staff

Primary prevention

Due to the scale of the Government's requirements for the completion of activities outlined in 'band 3' above, all the members of the practice team will be involved in collecting data. This will be stored in the patients' records and on the computer database.

Healthy individuals with no history of CHD will have their height, weight, body mass index, blood pressure, smoking habits, alcohol intake, family history and physical activity recorded. Through protocols the nurse can implement intervention to a high degree before referring the patient to another colleague or agency. In the case of elevated blood pressure, most health boards/family health services authorities (FHSAs) will have recognized protocols detailing the follow-up of patients. Use of protocols can standardize treatment for all patients. Dietary advice can be structured using a protocol available from the dietetic department of the local hospital. This may suggest that the nurse should refer the patient to the dietitians if a reduction of weight is not apparent after 3 months. This agreement would be included in the initial interview with the patient.

Women attending for pre-conceptual advice can be informed of the importance of dietary intake, the advantages of breast-feeding and the use of folic acid before and after conception. Information on infant weaning can be provided by the health visitor.

Protocols also exist for the management of plasma lipids. A referral to a dietitian if a reduction in lipid levels is not being achieved within a certain time span is often advised. Smoking cessation advice can be offered by all members of the team, either as a one-to-one consultation or with a group of similarly interested patients. It is important that all practitioners give a consistent message. Exercise is an important part of a patient's lifestyle, not only keeping the patient active and providing relaxation but also enabling social contact. Many areas of the country already offer exercise prescriptions or even hold aerobic classes within the surgery premises (Dunne 1995). It is useful to know what is offered in a particular area or have booklets available which may be used to encourage the patient to walk to the shops or get off the bus at an earlier stop every day, so fitting exercise into the patient's daily

---

Case Study 14.1

Mr Wilson, aged 34 years, attends the nurse to have his ears syringed. On checking the patient's notes the nurse notices that Mr Wilson rarely attends the surgery and so he is offered a well-man check. Mr Wilson's check highlights the following:

- Blood pressure 140/105
- Height 1.74 metres
- Weight 108 kg
- Smokes 15 cigarettes per day
- Drinks 6 units alcohol per day
- His mother developed angina aged 53 years
- He rarely takes exercise and drives a heavy goods vehicle.

The nurse will be able to assess the patient's risk factors using an agreed method of assessment. By allowing the patient time to discuss the findings and listening to him, the nurse discovers that Mr Wilson has recently separated from his wife and family and has also become unemployed. Due to the family breakdown, he feels unable to stop smoking at the present time but admits that his consumption of alcohol has increased recently. As a measure—to save money at least—Mr Wilson offers to cut back on his intake of alcohol.

The nurse can encourage this while offering to monitor his blood pressure over the next few weeks. This will give the nurse the opportunity to follow-up a patient who not only needs health education but also is having problems which are likely to be more immediately important to him than losing weight or stopping smoking. The risk factors can be addressed gradually and then the patient is likely to be more receptive. The patient has offered a compromise which may be more achievable for him at the present time.

---

routine. Alcohol advice can again be given by the nurse though in more extreme cases an outside agency may be suggested.

Two examples of primary prevention may present as described in Case Studies 14.1 and 14.2.

Secondary prevention

Secondary prevention aims to reduce occurrence of further coronary events in those patients with established CHD. Patients in this group are often anxious and well-motivated to make changes to their lifestyle in order to improve their longer-term health. Many will use the period immediately following their diagnosis of CHD as a time to reflect on their lifestyle and may self-refer to the nurse for advice and support.

With the introduction of chronic disease management clinics within the practice setting, patients may already be attending the nurse at the Hypertension Clinic, Diabetic Clinic or even at the Asthma Clinic. These clinics all give the nurse an opportunity to motivate change in the patient's lifestyle and, by including family members, the modifications can be beneficial to all in the family. For example, smoking cessation may prove more successful

---

Case Study 14.2

Mrs Wells attends for her holiday immunization. The patient's blood pressure, height, weight and BMI are all within normal limits. Mrs Wells is a non-smoker, drinks alcohol within normal limits and takes plenty of exercise. On checking the records, the nurse notices that Mrs Wells had a hysterectomy at the age of 31 years for fibroids. At the time, the doctors had told her that both ovaries were left intact, but that was 18 years ago. The nurse explains the implications of this and offers to do a blood test to check Mrs Wells' FSH and LH level. The nurse introduces the subject of hormone replacement therapy (HRT) and its role in CHD prevention, allowing time to discuss any fears related to HRT. Mrs Wells is then offered an appointment at the Well-Women Clinic if the blood test indicates this. The patient is provided with a booklet about the menopause which will allow her time to read the information and make her own informed decision about HRT. For a more detailed discussion of HRT, see Chapter 13.

---

if the patient's spouse also wants to stop smoking. Health promotion sessions should allow the patient time to voice fears about the future and gain more information about the disease. This may range from increasing the amount of fish, fruit and vegetables consumed on average in a week to discussing health-related activities that the patient enjoys. Counselling and recommendations should be tailored to individual preferences.

Medical therapies to treat symptoms and improve the prognosis of patients with CHD have been discussed in detail in Chapters 9, 10 and 11.

The nurse may be required to identify patients who should be screened. These patients can be selected from other clinics as, for example, in Case Studies 14.3 and 14.4.

As major studies reveal the long-term benefits of intervention for 'high-risk patients', the nurse in general practice will be spending more time identifying such patients for screening, management and follow-up (Fowkes 1995). Shared cardiac care, unlike diabetic care, is not available in all areas. It would be to the benefit of patient care if there were a more integrated care programme between primary and secondary care.

The concept of shared care is being introduced but this is in its infancy (Lindsay 1995). Health care practices are in a state of great flux. In the future, we can expect 40% of outpatient consultations with specialist medical staff to occur in locations other than in hospital and GPs to refer 20% fewer patients to specialist medical services. This would have implications for nurses with a specialist interest in cardiac rehabilitation, who may extend the service into the community (DoH 1993). There is certainly plenty of scope for nurses to develop professional practice in this area.

CONCLUSIONS

Increasingly, patient care is being returned to the community, and the workload of nurses in all specialities is increasing as health care expectations

---

Case Study 14.3

Mr Miller attends the nurse-led Asthma Clinic. The patient happens to mention that he has shortness of breath on exertion. The nurse checks his notes and notices:

- Previous MIs in 1985 and 1991
- Right temporal lobe CVA, 1991
- Pulmonary embolism, 1991
- Hypertension.

This patient has never been offered echocardiography and so he is informed of this service and the nurse asks the GP to refer the patient. The echocardiography shows impaired systolic left ventricular function. His atenolol medication is discontinued and the patient is commenced on an ACE inhibitor, and isosorbide mononitrate SR 60 mg daily. This appears successful and relieves the dyspnoea and chest pain. It is also suggested that the patient should have his lipid profile checked. His plasma total cholesterol is 5.9 mmol/l, which in the light of the findings of the 4S (Ch. 3) should be regarded as a level worthy of intervention. He is given detailed, tailored dietary advice and his cholesterol level should be re-checked in approximately 3 months. The patient is then discharged to the care of the practice for routine follow-up, his medication regimen including aspirin, warfarin, GTN, ACE inhibitor and isosorbide mononitrate SR. His raised lipid levels require careful follow-up.

Case Study 14.4

Mr Smith attends the nurse for a dressing. The nurse knows that he is a diabetic and checks his notes to review his past history. The patient has previously had CABG surgery 12 years ago. Other history includes peripheral vascular disease, ischaemic disease and CVA in 1993 (followed up by a stroke family support worker for 6 months) and non-insulin dependent diabetes mellitus. The GP refers this patient for an echocardiograph, the result of which is normal. Lipid levels checked by the nurse show a level of 6.2 mmol/l for cholesterol. The patient does eat healthily but admits to enjoying cheese. The fat content of this is explained and after attending the dietitian, who agrees that the patient is well motivated and understands his diet, his cholesterol level remains elevated. This prompts the GP to introduce bezafibrate 400 mg, one tablet daily. 3 months later, the patient's cholesterol level has fallen to 4.5 mmol/l.

---

rise. Close monitoring of these community-based activities is essential to ensure that the needs of our patients continue to be met and that a high standard of patient care is delivered. Nurses in all specialities in the community are working to promote a healthy lifestyle and reduce the incidence of CHD. General practices are concentrating on those aged between 15 and 74 years, while children are being provided with health education programmes at school. Secondary prevention may be considered to be the way forward and may be both identified and managed within primary care. Teams of practice nurses, district nurses, health visitors and GPs may identify and manage CHD risk factors. Through closer communication with hospital colleagues, a shared care service may be developed that focuses on the needs of the patient.

■ KEY POINTS

• Nurses are key members of the multidisciplinary health care team involved in the prevention of CHD.

• Shared care planning provides a basis for improved communication and the development of comprehensive health care.

• Identification of a pathway of care and the key elements of care are necessary in order to ensure a high standard and quality of care delivery.

• Health promotion activities have been outlined in British Government directives.

• The health care team have a clear mandate to improve CHD mortality and morbidity through these screening and health promotional activities.

• Clinical practice should be 'evidence-based'.

• Protocols based on clinical guidelines should be integrated into practice.

Case Study 14.5

Mr Green makes an appointment to see the nurse. He has complained of 'tightness in his chest while walking to the bowling club and also of having to get up at night to drink water'.

You have interviewed the patient and found his blood pressure to be within normal limits as he is already on anti-hypertensive treatment; he has never smoked and drinks moderate amounts of alcohol. His prescribed drugs include bendrofluazide.

How would you assess this patient? What tests would you suggest and which members of the team would you expect to be included in this patient's care?

Answers

The nurse finds that he has glycosuria and contacts the GP, who arranges for the patient to have an exercise tolerance test completed by the cardiologists at the local hospital. In the interim, the GP changes the patient's drug treatment to a calcium antagonist, as bendrofluazide may be diabetogenic and the calcium antagonists would give both anti-anginal and anti-hypertensive treatment.

The nurse arranges for the patient to have a glucose tolerance test at the surgery. This confirms that the patient has diabetes. The nurse discusses the results with the patient, providing an interim diabetic diet advice sheet and diabetic advice booklet. The patient is referred to the diabetic outpatient clinic for an initial assessment by the dietitian.

PRACTICAL EXERCISE

What protocols exist for the management of patients with established CHD? Are there any such protocols used in your practice? How would you go about integrating a new protocol into your health care team's practice?

REFERENCES

Badenhausen W E 1993 Improving patient outcomes following joint replacement surgery at Methodist Evangelical Hospital. The Quality Letter (June): 11–13

Buchanan L, Smith J 1993 Pathway to recovery—using anticipated recovery paths (ARP). Healthcare Today 8: 2–4

Department of Health (DoH) 1992 The health of the nation: a strategy for health in England. HMSO, London, pp 46–47, 62–64

Department of Health (DoH) 1993 The challenges to nursing and midwifery in the 21st century (the Heathrow debate). HMSO, London

Dunne F 1995 Exercising change. Practice Nursing 6(8): 11–13

Ellis N, Chisholm J 1993 Making sense of the Red Book. Radcliffe Medical Press, Oxford

Fowkes P 1995 Quality care in coronary heart disease. Primary Health Care 5(5): 3

General Medical Services Committee 1993 The new health promotion package. BMA, London

Lindsay G M 1995 Sharing coronary heart disease. Practice Nursing 6(7): 28–30

NHS Management Executive 1991 Integrated primary and secondary health care. Department of Health, London

OXCHECK Study 1995 Effectiveness of health checks conducted by nurses in primary care. British Medical Journal 310: 1099–1104

Parker S 1994 Protocols—protection or penalty? Medical Defence Union Nurse 4: 1–3

United Kingdom Central Council for Nursing, Midwifery and Health Visiting (UKCC) 1994 The future of professional practice—the Council's standards for education and practice following registration. UKCC, London

FURTHER READING

Department of Health, General Medical Service Committee and Royal College of General Practitioners Working Group on Health Promotion 1993 Better living, better life. Knowledge House, Henley-on-Thames

A useful loose-leaf book aimed at the multidisciplinary team, discussing all aspects of lifestyle interventions for CHD and stroke prevention.

Ewles L, Simnett I 1995 Promoting health—a practical guide. Scutari Press, London

A practical self-teaching aid for those working in health promotion, with useful case studies and exercises, and with relevant up-to-date information on 'The health of the nation' (DoH 1992).

Fowler G, Gray M, Anderson P 1993 Prevention in general practice. Oxford University Press, Oxford

This book addresses the effectiveness of prevention with practical information on how this should be carried out.

Index